Management of Urology

Series Editors

Sanchia S. Goonewardene, Princess Alexandra Hospital, Harlow, UK
Raj Persad, North Bristol NHS Trust, Bristol, UK

This series addresses the need for an increase in the quantity of literature focused upon the effects of cancer in urology. Books within it will draw attention to the management of subtype specific urology cancer patients at each step of their pathway with suggestions on how care can potentially be improved. Therefore, it is of interest to a range of trainee and practicing physicians in a range of disciplines including urology oncology, specialist nurse and general practitioners.

Sanchia S. Goonewardene · Raj Persad ·
David Albala
Editors

Robotic Surgery for Renal Cancer

Submitted on behalf of European Association of Urology
(EAU) Young Academic Urologists (YAU) Robotic Urology
Section

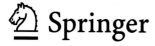

Editors
Sanchia S. Goonewardene
Princess Alexandra Hospital
Harlow, UK

Raj Persad
North Bristol NHS Trust
Bristol, UK

David Albala
Syracuse, NY, USA

ISSN 2730-6372   ISSN 2730-6380 (electronic)
Management of Urology
ISBN 978-3-031-10999-7   ISBN 978-3-031-11000-9 (eBook)
https://doi.org/10.1007/978-3-031-11000-9

© The Editor(s) (if applicable) and The Author(s), under exclusive license to Springer Nature Switzerland AG 2022
This work is subject to copyright. All rights are solely and exclusively licensed by the Publisher, whether the whole or part of the material is concerned, specifically the rights of translation, reprinting, reuse of illustrations, recitation, broadcasting, reproduction on microfilms or in any other physical way, and transmission or information storage and retrieval, electronic adaptation, computer software, or by similar or dissimilar methodology now known or hereafter developed.
The use of general descriptive names, registered names, trademarks, service marks, etc. in this publication does not imply, even in the absence of a specific statement, that such names are exempt from the relevant protective laws and regulations and therefore free for general use.
The publisher, the authors, and the editors are safe to assume that the advice and information in this book are believed to be true and accurate at the date of publication. Neither the publisher nor the authors or the editors give a warranty, expressed or implied, with respect to the material contained herein or for any errors or omissions that may have been made. The publisher remains neutral with regard to jurisdictional claims in published maps and institutional affiliations.

This Springer imprint is published by the registered company Springer Nature Switzerland AG
The registered company address is: Gewerbestrasse 11, 6330 Cham, Switzerland

Preface

On behalf of my team and the YAU ERUS Board, it has been a pleasure to put this book together for you. Upper tract surgery can be fraught with a myriad of dangers. When I was a young registrar at Guys and St. Thomas Hospitals, my trainers taught me the intricacies and technicalities of upper tract surgery, more specifically, renal cancer surgery. The world of major surgery has changed from open, to laparoscopic, and now to robotic.

Additionally, new robots have been developed that completely change the way that we operate and our ergonomics have to adapt as a result. With the advent of new robots, come new technologies, such as ICG, which again require our application of knowledge to detail.

This book covers operative skills for robotic surgery in renal cancer, in addition to groundbreaking work, such as IVC thrombectomy, 3D models in renal surgery, use of ICG and how to be a left-handed surgeon, in a right-handed world. The key is to always keep pushing your boundaries to make yourselves the very best you can be for your patients.

Harlow, UK   Sanchia S. Goonewardene
Bristol, UK   Raj Persad
Syracuse, USA   David Albala

Acknowledgements

For my family and friends, and work family, for always supporting me in what I do.

For all the Superheroes in my life, you have and always will be truly inspirational.

For my team at Springer Nature, for always giving myself and my team a chance to get published.

For my YAU—ERUS Board, a truly amazing bunch of Surgeons, Chairs and Mates.

For the amazing Prof. Raj Persad, still going strong, almost a decade down the line.

For my mentor and Editor-in-Chief, Prof. David Albala, I could not have achieved all of this without you.

Contents

1	**Suturing Techniques in Robot-Asssisted Partial Nephrectomy (RAPN)**	1
	Hannah Van Puyvelde and Ruben De Groote	
2	**Resection Techniques Robotic-Assisted Partial Nephrectomy**	7
	Sophie Knipper, Ruben De Groote, and Alexandre Mottrie	
3	**Clamping Techniques for Partial Nephrectomy**	9
	Ruben De Groote, Pietro Piazza, Rui Farinha, and Alexandre Mottrie	
4	**Robotic Retroperitoneal Partial Nephrectomy**	15
	Joseph Hon-Ming Wong, Peng-Fei Shao, and Jeremy Yuen-Chun Teoh	
5	**Robotic Partial Nephrectomy**	31
	Riccardo Campi, Selcuk Erdem, Onder Kara, Umberto Carbonara, Michele Marchioni, Alessio Pecoraro, Riccardo Bertolo, Alexandre Ingels, Maximilian Kriegmair, Nicola Pavan, Eduard Roussel, Angela Pecoraro, and Daniele Amparore	
6	**Pushing the Boundaries in Robot—Assisted Partial Nephrectomy for Renal Cancer**	43
	Charles Van Praet, Pieter De Backer, Riccardo Campi, Pietro Piazza, Alessio Pecoraro, Alexandre Mottrie, Andrea Minervini, and Karel Decaestecker	
7	**Perioperative Surgical Complications in Robotic Partial Nephrectomy**	63
	Riccardo Tellini, Giovanni Enrico Cacciamani, Michele Marchioni, Andrea Minervini, and Andrea Mari	
8	**Renal Robotic Surgery for Lefties: Left-Handedness in Upper Tract Robotic Surgery**	79
	Mylle Toon, Challacombe Ben, Uvin Pieter, and Mottrie Alexandre	

9	Training with New Robots and How to Transition from One System to the Next in Renal Cancer Surgery	87
	Kenneth Chen, Kae Jack Tay, John Shyi Peng Yuen, and Nathan Lawrentschuk	
10	New Robots and How this has Changed Operative Technique in Renal Cancer Surgery	99
	Christopher Soliman, Marc A. Furrer, and Nathan Lawrentschuk	
11	Use of Indocyanine Green (ICG) During Robotic Surgery for Renal Cancer	111
	Geert De Naeyer, Carlo Andrea Bravi, and Alexandre Mottrie	
12	3D Virtual Models and Augmented Reality for Robot-Assisted Partial Nephrectomy	119
	E. Checcucci, P. Verri, G. Cacciamani, S. Pulliatti, M. Taratkin, J. Marenco, J. Gomez Rivas, D. Veneziano, and F. Porpiglia	
13	Open Partial Nephrectomy: Current Status in the Minimally-Invasive Surgery Era	135
	Riccardo Campi, Selcuk Erdem, Onder Kara, Umberto Carbonara, Michele Marchioni, Alessio Pecoraro, Riccardo Bertolo, Alexandre Ingels, Maximilian Kriegmair, Nicola Pavan, Eduard Roussel, Angela Pecoraro, and Daniele Amparore	
14	Decision-Making for Patients with Localized Renal Masses	145
	Riccardo Campi, Selcuk Erdem, Onder Kara, Umberto Carbonara, Michele Marchioni, Alessio Pecoraro, Riccardo Bertolo, Alexandre Ingels, Maximilian Kriegmair, Nicola Pavan, Eduard Roussel, Angela Pecoraro, and Daniele Amparore	
15	Management of Localized Renal Masses: The European Association of Urology (EAU), American Urological Association (AUA) and American Society of Clinical Oncology (ASCO) Guidelines' Perspective	151
	Riccardo Campi, Selcuk Erdem, Onder Kara, Umberto Carbonara, Michele Marchioni, Alessio Pecoraro, Riccardo Bertolo, Alexandre Ingels, Maximilian Kriegmair, Nicola Pavan, Eduard Roussel, Angela Pecoraro, and Daniele Amparore	

16	**Active Surveillance and Watchful Waiting in Renal Cancer**	155
	Riccardo Campi, Selcuk Erdem, Onder Kara, Umberto Carbonara, Michele Marchioni, Alessio Pecoraro, Riccardo Bertolo, Alexandre Ingels, Maximilian Kriegmair, Nicola Pavan, Eduard Roussel, Angela Pecoraro, and Daniele Amparore	
17	**Ablative Therapies in Renal Cancer**	159
	Riccardo Campi, Selcuk Erdem, Onder Kara, Umberto Carbonara, Michele Marchioni, Alessio Pecoraro, Riccardo Bertolo, Alexandre Ingels, Maximilian Kriegmair, Nicola Pavan, Eduard Roussel, Angela Pecoraro, and Daniele Amparore	
18	**Open Radical Nephrectomy**	167
	Riccardo Campi, Selcuk Erdem, Onder Kara, Umberto Carbonara, Michele Marchioni, Alessio Pecoraro, Riccardo Bertolo, Alexandre Ingels, Maximilian Kriegmair, Nicola Pavan, Eduard Roussel, Angela Pecoraro, and Daniele Amparore	
19	**Transperitoneal and Retroperitoneal Port Placement**	173
	Alireza Ghoreifi, Hooman Djaladat, and Andre Luis Abreu	
20	**Robot Assisted Laparoscopy for Renal Cancer: Transperitoneal Versus Retroperitoneal Approach**	185
	Vidyasagar Chinni, Zein Alhamdani, Damien Bolton, Nathan Lawrentschuk, and Greg Jack	
21	**Robotic Radical Nephrectomy**	213
	Riccardo Campi, Selcuk Erdem, Onder Kara, Umberto Carbonara, Michele Marchioni, Alessio Pecoraro, Riccardo Bertolo, Alexandre Ingels, Maximilian Kriegmair, Nicola Pavan, Eduard Roussel, Angela Pecoraro, and Daniele Amparore	
22	**Preoperative Setting-Up of Patients Undergoing Robotic Inferior Vena Cava Thrombectomy**	217
	Raj Kumar, Nima Nassiri, Daniel Park, Vinay Duddalwar, Inderbir Gill, and Giovanni Cacciamani	
23	**Renal Cell Carcinoma with Tumor Thrombus: A Review of Relevant Anatomy and Surgical Techniques for the General Urologist**	227
	Christian A. Dewan, Joseph P. Vaughan, Ian C. Bennie, and Maurizio Buscarini	

24 **Cytoreductive Nephrectomy in Metastatic Renal Cell Carcinoma** 237
Roser Vives Dilme, Juan Gómez Rivas, Riccardo Campi, Javier Puente, and Jesús Moreno Sierra

About the Editors

Miss Sanchia S. Goonewardene MBChB (Hons.Clin.Sc), B.Med. S.c, PGCGC, Dip.SSc, MRCS, MPhil

Urology Registrar, The Princess Alexandra Hospital, Harlow

Sanchia S. Goonewardene qualified from Birmingham Medical School with Honours in Clinical Science and a B.Med. S.c Degree in Medical Genetics and Molecular Medicine. She has a specific interest in academia during her spare time, with over 733 publications to her name with 2 papers as a number 1 most cited in fields (Biomedical Library) and has significantly contributed to the Urological Academic World—she has since added a section to the European Association of Urology Congress on Prostate Cancer Survivorship and Supportive Care and has been an Associate Member of an EAU Guidelines Panel on Chronic Pelvic Pain (2015–2021). She is an EAU Abstract Reviewer and is part of the EAU Young Leaders Programme. She has been the UK lead in an EAU led study on Salvage Prostatectomy. She has also contributed to the BURST IDENTIFY study as a collaborator.

Her background with research entails an M.Phil., the work from which went on to be drawn up as a document for Prostate Cancer UK then endorsed by The National Institute of Clinical Excellence. She gained funding from the Wellcome Trust for her Research Elective. She is also an Alumni of the Urology Foundation, who sponsored a trip to USANZ trainee week. She also has 8 books published—Core Surgical Procedures for Urology Trainees (Ranked third on Book Authorities' 100 Best Urology Books of all Time), Prostate Cancer Survivorship, Basic Urological Management, Management of Non-Muscle Invasive Bladder Cancer, Salvage Therapy in Prostate Cancer, Management of Muscle Invasive Bladder Cancer, Surgical Strategies in Endourology for Stone Disease and Mens' Health and Wellbeing.

She has supervised her first thesis with Kings College London and Guys Hospital (BMedSci Degree gained first class, students' thesis score 95%). She is an Associate Editor for the Journal of Robotic Surgery and is responsible as Urology Section Editor. She is an Editorial Board Member of the World Journal of Urology and was invited to be Guest Editor for a Special Issue on Salvage Therapy in Prostate Cancer. She is also a review board member for BMJ case reports. Additionally, she is on The International Continence Society Panel on Pelvic Floor

Dysfunction, Good Urodynamic Practice Panel, is an ICS abstract reviewer and has been an EPoster Chair at ICS. More recently she has been an ICS Ambassador and is an ICS Mentor. She has also chaired semi-live surgery at ERUS and presented her work as part of the Young Academic Urology Section at ERUS. In her spare time, she enjoys fundraising for Rotary International and is Secretary and Vice-President (President Elect 2022–2023) for the Rotary Club of Hampstead. In addition, she is mentoring a Ph.D. student, from Roteract.

Prof. Raj Persad MB, BS, ChM, FRCS (Eng), FRCS (Urol), FEBU

Raj Persad, appointed in 1996, is a Consultant Urological Surgeon and Andrologist in Bristol.

In his clinical role, he is one of the most experienced pelvic cancer surgeons in the UK and was one of the first in the UK to practice female neobladder reconstruction following cystectomy for invasive bladder cancer. He has subspecialized over many years in precise surgical techniques which improve both oncologic and functional outcomes. This includes techniques ranging from (1) the use of the Da Vinci Robot for performing robot-assisted laparoscopic radical prostatectomy, (2) high-intensity focused ultrasound for minimally invasive non-surgical treatment of prostate cancer and (3) rectal spacer and fiducial marker precision placement for optimizing the outcomes of image-guided radiotherapy for prostate cancer.

In the field of diagnostics, he has been one of the National Leads in developing the prostate pre-biopsy MRI pathway for patients with elevated PSA. This has optimized the accuracy of cancer diagnosis minimized clinical risk and sepsis associated with transrectal biopsy. He has developed to a fine art both cognitive transperineal biopsies of the prostate and fusion biopsy of the prostate.

Professor Persad has been a national pioneer in minimally invasive techniques for the treatment of symptomatic benign prostatic as an alternative to transurethral prostatectomy (TURP). These techniques include Urolift (prostatic urethral lift) procedure which he does under general or local anaesthetic depending on patient preference as well as REZUM, steam treatment of the prostate. He also treats BPH with Green Light Laser. All these techniques are offered by him for BPH as well as traditional TURP if tablet therapy has failed or cannot be tolerated by the patient.

Professor Persad is also a National Authority in the treatment of Erectile Dysfunction. He practices optimum medical therapies for all male patients and has a large cohort of patients who are diabetic or who have had prostatectomy and in need of erectile function restoration. If conservative therapy fails with erectogenic pharmacotherapy or use of medical devices he can offer the insertion of state-of-the-art penile prosthetic devices. He also treats deformity due to Peyronie's disease across a range of severity, offering therapeutic injection in its early phases and various types of surgical correction if this fails according to patient needs.

Professor Persad has a 25-year experience in the restoration of fertility through microsurgical reversal of vasectomy and has some of the best results nationally. He also for more complex cases offers epidydimo-vasovasostomy. In combination with the Bristol Centre for Reproductive Medicine, he will soon be offering male infertility procedures such as micro-TESE (testicular extraction of sperm) in order to optimize assisted conception techniques.

Academically, Prof. Persad is involved in an extensive range of research with the Universities of Bristol, Pittsburgh, London and Oxford. These include the detection of early bladder and prostate cancer and novel imaging and treatment strategies for these diseases. He formerly led a team of researchers engaged in improving strategies for treatment of advanced prostate cancer in areas of hormonal treatment and immunotherapy (BPCRN). He has been Principal Investigator, Chief Investigator and Collaborator in many national and international studies sponsored by the MRC, EORTC, CRUK and NCRN. He has been a recipient of £4.5m research grants from UK bodies as well as the NIH USA, and has published over 300 scientific articles and 7 books in the field of Urology.

Together with scientists and clinicians in Bristol he is part of the productive BRC (Biomed Research Centre), which has a number of far-reaching clinical and scientific goals in the field of cancer and is Surgical Principle Investigator for the PreVent and Pre-Empt trials of lifestyle intervention in prostate cancer. He has an innovative research programme with Prof. Chris Melhuish in Medical Robotics to enhance surgery and radiotherapy modalities with robotic assistance.

In addition to his University and NHS Clinical commitments, he spends time visiting hospital units in the developing world (e.g. Tanzania), where he helps to train junior doctors and other healthcare professionals.

Dr. David Albala MD, Associated Medical Professionals

Dr. David Albala graduated with a geology degree from Lafayette College in Easton, Pennsylvania. He completed his medical school training at Michigan State University and went on to complete his surgical residency at the Dartmouth-Hitchcock Medical Centre. Following this, he was an endourology fellow at Washington University Medical Centre under the direction of Ralph V. Clayman. He practised at Loyola University Medical Centre in Chicago and rose from the ranks of Instructor to full Professor in Urology and Radiology in 8 years. After 10 years, he became a tenured Professor at Duke University Medical Centre in North Carolina. At Duke, he was Co-Director of the Endourology fellowship and Director for the Centre of Minimally Invasive and Robotic Urological Surgery. He has over 180 publications in peer-reviewed journals and has authored six books in endourology and general urology. He is the Editor-in-Chief of the Journal of Robotic Surgery. He serves on the editorial board for Medical Reviews in Urology, Current Opinions in Urology and Urology Index and Reviews. He serves as a reviewer for eight surgical journals.

Presently, he is Chief of Urology at Crouse Hospital in Syracuse, New York, and a Physician at Associated Medical Professionals (a group of 33 urologists). He is considered a national and international authority in laparoscopic and robotic urological surgery and has been an active teacher in this area for over 20 years. His research and clinical interests have focused on robotic urological surgery. In addition, other clinical interests include minimally invasive treatment of benign prostatic hypertrophy (BPH), stone disease and the use of fibrin sealants in surgery.

He has been a Visiting Professor at numerous institutions across the United States as well as overseas in countries such as India, China, England, Iceland, Germany, France, Japan, Brazil, Australia and Singapore. In addition, he has done operative demonstrations in over 32 countries and 23 states. He has trained 16 fellows in endourology and advanced robotic surgery.

In addition, he is a past White House Fellow who acted as a special assistant to Federico Pena, Secretary of Transportation, on classified and unclassified public health-related issues.

Abbreviations

AI	Artificial Intelligence
AJCC	American Joint Committee on Cancer
AKI	Acute Kidney Injury
AO	Arterial Only
AR	Augmented Reality
AS	Active Surveillance
ASCO	American Society of Clinical Oncology
AUA	American Association of Urology
AVF	Arteriovenous Fistula
BMI	Body Mass Index
CPB	Cardiopulmonary Bypass
CKD	Chronic Kidney Disease
CN	Cytoreductive Nephrectomy
CRA	Cryoablation
CSA	Contact Surface Area
CSS	Cancer-Specific Survival
CT	Computerized Tomography
CTA	Computed Tomography of Renal Angiogram
DFS	Disease-Free Survival
DHCA	Deep Hypothermic Circulatory Arrest
DI	Delayed Intervention
DISSRM	Delayed Intervention and Surveillance for Small Renal Masses
DVSS	DA Vinci Skills Simulator
EAU	European Association of Urology
EAUIAIC	Intraoperative Adverse Incident Classification
EGFR	Estimated Glomerular Filtration Rate
EORTC	European Organisation for Research and Treatment of Cancer
FEM	Finite Element Model
GEARS	Global Evaluative Assessment of Robotic Skills
HA3D™	Hyper-accuracy Three-Dimensional
IC	Intraoperative Complication
ICG	Indocyanine Green
ICI	Immune Checkpoint Inhibitors

IMDC	International Metastatic Renal Cell Carcinoma Database Consortium
I/R	Ischaemia and Reperfusion
ITV	Intraoperative Tumour Violation
IVC	Inferior Vena Cava
LPN	Laparoscopic Partial Nephrectomy
LRM	Localized Renal Masses
MRCC	Metastatic Renal Cell Carcinoma
METASTASES	Free Survival
MIC	Score-Margin, Ischaemia and Complication Rate
MIPN	Minimally Invasive Partial Nephrectomy
MRI	Magnetic Resonance Imaging
MR	Mixed Reality
MSKCC	Memorial Sloan Kettering Cancer Center
MVA	Microwave Ablation
NCCN	National Comprehensive Cancer Network
NIRF	Near-Infrared Fluorescence Imaging
NSS	Nephron Sparing Surgeries
OPN	Open Partial Nephrectomy
ORN	Open Radical Nephrectomy
OS	Overall Survival
PN	Partial Nephrectomy
PSM	Positive Surgical Margins
RAE	Renal Artery Embolization
RAP	Renal Artery Pseudo-aneurysms
RAPN	Robot-Assisted Partial Nephrectomy
RARP	Robot-Assisted Radical Prostatectomy
RCC	Renal Cell Carcinoma
RCTS	Randomized Controlled Trials
RFA	Radiofrequency Ablation
RIVCT	Robotic IVC Thrombectomy
RN	Radical Nephrectomy
ROSS	Robotic Surgical Simulator
SIB	Surface-Intermediate-Base
SEP	Simsurgery Educational Platform
SRBS	Self-retaining Barbed Suture
SRM	Small Renal Masses
STRAPN	Standard RAPN
SURAPN	Sutureless RAPN
SWOG	Southwest Oncology Group
TA	Tumour Ablation
TEE	Transesophageal Echocardiogram
TE	Tumour Enucleation
TKI	Tyrosine Kinase Inhibitors
TUM	Techno Urology Meeting

URINARY	Collecting System UCS
UL	Urinary Leak
US	Ultrasound
VVB	Venovenous Bypass
VHL	Von Hippel-Lindau
VR	Virtual Reality
WIT	Warm Ischaemia Time
YAU	Young Academic Urologists

Suturing Techniques in Robot-Asssisted Partial Nephrectomy (RAPN)

1

Hannah Van Puyvelde and Ruben De Groote

1.1 Introduction

Over the years, there has been an evolution in renorrhapy techniques in minimally invasive partial nephrectomy (MIPN). Earlier, the approach was to minimize intraoperative complications (avoid blood loss, avoid urine leakage when opening the collecting system). Nowadays, we try to minimize the ischaemic effect of our renorrhaphy technique to optimize renal function [5].

Unfortunately there is no consensus about the best renorrhaphy technique. Studies are limited, most of them without information on the tumor complexity and only assessing the early postoperative functional outcome. In the following content, we'll try to summarize the variety of techniques.

1.2 Classic Renorrhaphy

A classical renorrhaphy typically consists of a double-layer technique with a medullary suture (inner layer) and a cortical suture (outer layer).

Depending on the lesion's growth pattern, it's important to be aware of the anatomy of the intraparenchymal arteries. With a deep resection, there needs to be attention for the radial anatomy of the renal lobe (the pyramid) and its respective interlobar arteries. The renal parenchyma will be devascularised when they have been included in the medullary suture [5]. With a deep needle passage, you also

H. Van Puyvelde (✉)
ZNA Jan Palfijn/Stuivenberg, Antwerp, Belgium
e-mail: hannah.vanpuyvelde@zna.be

R. De Groote
OLV Hospital Aalst, Aalst, Belgium

© The Author(s), under exclusive license to Springer Nature Switzerland AG 2022
S. S. Goonewardene et al. (eds.), *Robotic Surgery for Renal Cancer*, Management of Urology, https://doi.org/10.1007/978-3-031-11000-9_1

should try to avoid the involvement of the urinary collecting system (UCS). When the UCS is opened during tumour excision, you should use superficial sutures or single re-absorbable clips to achieve a watertight closure of the defect [2].

The medullary suture is often performed in a knotless fashion using a running suture fixed by clips. These clips better be re-absorbable to avoid decubitus and potential migration into the UCS [2].

When performing the cortical suture, the orientation of the needle should be at right angles with respect to the line of the arcuate arteries. If the suture has been performed superficial enough in order to avoid the involvement of the arcuate arteries: the blood supply to the medullar parenchyma by the vasa recta is spared [5]. The cortical suture is used to re-approximate the renal defect, often performed using a sliding-clip technique. With this techniques it's possible to allow more precise control and readjustment of the tension placed during suturing, reducing both warm ischaemia time (WIT) and risk of the 'cheese-cutting effect' associated with conventional parenchymal sutures [3].

1.3 Single Versus Double Layer

In the systematic review of Bertolo et al. [2], a comparison was made between single-layer vs double-layer groups. There was a significant advantage in terms of operating time (mean difference -11.13 min [95% CI -20.14, -2.13]) and WIT (-3.39 min [95% CI -4.53, -2.24]) favouring the single-layer technique. Conversely, no significant differences were found in terms of blood loss, postoperative complications and urinary leakages.

Renal function (pre- and postoperative estimated glomerular filtration rate (eGFR)) was analysed, comparing single-layer versus double-layer groups. There was a benefit in functional outcome in favor of the single-layer technique (3.19 ml/min, 95% CI 8.09; 1.70, $p = 0.2$ versus -6.07 ml/min, 95% CI 10.75; 1.39, $p = 0.01$) [3].

Bahler et al. [1] investigated the feasibility and safety of omitting cortical renorrhaphy during robot assisted partial nephrectomy (RAPN). Without differences in postoperative complications, they found a significantly higher renal volume loss if cortical renorrhaphy was performed (assessed by software-based volumetric assessment on computed tomography scans). This finding was suggested to be secondary to the hypoperfusion of the parenchyma that occurs during cortical renorrhaphy.

Overall, a single-layer renorrhaphy technique appears to be feasible and safe in selected cases of MIPN, with clear advantages in terms of reduced WIT. According to the available evidence and expert opinion, when single-layer renorrhaphy is attempted, the cortical rather than the medullary layer should be omitted [3].

1.4 Running Versus Interrupted Suture

The systematic review of Bertolo et al. [2], found six studies that compared running vs interrupted suture. The groups were comparable in terms of age, body mass index (BMI) and tumour size. A running suture resulted in a significant advantage in terms of operating time (mean difference −17.12 min [95% CI −24.30, −9.94]), WIT (mean difference −8.73 min [95% CI −12.41, −5.06]) and occurrence of postoperative complications (odds ratio 0.54 [95% CI 0.32, 0.89]) and transfusions (odds ratio 0.30 [95%CI 0.15, 0.59]).

No significant differences were found between pre- and postoperative eGFR in both patients who received an interrupted suture (WMD −4.88 ml/min, 95% confidence interval [CI] −11.38; 1.63, $p = 0.14$) or those who received a running suture (−3.42 ml/min, 95% CI −9.96; 3.12, $p = 0.31$) [3].

1.5 Barbed Versus Nonbarbed Suture

The introduction of barbed sutures further reduced operating time and WIT (as compared with non-barbed sutures), with the added advantages of reduced blood loss [2].

The systematic review of Zhan et al. [6], compared the use of a self-retaining barbed suture (SRBS) with a non-SRBS for parenchymal repair during laparoscopic partial nephrectomy (LPN). They found a shorter WIT ($P < 0.00001$), a shorter overall operative time ($P < 0.00001$), a lower estimated blood loss ($P = 0.02$) and better renal function preservation ($P = 0.001$) with a SRBS. There was no significant difference between both sutures with regard to complications ($P = 0.08$) and length of hospital stay ($P = 0.25$).

Not only during cortical renorrhaphy, but also for inner-layer renorrhaphy, some authors reported a reduced renorrhaphy time while using a SRBS [2].

1.6 Hemostatic Agents

To complete haemostasis, some surgeons prefer the use of haemostatic agents (fibrin glues, gelatin-based sealants (i.e. FloSeal; Baxter Healthcare, i.e. Veriset; Medtronic) or human fibrinogen and thrombin fleece (i.e. TachoSil; Nycomed). In the early robotic experiences, surgical bolsters were used to fill the renal defect after inner-layer renorrhapy. Nowadays they are rarely used [2].

In the systematic review of Bertolo et al. [3], there were no studies who compared the differential role of renorrhaphy techniques and haemostatic agents on PN outcomes.

1.7 Selective Suturing—Sutureless Technique

The sutureless technique was developed to retain more renal parenchyma and protect renal function. After excision of the tumour (if possible clampless), forced bipolar or monopolar coagulation is carried out on the tumour bed. When persistent arterial bleeding is observed, a selective suturing is achieved. If not, then it is possible to perform a sutureless technique. A hemostatic agent is then applied to the tumour bed.

Farihna et al. [4], compared selective-suturing or sutureless RAPN (suRAPN) and standard RAPN (stRAPN). Overall, 29 patients (31%) were treated with suRAPN. Only one suRAPN patient experienced intraoperative complications ($p = 0.9$). Two suRAPN patients (6.9%) and four stRAPN patients (13.8%) experienced 30-d postoperative complications ($p = 0.3$). Operative time (110 vs 150 min; $p < 0.01$) and length of stay (2 vs 3 d; $p = 0.02$) were shorter for suRAPN than for stRAPN. The trifecta outcome (warm ischemia time < 25 min, negative surgical margins, and no perioperative complications) was achieved in 25 suRAPN patients (86%) and 20 stRAPN patients (70%; $p = 0.1$). Specifically, WIT < 25 min was reported for 28 (97%) suRAPN patients versus 25 (86%) stRAPN patients. Negative surgical margins were reported for 28 (97%) suRAPN patients versus 28 (97%) stRAPN patients. Finally, only one suRAPN patient (3.4%) versus five stRAPN patients (17%) experienced postoperative AKI ($p = 0.2$). At 6-mo follow-up, the median eGFR decrease was −5.6 (IQR: −3.4–8.3) for the suRAPN group versus −9.1% (IQR: −7.3–11) for the stRAPN group ($p < 0.01$).

1.8 Conclusion

This chapter provides an overview of the different renorraphy methods during MIPN. Over the last decade a transition from double-layer renorraphy towards single layer and sutureless renorraphy can be noted in order to optimally preserve residual kidney parenchyma. Existing evidence indicates that this might lead to better kidney function preservation without increasing peri-operative complications.

References

1. Bahler CD, Dube HT, Flynn KJ, et al. Feasibility of omitting cortical renorrhaphy during robot-assisted partial nephrectomy: a matched analysis. J Endourol. 2015;29:548–55.
2. Bertolo R, Campi R, Klatte T, Kriegmair MC, Mir MC, Ouzaid I, Salagierski M, Bhayani S, Gill I, Kaouk J, Capitanio U. Young Academic Urologists (YAU) Kidney Cancer working group of the European Urological Association (EAU). Suture techniques during laparoscopic and robot-assisted partial nephrectomy: a systematic review and quantitative synthesis of peri-operative outcomes. BJU Int. 2019;123(6):923–946. https://doi.org/10.1111/bju.14537. Epub 2018 Nov 19. PMID: 30216617.

3. Bertolo R, Campi R, Mir MC, Klatte T, Kriegmair MC, Salagierski M, Ouzaid I, Capitanio U. Young academic urologists kidney cancer working group of the european urological association. Systematic review and pooled analysis of the impact of renorrhaphy techniques on renal functional outcome after partial nephrectomy. Eur Urol Oncol. 2019;2(5):572–575. https://doi.org/10.1016/j.euo.2018.11.008. Epub 2018 Dec 9. PMID: 31412012.
4. Farinha R, Rosiello G, Paludo AO, Mazzone E, Puliatti S, Amato M, De Groote R, Piazza P, Berquin C, Montorsi F, Schatteman P, De Naeyer G, D'Hondt F, Mottrie A. selective suturing or sutureless technique in robot-assisted partial nephrectomy: results from a propensity-score matched analysis. Eur Urol Focus. 2021;25:S2405–4569(21)00098–5. https://doi.org/10.1016/j.euf.2021.03.019. Epub ahead of print. PMID: 33775611.
5. Porpiglia F, Bertolo R, Amparore D, Fiori C. Nephron-sparing suture of renal parenchyma after partial nephrectomy: which technique to go for? Some best practices. Eur Urol Focus. 2017. In Press. https://doi.org/10.1016/j.euf.2017.08.006.
6. Zhan H, Huang C, Li T, Yang F, Cai J, Li W, Mao Y, Zhou X. The self-retaining barbed suture for parenchymal repair in laparoscopic partial nephrectomy: a systematic review and meta-analysis. Surg Innov. 2019;26(6):744–52. https://doi.org/10.1177/1553350619856167. Epub 2019 Jun 19 PMID: 31215335.

Resection Techniques Robotic-Assisted Partial Nephrectomy

2

Sophie Knipper, Ruben De Groote, and Alexandre Mottrie

After dissection and control of the hilar vessels, as well as incision of the Gerota's facia, the tumour and the surrounding renal capsule is exposed [7]. Depending on the anatomy of the tumour, use of intraoperative ultrasound may be helpful. This is particularly advantageous for neoplasms with substantial endophytic growth and/or hilar location [6]. Here, robotic drop-in ultrasound probes, which are directly controlled by the console surgeon, can be used, displaying the live intraoperative images as a picture on picture display on the console screen [1, 7]. However, intraoperative ultrasound is not mandatory in the case of primarily exophytic tumours as identification is usually easily feasible.

After clear identification of the mass, the resection margins are marked with cautery. Depending on the tumour anatomy, there are several resection techniques available:

1. Resection
2. Enucleoresection
3. Enucleation.

In case of resection, the tumour is excised sharply with a rim of healthy renal parenchyma. During tumour resection, the assistant applies counter traction with the suction to ensure adequate visualization. Ideally, mainly cold scissors are used to better visualize the healthy parenchyma surrounding the tumour and to minimize the risk of positive surgical margins [6].

S. Knipper (✉) · R. De Groote · A. Mottrie
Department of Urology, Onze-Lieve-Vrouwziekenhuis, Aalst, Belgium
e-mail: a.knipper@uke.de

A. Mottrie
e-mail: alex.mottrie@olvz-aalst.be

© The Author(s), under exclusive license to Springer Nature Switzerland AG 2022
S. S. Goonewardene et al. (eds.), *Robotic Surgery for Renal Cancer*,
Management of Urology, https://doi.org/10.1007/978-3-031-11000-9_2

In case of enucleoresection, the capsule of the kidney is incised circular about 5 mm around the tumour. A pseudocapsule of compressed healthy tissue around the tumour is found and mainly blunt dissection is done with cold scissors. At the base of the dissection, the resection is completed sharply [5].

In case of enucleation, the kidney capsule is again sharply incised close to the tumour, the pseudocapsula is found and the tumour is enucleated by blunt dissection, with no visible rim of healthy parenchyma around the tumour [4].

Recently, a prospective multicentre study described the resection technique to be an important predictor of surgical complications, early functional outcomes, as well as positive surgical margins [3]. Here, enucleation and resection showed to be superior in achieving the trifecta outcomes (no major complications, no acute kidney failure, negative surgical margins) compared to enucleoresection. However, suturing techniques for renorrhaphy were not considered in this analysis.

Since renal parenchyma preservation is one of the strongest predictors of functional outcomes following partial nephrectomy, the amount of healthy tissue excised during surgery should be carefully weighed by the surgeon's judgment based on patient and tumour characteristics [2].

References

1. Kaczmarek BF, Sukumar S, Petros F, Trinh Q-D, Mander N, Chen R, Menon M, Rogers CG. Robotic ultrasound probe for tumor identification in robotic partial nephrectomy: initial series and outcomes. Int J Urol Off J Jpn Urol Assoc. 2013;20:172–6. https://doi.org/10.1111/j.1442-2042.2012.03127.x.
2. Maurice MJ, Ramirez D, Malkoç E, Kara Ö, Nelson RJ, Caputo PA, Kaouk JH. Predictors of excisional volume loss in partial nephrectomy: is there still room for improvement? Eur Urol. 2016;70:413–5. https://doi.org/10.1016/j.eururo.2016.05.007.
3. Minervini A, Campi R, Lane BR, De Cobelli O, Sanguedolce F, Hatzichristodoulou G, Antonelli A, Noyes S, Mari A, Rodriguez-Faba O, Keeley FX, Langenhuijsen J, Musi G, Klatte T, Roscigno M, Akdogan B, Furlan M, Karakoyunlu N, Marszalek M, Capitanio U, Volpe A, Brookman-May S, Gschwend JE, Smaldone MC, Uzzo RG, Carini M, Kutikov A. Impact of resection technique on perioperative outcomes and surgical margins after partial nephrectomy for localized renal masses: a prospective multicenter study. J Urol. 2020;203:496–504. https://doi.org/10.1097/JU.0000000000000591.
4. Minervini A, di Cristofano C, Lapini A, Marchi M, Lanzi F, Giubilei G, Tosi N, Tuccio A, Mancini M, della Rocca C, Serni S, Bevilacqua G, Carini M. Histopathologic analysis of peritumoral pseudocapsule and surgical margin status after tumor enucleation for renal cell carcinoma. Eur Urol. 2009;55:1410–8. https://doi.org/10.1016/j.eururo.2008.07.038.
5. Mottrie A, Koliakos N, DeNaeyer G, Willemsen P, Buffi N, Schatteman P, Fonteyne E. Tumor enucleoresection in robot-assisted partial nephrectomy. J Robot Surg. 2009;3:65–9. https://doi.org/10.1007/s11701-009-0136-8.
6. Novara G, La Falce S, Kungulli A, Gandaglia G, Ficarra V, Mottrie A. Robot-assisted partial nephrectomy. Int J Surg Lond Engl. 2016;36:554–9. https://doi.org/10.1016/j.ijsu.2016.05.073.
7. Sukumar S, Rogers CG. Robotic partial nephrectomy: surgical technique. BJU Int. 2011;108:942–7. https://doi.org/10.1111/j.1464-410X.2011.10457.x.

Clamping Techniques for Partial Nephrectomy

3

Ruben De Groote, Pietro Piazza, Rui Farinha, and Alexandre Mottrie

3.1 Introduction

Hilum identification, isolation and control is a core step of nephron sparing surgery. Having a proper control of the renal hilum is of utmost importance in order to provide patients with a safer procedure. Before beginning the excision of the tumor, the renal hilum is usually clamped. Arterial clamping is associated with a more precise tumor resection, allowing an improved visualization of the tumor pseudo capsule, reducing the amount of health parenchyma resected and decreasing the blood loss. The role of renal ischemia on subsequent acute kidney injury (AKI) or with development of chronic kidney disease (CKD) has been deeply investigated and, despite being recognized as a major risk factor for renal function loss, a significantly higher importance has been granted to preoperative kidney function and remaining vascularized parenchyma [20]. Recent studies suggested that renal parenchyma is able to withstand prolonged ischemia, especially in case of healthy kidneys [1], therefore transforming the concept of a "safe ischemia time" limited to 20–30 min into a dogma [16]. Nonetheless, ischemia remains

R. De Groote (✉) · P. Piazza · A. Mottrie
Department of Urology, Onze-Lieve-Vrouw Hospital, Aalst, Belgium
e-mail: degroote.ruben@gmail.com

A. Mottrie
e-mail: alex.mottrie@olvz-aalst.be

R. De Groote · P. Piazza · R. Farinha · A. Mottrie
ORSI Academy, Melle, Belgium

P. Piazza
Division of Urology, IRCCS Azienda Ospedaliero-Universitaria di Bologna, Bologna, Italy

R. Farinha
Urology Department, Lusíadas Hospital, Lisbon, Portugal

© The Author(s), under exclusive license to Springer Nature Switzerland AG 2022
S. S. Goonewardene et al. (eds.), *Robotic Surgery for Renal Cancer*,
Management of Urology, https://doi.org/10.1007/978-3-031-11000-9_3

one of the few modifiable factors for parenchymal preservation. Therefore, several techniques have been developed over the course of the last two decades as an alternative to the classical arterial only or arteriovenous clamping.

3.2 Warm-Ischemia Resection

Warm ischemia resection is defined as a renal tumorectomy performed while actively obstructing the vascular flow to the organ. Historically, warm-ischemia resections have been performed while clamping both main renal artery and main renal vein. This approach provides surgeons with a bloodless surgical field, limiting both the in-flow as the backflow from the renal veins. In order to try minimizing the ischemic renal damage associated with the technique, artery-only clamping has been proposed. However, a recent systematic review and meta-analysis showed no significant difference in renal function preservation at short term follow-up. Despite this finding, the author suggested that arterial-only (AO) clamping might produce less ischemia damage in a long-term setting, therefore suggesting the use of an AO technique, considering that this approach is not associated with an increased difficulty in performing the resection step of the procedure [7].

3.3 Off-Clamp Resection

Off clamp resection technique is characterized by a complete lack of hilar clamping. The whole renal parenchyma, and the tumor, maintain a complete vascularization during the entire surgery.

Several studies compared on and off clamp partial nephrectomies, still providing controversial and contradictory results. A recent systematic review and meta-analysis reported similar perioperative and oncological outcomes, despite a slightly higher blood loss was described for off-clamp RAPN. The off-clamp group, however, showed a superior renal function preservation, both in the short (+7%) as in the long-term follow-up (+4%), when compared with patient undergoing warm-ischemia RAPN [6].

Two randomized controlled trials (RCTs) compared off-clamp partial nephrectomy with the standard technique. The CLOCK trial randomized patients with bilateral kidneys, normal kidney function and single renal tumor (RENAL score $\leq$ 10) to receive either an on-clamp or an off-clamp RAPN [2]. No significant differences were recorder in terms of perioperative outcomes, nor in terms of postoperative kidney function at 6, 12, 18 and 24 months. Current evidence suggests that in case of healthy patients with normal preoperative renal function, the choice between on- or off-clamp partial nephrectomy might have limited impact on clinical outcome. However, this statement may not be applicable to patients with a solitary kidney, complex tumors, or pre-existing CKD, since reliable data regarding these frail patients are lacking.

3.4 Early Unclamping

Early unclamping partial nephrectomy is characterized by the restoration of vascularization of the renal parenchyma after the inner renorraphy, requiring the completion of the double-layer renorraphy with a perfused kidney [3]. According to previous studies, early unclamping can provide up to 6 min less warm ischemia time, when compared with traditional partial nephrectomy [17]. Moreover, a recent meta-analysis suggested that early unclamping is associated only with a modest increase in blood loss, when compared with the standard of care (+37 mL), without significant differences in transfusion rates or adverse events [6]. Finally, only one study compared changes in postoperative renal function between the two techniques, founding no significant differences [17]. As sidenote, early unclamping can be useful for the surgeons, hence it provides prompt feedback on the quality of the hemostatic inner renorraphy.

3.5 Superselective Clamping

Superselective clamping, also known as the "zero-ischemia" technique, is defined by the temporary clamping of only the tumor-feeding renal vessels. This allows to reduce the ischemic insult to healthy parenchyma while minimizing the risk of complications due to excessive bleeding. The technique was firstly described by Gill et al. [11], requiring the isolation and dissection of tertiary or higher order branches of the renal artery. One of the main drawbacks associated with this technique is how to properly determine preoperatively which vessels need to be clamped, and if the clamping of the expected vessels will indeed provide a dry surgical. Gill et al. suggested that these problems could be overcome by using 3D models [12]. Several studies, however, have shown how a purely cognitive estimation does not always allow the achievement of an avascular resection [5]. Lateral rim tumors vascularization estimation, for example, is quite challenging due to limits in CT imaging resolution.

Several perfusion models have been proposed in the last 5 years. Porpiglia et al. proposed a 3D based perfusion model in 2018; the major limitation of the algorithm was due to the estimation that each vessel was perfusing the same volume of parenchyma, therefore producing perfusion areas separated by straight planes [18].

Recently, De Backer et al. proposed a novel perfusion algorithm based on mathematical models, evaluating several specific arterial features [10], showing an higher accuracy in predicting the perfused parenchyma associated with each vessel. Finally, the use of Near-infrared imaging and indocyanine green (ICG) as proven a paramount role in the diffusion of "zero-ischemia" PN, allowing the surgeon to determine the success of the selective clamping prior to the start of the resection [19].

3.6 Cold Ischemia

When ischemia times >30 min are expected, cold ischemia techniques may be applied in order to limit the renal parenchyma damage. Cold ischemia use in minimally invasive surgery has been limited by its complex realization [4]. Several techniques, such as cold saline surface irrigation [15], retrograde cooling through the ureter [9] and intra-arterial cold perfusion [14] have been proposed for laparoscopic surgery. These techniques, however, have never been compared in terms of functional outcomes or kidney's temperature.

This lack of minimally invasive 'ideal' cooling systems has severely limited the adoption of cold ischemia in RAPN. The use of this technique could improve our clinical practice, as recent studies with high level of evidence suggested that no significant differences exist between cold and warm ischemia in terms of perioperative outcomes, positive margins and postoperative kidney function preservation [13].

3.7 Reclamping

Reclamping during kidney conservative surgery can lead to ischaemia–reperfusion syndrome. The microvascular dysfunction presents iteself as an impaired endothelium-dependent dilation in arterioles, enhanced fluid filtration and leukocyte plugging in capillaries and plasma protein extravasation in postcapillary venules. Activated endothelial cells in all segments of the microcirculation produce more oxygen radicals, but less nitric oxide, in the initial period following reperfusion. The resulting imbalance between superoxide and nitric oxide in endothelial cells leads to the production and release of inflammatory mediators and enhances the biosynthesis of adhesion molecules that mediate leukocyte–endothelial cell adhesion. Some of the known risk factors for cardiovascular disease (hypercholesterolaemia, hypertension, and diabetes) appear to exaggerate many of the microvascular alterations caused by ischaemia and reperfusion (I/R). The inflammatory mediators released as a consequence of reperfusion also appear to activate endothelial cells in remote areas not exposed to the initial ischemic insult [8].

3.8 Summary

Currently, no evidence suggests the superiority of any no ischemia technique (off-clamp, on-clamp, superselective clamping or cold ischemia) over the other.

An adequate balance between ischemia time, limited ischemic parenchymal zone, risk of intraoperative complications and oncological safety is of paramount importance when performing nephron sparing surgery. The use of technological aids, such as 3D models, perfusion algorithms and augmented reality could improve our knowledge of the case and help surgeons to choose the most suited strategy.

References

1. Abdel Raheem A, Alowidah I, Capitanio U, Montorsi F, Larcher A, Derweesh I, Ghali F, Mottrie A, Mazzone E, DE Naeyer G, Campi R, Sessa F, Carini M, Minervini A, Raman JD, Rjepaj CJ, Kriegmair MC, Autorino R, Veccia A, Mir MC, Claps F, Choi YD, Ham WS, Tadifa JP, Santok GD, Furlan M, Simeone C, Bada M, Celia A, Carrion DM, Aguilera Bazan A, Ruiz CB, Malki M, Barber N, Hussain M, Micali S, Puliatti S, Alwahabi A, Alqahtani A, Rumaih A, Ghaith A, Ghoneem AM, Hagras A, Eissa A, Alenzi, MJ, Pavan N, Traunero F, Antonelli A, Porcaro AB, Illiano E, Costantini E, Rha KH. Warm ischemia time length during on-clamp partial nephrectomy: dose it really matter? Minerva Urol Nephrol. 2021. https://doi.org/10.23736/S2724-6051.21.04466-9.
2. Antonelli A, Cindolo L, Sandri M, Veccia A, Annino F, Bertagna F, Carini M, Celia A, D'Orta C, De Concilio B, Furlan M, Giommoni V, Ingrosso M, Mari A, Nucciotti R, Olianti C, Porreca A, Primiceri G, Schips L, Sessa F, Bove P, Simeone C, Minervini A, AGILE Group (Italian Group for Advanced Laparo-Endoscopic Surgery). Is off-clamp robot-assisted partial nephrectomy beneficial for renal function? Data from the CLOCK trial. BJU Int. 2021. https://doi.org/10.1111/bju.15503.
3. Baumert H, Ballaro A, Shah N, Mansouri D, Zafar N, Molinié V, Neal D. Reducing warm ischaemia time during laparoscopic partial nephrectomy: a prospective comparison of two renal closure techniques. Eur Urol. 2007;52:1164–9. https://doi.org/10.1016/j.eururo.2007.03.060.
4. Becker F, Van Poppel H, Hakenberg OW, Stief C, Gill I, Guazzoni G, Montorsi F, Russo P, Stöckle M. Assessing the impact of ischaemia time during partial nephrectomy. Eur Urol. 2009;56:625–34. https://doi.org/10.1016/j.eururo.2009.07.016.
5. Borofsky MS, Gill IS, Hemal AK, Marien TP, Jayaratna I, Krane LS, Stifelman MD. Near-infrared fluorescence imaging to facilitate super-selective arterial clamping during zero-ischaemia robotic partial nephrectomy. BJU Int. 2013;111:604–10. https://doi.org/10.1111/j.1464-410X.2012.11490.x.
6. Cacciamani GE, Medina LG, Gill TS, Mendelsohn A, Husain F, Bhardwaj L, Artibani W, Sotelo R, Gill IS. Impact of renal hilar control on outcomes of robotic partial nephrectomy: systematic review and cumulative meta-analysis. Eur Urol Focus. 2019;5:619–35. https://doi.org/10.1016/j.euf.2018.01.012.
7. Cao J, Zhu S, Ye M, Liu K, Liu Z, Han W, Xie Y. Comparison of renal artery vs renal artery-vein clamping during partial nephrectomy: a system review and meta-analysis. J Endourol. 2020;34:523–30. https://doi.org/10.1089/end.2019.0580.
8. Chatauret N, Badet L, Barrou B, Hauet T. Ischemia-reperfusion: from cell biology to acute kidney injury. Progres En Urol J Assoc Francaise Urol. Soc Francaise Urol. 2014;24(Suppl)1:S4–12. https://doi.org/10.1016/S1166-7087(14)70057-0.
9. Crain DS, Spencer CR, Favata MA, Amling CL. Transureteral saline perfusion to obtain renal hypothermia: potential application in laparoscopic partial nephrectomy. JSLS. 2004;8:217–22.
10. De Backer P, Vangeneugden J, Van Praet C, Lejoly M, Vermijs S, Vanpeteghem C, Decaestecker K. V04-12 Robot-assisted partial nephrectomy using intra-arterial renal hypothermia for highly complex endophytic or hilar tumors. J Urol. 2021;206. https://doi.org/10.1097/JU.0000000000002000.12.
11. Gill IS, Eisenberg MS, Aron M, Berger A, Ukimura O, Patil MB, Campese V, Thangathurai D, Desai MM. "Zero ischemia" partial nephrectomy: novel laparoscopic and robotic technique. Eur Urol. 2011;59:128–34. https://doi.org/10.1016/j.eururo.2010.10.002.
12. Gill IS, Patil MB, Abreu AL de C, Ng C, Cai J, Berger A, Eisenberg MS, Nakamoto M, Ukimura O, Goh AC, Thangathurai D, Aron M, Desai MM. Zero ischemia anatomical partial nephrectomy: a novel approach. J Urol. 2012;187:807–14.https://doi.org/10.1016/j.juro.2011.10.146.

13. Greco F, Autorino R, Altieri V, Campbell S, Ficarra V, Gill I, Kutikov A, Mottrie A, Mirone V, van Poppel H. Ischemia techniques in nephron-sparing surgery: a systematic review and meta-analysis of surgical, oncological, and functional outcomes. Eur Urol. 2019;75:477–91. https://doi.org/10.1016/j.eururo.2018.10.005.
14. Janetschek G, Abdelmaksoud A, Bagheri F, Al-Zahrani H, Leeb K, Gschwendtner M. Laparoscopic partial nephrectomy in cold ischemia: renal artery perfusion. J Urol. 2004;171:68–71. https://doi.org/10.1097/01.ju.0000101040.13244.c4.
15. Kijvikai K, Viprakasit DP, Milhoua P, Clark PE, Herrell SD. A simple, effective method to create laparoscopic renal protective hypothermia with cold saline surface irrigation: clinical application and assessment. J Urol. 2010;184:1861–6. https://doi.org/10.1016/j.juro.2010.06.100.
16. Nahar B, Bhat A, Parekh DJ. Does every minute of renal ischemia still count in 2019? unlocking the chains of a flawed thought process over five decades. Eur Urol Focus. 2019;5:939–42. https://doi.org/10.1016/j.euf.2019.03.019.
17. Peyronnet B, Baumert H, Mathieu R, Masson-Lecomte A, Grassano Y, Roumiguié M, Massoud W, Abd El Fattah V, Bruyère F, Droupy S, de la Taille A, Doumerc N, Bernhard J-C, Vaessen C, Rouprêt M, Bensalah K. Early unclamping technique during robot-assisted laparoscopic partial nephrectomy can minimise warm ischaemia without increasing morbidity. BJU Int. 2014;114:741–7. https://doi.org/10.1111/bju.12766.
18. Porpiglia F, Fiori C, Checcucci E, Amparore D, Bertolo R. Hyperaccuracy three-dimensional reconstruction is able to maximize the efficacy of selective clamping during robot-assisted partial nephrectomy for complex renal masses. Eur Urol. 2018;74:651–60. https://doi.org/10.1016/j.eururo.2017.12.027.
19. Simone G, Tuderti G, Anceschi U, Ferriero M, Costantini M, Minisola F, Vallati G, Pizzi G, Guaglianone S, Misuraca L, Gallucci M. "Ride the Green Light": indocyanine green-marked off-clamp robotic partial nephrectomy for totally endophytic renal masses. Eur Urol. 2019;75:1008–14. https://doi.org/10.1016/j.eururo.2018.09.015.
20. Thompson RH, Lane BR, Lohse CM, Leibovich BC, Fergany A, Frank I, Gill IS, Blute ML, Campbell SC. Renal function after partial nephrectomy: effect of warm ischemia relative to quantity and quality of preserved kidney. Urology. 2012;79:356–60. https://doi.org/10.1016/j.urology.2011.10.031.

Robotic Retroperitoneal Partial Nephrectomy

4

Joseph Hon-Ming Wong, Peng-Fei Shao, and Jeremy Yuen-Chun Teoh

4.1 Introduction

Robot-assisted partial nephrectomy has rapidly gained popularity in urology to treat localized renal tumours in this decade because of the improved precision and ease of suturing compared to the laparoscopic approach. While a transperitoneal approach allows good exposure of the kidney, it might be technically difficult in patients with anticipated intra-abdominal adhesions. Renal tumours located posteriorly will also require extensive mobilisation of the kidney upon a transperitoneal approach, and sometimes visualisation can still be difficult. Robotic retroperitoneal partial nephrectomy has been shown to be a highly feasible surgery in treating renal tumours. In this chapter, we shall discuss how to plan and perform robotic retroperitoneal partial nephrectomy in a step-by-step manner, and summarize the latest evidence that is available in the literature.

J. H.-M. Wong (✉) · J. Y.-C. Teoh
S.H. Ho Urology Centre, The Chinese University of Hong Kong, Hong Kong, China
e-mail: hmwong@surgery.cuhk.edu.hk

J. Y.-C. Teoh
e-mail: jeremyteoh@surgery.cuhk.edu.hk

P.-F. Shao
The First Affiliated Hospital of Nanjing Medical University, Nanjing, China
e-mail: spf032@hotmail.com

J. Y.-C. Teoh
European Association of Urology – Young Academic Urologist (EAU-YAU), Hong Kong, China

4.2 Patient Selection

Retroperitoneal approach is ideal for posteriorly or laterally located tumours; or if the target segmental arterial branch is posterior to the renal vein when selective arterial clamping is contemplated; or in patients who had previous transperitoneal surgery. On the other hand, retroperitoneal approach is not recommended for anteriorly located tumours, large tumour (e.g. >4 cm), or morbidly obese patients, because of the relatively smaller working space compared to transperitoneal approach.

4.3 Pre-operative Evaluation and Preparation

Pre-operative evaluations including a thorough workup of the tumour and renal vascular anatomies, as well as assessment of patients' medical fitness are necessary. A computed tomography of renal angiogram (CTA) with 3D reconstruction of tumour location and vascular anatomy is recommended (Fig. 4.1). It is important to visualize the tumour in all three planes (axial, coronal and sagittal), as it is often misleading by studying one plane alone. Furthermore, a 3D reconstructed digital kidney model allows firstly a realistic tumour visualization and hence its localization in the kidney, and secondly an accurate depiction of renal vascular anatomy, which is crucial in situations of complex vascular anatomy and when selective arterial clamping is planned.

All anticoagulants and antiplatelets (except low-dose aspirin) need to be withheld before operation, the duration of which depend on the individual drug profile. Bowel preparation is usually not needed. Informed consent is taken with patient

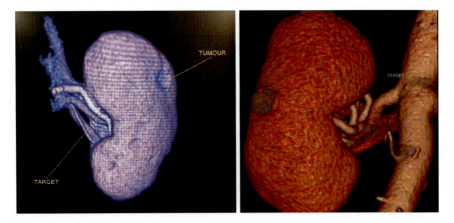

Fig. 4.1 CT renal angiograms depicting tumour location and vascular anatomy, with the segmental artery supplying the tumours labelled

counselled on the potential surgical complications, as well as the uncommon situations of open conversion and total nephrectomy. Prophylactic intravenous antibiotic (e.g. penicillin class with beta-lactamase inhibitor) is administered on induction of operation.

4.4 Patient Position

After general anaesthesia and insertion of 16 French Foley catheter, the patient is put in full lateral position. All pressure points are carefully padded, and sequential compression stockings are worn. The table is then broken and flexed slowly to 60° to expand the ipsilateral flank space for optimal trocar placement and hence reduce risk of instruments collision (Fig. 4.2).

4.5 Obtaining Access

Obtaining access to the retroperitoneal space and good trocar placements are the critical steps for robotic retroperitoneal partial nephrectomy. Five ports (with 4 robotic arms) configuration is recommended. First, a 2 cm skin incision is made at 2 cm above the iliac crest at the mid axillary line for the camera port. External oblique muscle is retracted, and lumbosacral fascia is punctured bluntly to enter the retroperitoneal space, which is confirmed by palpation of psoas muscles posteriorly and lower pole of kidney superiorly. The retroperitoneal space is dilated using a balloon dilator (Spacemaker™ Plus Dissector System) with 700 cc of air under

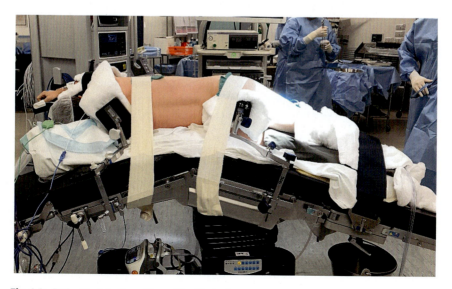

Fig. 4.2 Patient in lateral position with table broken

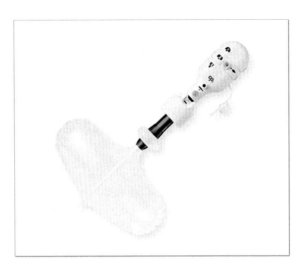

Fig. 4.3 Spacemaker™ Plus Dissector System which comprises of a balloon dilator and a balloon trocar

laparoscopic guidance (Figs. 4.3 and 4.4). Two robotic ports are then inserted at 8 cm on either side of the camera port under finger guidance. A 12 mm assistant port is inserted inferiorly on the abdominal side, and carbon dioxide insufflation into the retroperitoneum follows. When the da Vinci Xi robotic system is used, the trocar-in-trocar technique is applied for the camera port by passing a robotic trocar into the balloon trocar. The balloon trocar helps to maximize the operative field while avoiding slippage of robotic trocar in the relatively small retroperitoneal space.

Utilization of the fourth robotic port is favoured, as it enables the operating surgeon to have self-controlled tissue retraction and hence rely less on the experience of assistant. Before its insertion, peritoneum is dissected carefully away from the rectus muscle by laparoscopic instruments. Subsequently, the fourth robotic port is inserted superiorly and more medially on the abdominal side at the mid-clavicular line, under laparoscopic visual guidance (Fig. 4.5). The five ports configuration is shown below (Fig. 4.6).

4.6 Robot Docking

The robot docking approach depends on the model that is used. When the da Vinci Xi robotic system is used, it is docked from the back of patient, with the overhead boom-mounted robotic arms rotated 90° caudally (Fig. 4.7). This overhead boom

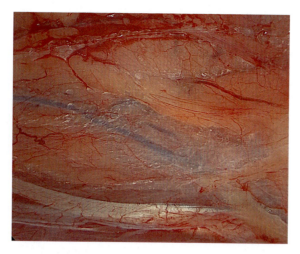

Fig. 4.4 Retroperitoneal space is dilated with balloon dilator under laparoscopic guidance

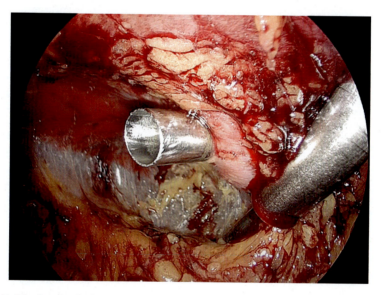

Fig. 4.5 The fourth robotic port is inserted after peritoneum is dissected away from the rectus muscle under laparoscopic guidance

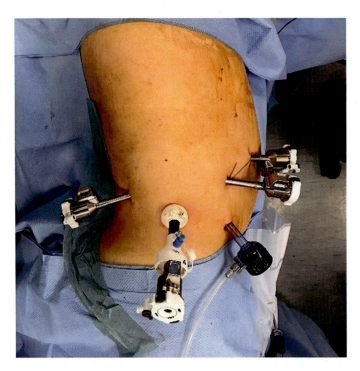

Fig. 4.6 Five ports configuration in robot-assisted retroperitoneal right partial nephrectomy (abdominal side on the right; cranial side on top). Note the trocar-in-trocar technique for the camera port

mount is advantageous because the endotracheal tube of patient is spared by the da Vinci Xi robotic system, in contrast to the previous models (e.g. da Vinci S or Si robotic systems), in which the robot would dock from the patient's head, and management with the endotracheal tube by the anaesthetist would be hindered.

4.7 Partial Nephrectomy: Techniques

In robotic retroperitoneal partial nephrectomy, a 30° downward-lens camera is favoured, with the kidney oriented vertically. The robotic instruments preferred are listed in Table 4.1.

The Gerota's fascia is incised to expose the kidney. Posterior aspect of kidney is then mobilized to expose the renal hilum. The fourth robotic arm helps to retract the kidney medially (Fig. 4.8). Careful and gentle tissue handling is essential in dissecting the renal vasculature. Identification of the renal pedicle is facilitated by maintaining adequate retraction on kidney. As renal artery is located posterior to the vein, the main renal artery is usually more readily identifiable than in

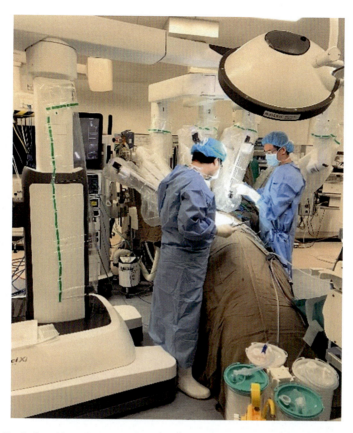

Fig. 4.7 Docked position of da Vinci Xi Robotic system in retroperitoneal right partial nephrectomy

Table 4.1 Robotic instruments used in different steps of partial nephrectomy

	Left arm	Right arm	Fourth arm
Kidney mobilization & vascular dissection	Maryland bipolar forceps	Monopolar curved scissors	ProGrasp™ forceps
Tumour excision & renorrhaphy	ProGrasp™ forceps	Monopolar curved scissors & Large needle driver	Maryland bipolar forceps

transperitoneal approach (Fig. 4.9). In selected cases in which selective clamping is contemplated, the segmental arterial branch or branches supplying the tumour are identified. In cases where the segmental arterial branch is anterior to the renal vein, anterior aspect of kidney is dissected to reach the target segmental arterial branch. Renal vein mobilization is done only for hilar tumours.

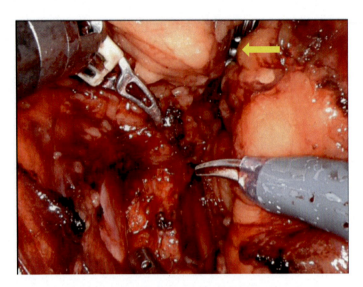

Fig. 4.8 The fourth robotic arm facilitates hilar dissection by retracting the kidney medially (yellow arrow)

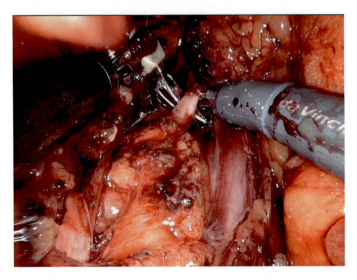

Fig. 4.9 The main renal artery, which is more readily identifiable due to its posterior location to the vein, is mobilized and slinged

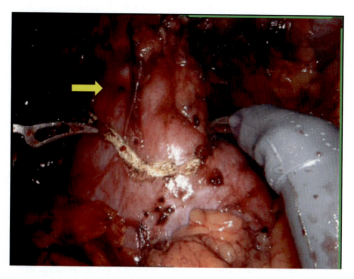

Fig. 4.10 The perinephric fat surrounding the tumour at upper pole of right kidney (yellow arrow) is excised with adequate margin for subsequent renorrhaphy

The kidney is then mobilized adequately to locate the tumour. The fourth robotic arm is used to retract the peritoneum medially, and care should be taken to avoid breaching the peritoneum into transperitoneal cavity. Perinephric fat surrounding the tumour is then excised with adequate margin for renorrhaphy (Fig. 4.10). It is not uncommon to encounter adhesive perinephric fat in particular of that near the tumour, therefore ample time should be reserved for meticulous fat dissection. If the perinephric fat is markedly adhesive, it is advisable to leave a thin strip of sticky fat on the kidney surface, rather than stripping off the kidney capsule. Intraoperative drop-in ultrasound probe is used to help define the tumour margin, especially for endophytic tumours.

The main renal artery or the target segmental arterial branch is then clamped by bulldog (Fig. 4.11). The perfusion deprivation of renal parenchyma surrounding the tumour is confirmed by a 2.5 mg intravenous bolus injection of indocyanine green (ICG) (Fig. 4.12). Clamping of renal vein is unnecessary in majority of cases, except for hilar tumours.

The techniques used for tumour excision and renorrhaphy in retroperitoneal partial nephrectomy are identical to transperitoneal approach. Renal tumour is enucleo-resected with athermal scissors, with care taken not to breach the tumour, at the same time, not to resect excessive normal renal parenchyma. The resected tumour is inspected for gross complete resection and put in an Endo catch™ bag. Frozen section of margin is not routinely taken unless in doubtful cases (Fig. 4.13).

After resecting the tumour, the renal defect is repaired in two layers. The renal defect bed, which includes bleeders & collecting system, is meticulously plicated

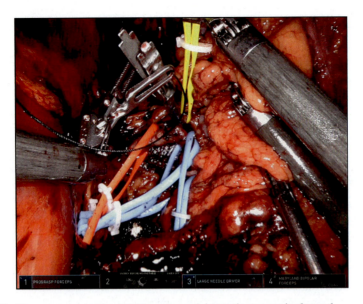

Fig. 4.11 The segmental renal arterial branch supplying to the tumour is clamped

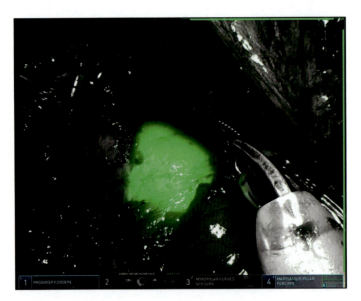

Fig. 4.12 Perfusion deprivation after segmental artery clamping is confirmed by indocyanine green (ICG), with absence of green colour on the parenchymal surface at the tumour site

4 Robotic Retroperitoneal Partial Nephrectomy

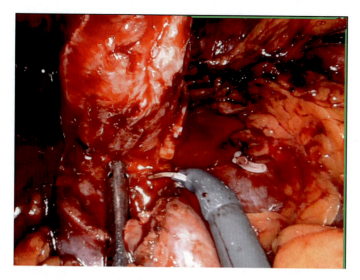

Fig. 4.13 The tumour is enucleo-resected with athermal scissors

with 3–0 barbed sutures, in continuous manner, with sliding-clip compression technique (inner layer). Absorbable clips (Absolok®) are preferred to avoid stone formation in case of migration into collecting system, and to reduce post-operative image artifacts. Early unclamping of renal artery is then done in most cases, which can significantly reduce the ischaemia time. Repair of the outer renal parenchyma subsequently follows with 2–0 barbed sutures using CT-1 needle, also in continuous manner, with similar sliding-clip compression technique (outer layer). This warm ischaemia time should be kept to minimum, to reduce ischaemia insult to the kidney. Ureteric stent is seldom required. Haemostatic agents e.g. Tisseel is applied to the site of repair in selected cases to reinforce haemostasis. A 12 French drain is inserted, and the specimen is retrieved through the camera port at the end of procedure (Figs. 4.14, 4.15 and 4.16).

4.8 Special Concerns

4.8.1 Breach of Peritoneum

If peritoneum is inadvertently opened, it should be clipped with hem-o-lok® immediately when the defect is small to maintain the retroperitoneal space. However, if the peritoneal defect is large, suture repair is often difficult, and retroperitoneal space may be maintained by using the robotic fourth arm to retract peritoneum medially, or alternatively, extend the peritoneal defect widely to convert to a flank transperitoneal approach.

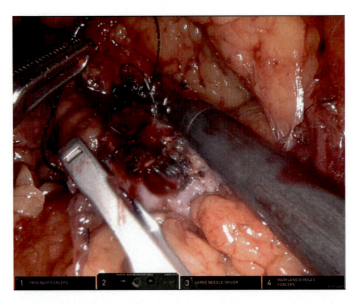

Fig. 4.14 Renorrhaphy is performed by two layers of barbed sutures in continuous manner. The inner layer repair is shown here

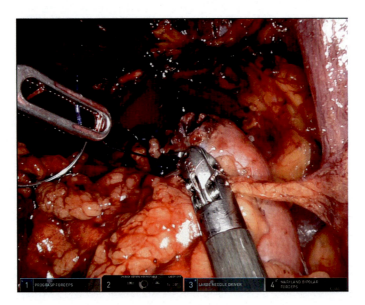

Fig. 4.15 The outer layer of parenchymal repair using barbed sutures with sliding-clips compression technique

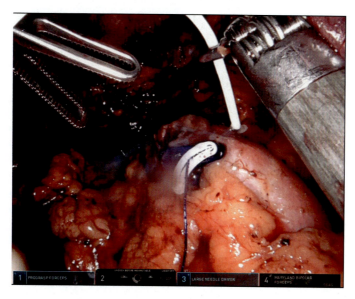

Fig. 4.16 Tisseel was applied to the defect to augment haemostasis

4.8.2 Selective Artery Clamping

While segmental arterial branch clamping limits ischaemia to renal parenchyma surrounding the tumour and helps to reduce ischaemic injury, it should be performed only in selected cases, preferably with pre-operative CTA and intra-operative ICG. Most suitable tumours are those small ones, or tumours that are supplied by a single segmental artery. It is not recommended for hilar tumours where renal vein may need to be controlled, or large tumours that are supplied by multiple segmental arteries.

4.8.3 Parenchyma Around Tumour Lights Up with ICG

Bulldog should be checked for any trapping of tissue adjacent to the artery, and proper clamping should be ensured. If bulldog is well positioned or fresh bleeding is observed upon commencement of tumour resection, then bulldog should be released, vascular anatomy in CTA re-studied, and additional renal artery should be looked for. Main renal artery clamping should be considered if selective artery clamping is initially planned. Parenchymal perfusion around the tumour may be re-checked by administering another intravenous dose of ICG (2.5 mg) after its washout 20 to 30 min later.

4.9 Literature Review

In 2009, Patel et al. described ten cases of robotic retroperitoneal renal surgeries, of which three of them were partial nephrectomies. For the three partial nephrectomy patients, tumour size ranged from 1.8–3.6 cm. The mean warm ischemia time was 17.3 min, and blood loss ranged from 50–100 mL only. The authors proposed that this approach might be preferred for posterior renal tumours, or for patients with prior abdominal surgery or on peritoneal dialysis. This report was instrumental in establishing the feasibility of using robotics for retroperitoneal partial nephrectomy. The technique has gradually gained interest and popularity in the past decade.

Recently, there was a meta-analysis comparing between robotic retroperitoneal and transperitoneal partial nephrectomy. A total of 11 studies with 2984 patients with localised renal tumour were included. Among them, 1715 underwent robotic transperitoneal and 1269 underwent robotic retroperitoneal partial nephrectomy. Among the studies, the mean tumour size ranged from 2.5 to 4.8 cm, and the mean RENAL score ranged from 6 to 8. Need of open conversion was only 0.8% in the patients undergoing robotic retroperitoneal partial nephrectomy. The key findings of the meta-analysis are summarised below.

4.9.1 Operative Time and Warm Ischemia Time

Among 10 studies with 2216 patients, retroperitoneal approach was associated with a shorter operative time than the transperitoneal approach (Mean difference 21.68 min, 95% CI 11.61–31.76, $p < 0.001$). Among 9 studies with 2003 patients, there was no significant difference in the warm ischemia time (Mean difference 0.17 min, 95% -0.80–1.14, $p = 0.73$). Overall, the difference in the operative time of 21.68 min may not be clinically important, especially when there was no significant difference in the warm ischemic time between the two groups.

4.9.2 Estimated Blood Loss and Length of Hospital Stay

Among 10 studies with 2216 patients, retroperitoneal approach was associated with lower amount of estimated blood loss (Mean difference 40.94 mL, 95% 14.87–67.01, $p = 0.002$). Among 9 studies with 2003 patients, the retroperitoneal group had a shorter hospital stay than the transperitoneal group (Mean difference 0.86 days, 95% 0.35–1.37, $p = <0.001$). Despite the apparent advantages being observed, we must acknowledge that the absolute differences were quite small and they might not be clinically important.

4.9.3 Clavien-Dindo Minor (Grade 1 to 2) and Major (Grade 3 to 5) Complications

Among 9 studies with 2113 patients, the rates of grade 1 to 2 complications were 8.1% in the retroperitoneal group and 10.8% in the transperitoneal group; the difference was statistically different (OR 1.39, 95% CI 1.01–1.91, $p = 0.04$). Among 10 studies with 2881 patients, the rates of grade 3 to 5 complications were 5.9% in the retroperitoneal group and 3.7% in the transperitoneal group; the different was not statistically different (OR 0.72, 95% CI 0.51–1.03, $p = 0.07$).

4.9.4 Decline in Estimated Glomerular Filtration Rate and Upstaging of Chronic Kidney Disease

Among 4 studies with 923 patients, there was no significant difference in the decline in estimated glomerular filtration rate (Mean difference -1.44 mL/min/1.73m^2, 95% CI -4.96–2.08, $p = 0.42$) between the two groups. Among 3 studies with 809 patients, there was also no significant difference in the risk of upstaging of chronic kidney disease (OR 1.07, 95% CI 0.74–1.56, $p = 0.72$) between the two groups. Both the retroperitoneal and transperitoneal approaches were equally effective in preserving kidney function upon robotic partial nephrectomy.

4.9.5 Positive Surgical Margin and Overall Tumour Recurrence

Among 10 studies with 2771 patients, the positive surgical margin rates were 2.9% in the retroperitoneal group and 2.7% in the transperitoneal group. There was no significant difference between the two groups (OR 1.04, 95% CI 0.65–1.65, $p = 0.87$). Among 3 studies with 564 patients, the tumour recurrence rates were 1.3% in the retroperitoneal group and 0.7% in the transperitoneal group. There was again no significant difference between the two groups (OR 0.50, 95% CI 0.02–10.84, $p = 0.66$). Both the retroperitoneal and transperitoneal approaches were equally effective in achieving a good oncological control in robotic partial nephrectomies.

4.9.6 Summary of Evidence

Robotic retroperitoneal partial nephrectomy is a highly feasible, safe and effective treatment for patients with localised renal tumour. Robotic retroperitoneal partial nephrectomy could have additional benefits including a shorter operative time, reduced estimated blood loss, and a lower rate of minor complications. Robotic retroperitoneal partial nephrectomy could achieve similar functional and oncological outcomes as compared to the robotic transperitoneal partial nephrectomy. Based on the current evidence, the retroperitoneal approach is at least equivalent, if not better, than the transperitoneal approach in performing robotic partial nephrectomy.

Robotic Partial Nephrectomy

Riccardo Campi, Selcuk Erdem, Onder Kara, Umberto Carbonara, Michele Marchioni, Alessio Pecoraro, Riccardo Bertolo, Alexandre Ingels, Maximilian Kriegmair, Nicola Pavan, Eduard Roussel, Angela Pecoraro, and Daniele Amparore

Partial nephrectomy (PN) is nowadays considered as the gold standard treatment for the management of clinical T1 renal masses [1]. Across the past decades, the surgical techniques for PN have evolved in parallel with the diffusion and accessibility to minimally-invasive approaches such laparoscopy and robotics. From the first description of robotic-assisted partial nephrectomy (RAPN) in 2004 [2], the wide and continuous spread of robotic platforms has led to increase the proportion of nephron sparing surgeries (NSS) performed with such apparoach [3]. Thanks to its 3D magnification and stereoscopic vision, as well as its extremely flexible manipulative robotic arms robotic technology has undoubted advantages of dexterity and visualization of the operative fields if compared to open and laparoscopic surgery, improving the precision of both extirpative and reconstructive phases of PN [4]; moreover, it has a shorter learning curve, justifying its progressive diffusion over the other approaches, and takes advantages of new technological

R. Campi (✉) · A. Pecoraro
Unit of Urological Robotic Surgery and Renal Transplantation, Careggi Hospital, University of Florence, Florence, Italy
e-mail: riccardo.campi@unifi.it

R. Campi
Department of Experimental and Clinical Medicine, University of Florence, Florence, Italy

S. Erdem
Division of Urologic Oncology, Department of Urology, Istanbul Faculty of Medicine, Istanbul University, Istanbul, Turkey

O. Kara
Department of Urology, School of Medicine, Kocaeli University, Kocaeli, Turkey

U. Carbonara
Department of Emergency and Organ Transplantation-Urology, Andrology and Kidney Transplantation Unit, University of Bari, Bari, Italy

tools, such TilePro, near-infrared fluorescence imaging and three-dimensional virtual models guidance, to push through the limits in treating tumors higher in complexity and larger in size [5].

5.1 Indications

Focusing on the indications, current EAU guidelines report that PN can be performed to treat clinical T1 tumors, either by open-, pure laparoscopic- or robot-assisted approach, based on surgeon's expertise and skills, underlying the last two that are associated with shorter length of hospital stay and lower blood loss compared to open surgery [1].

Indeed, if compared to open PN, RAPN shows decreased morbidity with lower complications rate [6], while similar rates of local recurrence, distant metastasis and cancer specific mortality were recorded for all the approaches [7].

Moreover, in comparison with pure laparoscopy, RAPN seems to offer lower rate of conversion to open surgery and to radical surgery, shorter warm ischaemia time (WIT) and smaller change in estimated glomerular filtration rate (eGFR) after surgery [8].

At last, as demonstrated analyzing over 18.000 patients in a retrospective study of a U.S. National Cancer Database, the prognostic outcomes of RAPN are

---

M. Marchioni
Laboratory of Biostatistics, Department of Medical, Oral and Biotechnological Sciences, University "G. D'Annunzio" Chieti-Pescara, Chieti, Italy

Department of Urology, SS Annunziata Hospital, "G. D'Annunzio" University of Chieti, Chieti, Italy

R. Bertolo
Department of Urology, San Carlo Di Nancy Hospital, Rome, Italy

A. Ingels
Department of Urology, University Hospital Henri Mondor, APHP, 51 Avenue du Maréchal de Lattre de Tassigny, 94010 Créteil, Biomaps, France

Biomaps, UMR1281, INSERM, CNRS, CEA, Université Paris Saclay, Villejuif, France

M. Kriegmair
Department of Urology, University Medical Centre Mannheim, Mannheim, Germany

N. Pavan
Department of Medical, Surgical and Health Science, Urology Clinic, University of Trieste, Trieste, Italy

E. Roussel
Department of Urology, University Hospitals Leuven, Leuven, Belgium

A. Pecoraro · D. Amparore
Division of Urology, Department of Oncology, School of Medicine, San Luigi Hospital, University of Turin, Orbassano (Turin), Italy

impacted by the hospital volume, showing better perioperative results and positive surgical margin rates if high-volume centers are considered [9].

More recent data, published by the Transatlantic Robotic Nephron-sparing Surgery study group, demonstrated the efficacy of such robotic approach considering 635 patients with clinically localized kidney cancer. The surgical outcome of RAPN, expressed as MIC score (margin, ischemia, and complication rate) reached 72%, with surgical complexity as the only independent risk factor for surgical outcomes [10].

Even if EAU guidelines discourage to perform minimally invasive surgery in case of risk of oncological, functional or perioperative outcomes compromission [1], nowadays many experiences of RAPN for complex or large renal tumors are reported in Literature [11].

A multicenter study considering 255 patients with complex renal masses with PADUA score ≥ 10 revealed optimal surgical outcomes (margins, ischemia, complication—MIC score achieved in 62% of the cases) [5]. Similarly, another study involving 144 RAPNs performed for renal masses with RENAL score ≥ 10, confirmed a Trifecta achievement rate of 61.8% [12].

In parallel with surgical complexity, also the large size of the tumor is a factor still under scrutiny when considering robotic approach [13]. The largest series of clinical T2 tumors treated with RAPN was reported by the ROSULA Collaborative Group, that analyzed data of 298 patients [14]. In 49% of them the Trifecta outcome was achieved, with pathological upstaging to pT3a as the only predictive factor of recurrence/metastasis (10%).

Even more controversial, but currently under investigation, the use of RAPN for clinical T3a renal masses. In a recent study involving 157 patients undergone RAPN for cT3a tumors, the Trifecta outcome was achieved in 64.3%, with negative surgical margins at final pathology in 150 patients (95.5%) and 5-yr recurrence-free survival, cancer-specific survival, and overall survival, of 82.1%, 93.3%, and 91.3%, respectively [15].

Among the indications to RAPN, it is worth to be mentioned its use in case of elderly patients presenting localized renal tumors. In this field of research some studies have been published. The results of the RESURGE collaborative database, including 216 patients aged 75 or older diagnosed with cT1-2 renal mass, confirmed that minimally-invasive PN is associated with acceptable perioperative outcomes. The use of a robotic approach over standard laparoscopy should be preferred when available, giving advantages with respect to clinically relevant outcomes such as postoperative eGFR [16].

5.2 Techniques

5.2.1 Approaches

RAPN can be performed by either transperitoneal and retroperitoneal approaches. Even if more often performed transabdominally, no consensus is reached about the best approach looking at the surgical outcomes. Transperitoneal approach has the advantages of the larger working space and familiar anatomical landmarks for the surgeon, whilst retroperitoneoscopy allows to avoid the incision of the peritoneum and the opening of the abdominal cavity [17]. Data from a study of the Vattikuti Collective Quality Initiative collaboration, showed that both the hospital length of stay and estimated blood loss were lower in the retroperitoneal-RAPN group as compared with the transperitoneal-RAPN group, with similar operative time, WIT and complications rate [18]. Also other studies confirmed the advantages of retroperitoneal approach [19], even if seems that the ultimate choice should be based on lesion features and surgeon comfort, not being clear advantages of an access over the other from studies specifically focused on tumor's location [11, 20].

The recent FDA approval of the da Vinci® SP robotic platform has led to its use in minimally invasive approaches to urologic malignancies. There are little data on its feasibility and safety for partial nephrectomy. One of the more recent experiences published in Literature included 14 consecutive patients with localized renal cancer who underwent SP RAPN at a single institution, with a Trifecta outcome achievement rate of 79%, but further studies are warranted [21].

5.2.2 Pedicle Management

Although most surgeons continue to perform main renal artery clamping during their RAPNs, producing global ischemia, recent studies evaluated the role of alternatives in terms of clamping technique, such as the clampless fashion (off-clamp), the early unclamping and the selective clamping [22].

The first prospective randomized trial comparing off-clamp and on-clamp RAPNs [23] included 80 patients and did not find significant differences in terms of eGFR rate or percentage split renal function between the techniques, confirming previous results [24, 25].

Moreover, of the 152 patients randomized to the off-clamp group in the ongoing prospective CLOCK trial [26], 40% were shifted to the on-clamp group, following intraoperative decision. Despite the high conversion rate, no significant differences in postoperative complications or renal function at six months follow-up were recorded.

In parallel to the concept of clampless technique, a great innovation in the history of clamping management during RAPN is represented by the zero-ischemia technique, reported for the first time by Gill et al. [27] and based on the principle of cutting the tumor with cold scissors or hemostatic instruments without clamping the main artery.

Similarly, also early unclamping techniques, based on the removal of clamping before the end of the renorraphy to reduce ischemic time, have been explored. A recently published retrospective study including 463 patients support the use of such technique, showing a 30-day complication rate of 14.7%, with 88% of patients experiencing low grade complications [28].

An alternative technique for the management of the renal pedicle during RAPN is the selective arterial clamping, based on the concept of clamping single or multiple branches of the artery directed towards the tumor, avoiding global ischemia. Even if associated with an improved postoperative renal function if compared with the clamping of the main renal artery, it requires distal dissection of the artery branches, increasing the risk of intraoperative bleedings [29, 30].

Recent systematic reviews and meta-analyses summarizing the available evidence on ischemia techniques did not found conclusive results, leading to the impossibility to recommend one technique over the other [22, 31].

5.2.3 Resection and Suture Techniques

Among the different techniques for the suture of the parenchyma in the setting of RAPN, running sutures for both medullary and cortical renorrhaphy are widely diffused, optimizing the WIT and the time of reconstructive phase of the surgery, as well as lowering the complication rate and facilitating the procedure itself from a technical point of view, if compared with interrupted suture [32]. Always in the setting of the renal defect closure during RAPN, it has to be mentioned the sliding-clip technique, described in 2009 by Benway et al. [33]. It is based on the use of of Weck Hem-O-Lock clips that are slid into place and secured with a LapraTy clip at the tail end, further shortening WIT and operative time. The last actor of this stage is the barbed suture, used for both inner- and outer-layer renorrhaphy, that seems to contribute in maximizing the above mentioned intraoperative outcomes [34].

5.2.4 Novel Technologies

In the last years, to improve the surgical outcomes of RAPN, novel technologies have been implemented, especially in the field of intraoperative image guidance. One of the most known is the administration of indocyanine green (ICG) to evaluate kidney perfusion intraoperatively. The results of the Transatlantic Robotic Nephron-sparing Surgery, including 318 patients undergone ICG-guided RAPN, confirmed the usefulness of such tool in the assessment of the vascular anatomy, especially in challenging cases [35].

In parallel, pilot experiences are testing the intraoperative use of three-dimensional virtual models in performing Augmented Reality (AR) procedures. Two studies already demonstrated that the real-time overlap of these virtual models to the in-vivo anatomy during AR-RAPN is useful for identifying vessels, complex endophytic lesions and intraparenchymal structures, optimizing the pedicle management as well as the quality of the resection phase, leading to a reduction in postoperative complications [36, 37], with better functional recovery [38].

5.3 Conclusions

Great innovations and technical improvements have been done in the last years to optimize the outcomes of RAPN (Figs. 5.1, 5.2, 5.3 and 5.4) [39–42]. Thanks to these efforts, indications to partial nephrectomy have expanded widely and are still evolving. The future of such highly technological surgery is going to be characterized by further steps forward, with the goals of maximizing as much as possible safety, oncological outcomes and functional recovery.

From left to right, from top to bottom: (a) Preoperative careful evaluation of computed tomography scans, revealing a large, mostly endophytic left renal mass involving the renal sinus; (b) Isolation of the kidney; (c) Delineation of the tumor's contours by means of intraoperative ultrasound; (d) clamping of the renal artery;

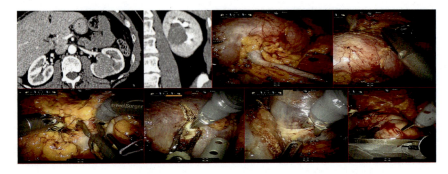

Fig. 5.1 Overview of the main surgical steps for robot-assisted partial nephrectomy

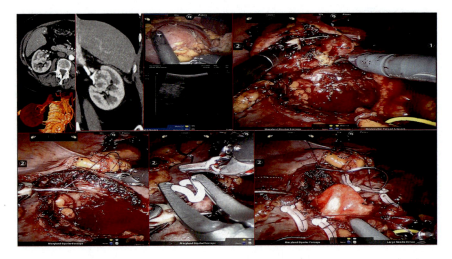

Fig. 5.2 Overview of the main steps for renal reconstruction after robot-assisted partial nephrectomy

5 Robotic Partial Nephrectomy

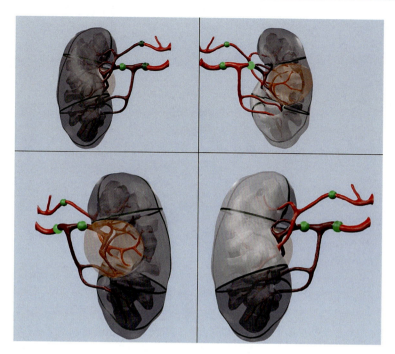

Fig. 5.3 Use of virtual 3D models to simulate the clamping strategy before a case of robot-assisted partial nephrectomy for a posterior, predominantly endophytic right renal mass

(e) circular nephrotomy along the tumor's contours; (f) tumor enucleation (or enucleoresection), following the dissection plane between the tumor and the peritumoral pseudocapsule (or macroscopically healthy renal parenchyma); (g) complete excision of the tumor and placement into an endobag for subsequent retrieval.

From left to right, from top to bottom: (a) Computed tomography scans revealing a large, completely endophytic right renal mass involving the renal sinus in a patient with a single kidney; (b) Delineation of the tumor's contours by means of intraoperative ultrasound; (c) tumor excision (please note the tumor resection bed after pure tumor enucleation; (d) inner-layer renorrhaphy using a continuous monofilament suture (sliding-clip technique); (e) use of hemostatic agents (in the figure, Floseal) before completing the renorrhaphy with the outer-layer suture.

As shown in the figure, different clamping strategy may lead to different degrees of ischemic insult to the renal parenchyma. As such, the surgeon may use 3D models to guide the choice of selective-clamping approaches during surgery in order to allow clear visualization of the tumor contours during tumor excision while minimizing the ischemic insult to the healthy renal parenchyma. In the figure, contrast-enhanced CT scan images in DICOM format were processed by MEDICS Srl (www.medics3d.com) using a dedicated software to achieve a Hyperaccuracy Three-Dimensional (HA3D) Virtual Model.

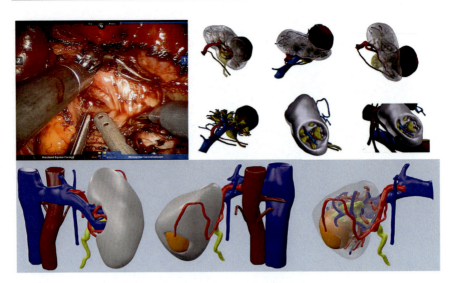

Fig. 5.4 Preoperative planning of robot-assisted partial nephrectomy using virtual 3D models

From left to right, from top to bottom: (a) intraoperative snapshot showing the dissection plane during a pure tumor enucleation, which aims to follow the natural cleavage plane between the tumor and the healthy renal parenchyma. The resection technique during robot-assisted partial nephrectomy may be tailored to the specific anatomical characteristics of the tumor through a comprehensive, detailed analysis of preoperative virtual 3D models (developed by specific software using DICOM images from computed tomography [CT] scans). 3D models allow the surgeon to appreciate the anatomy and topographical characteristics of each tumor, and its relationships with the urinary collecting system and renal vasculature. This allows precise preoperative planning of both resection and reconstruction techniques during robot-assisted partial nephrectomy. In the figure, contrast-enhanced CT scan images in DICOM format were processed by MEDICS Srl (www.medics3d.com) using a dedicated software to achieve a Hyperaccuracy Three-Dimensional (HA3D) Virtual Model.

References

1. Ljungberg B, Albiges L, Bedke J, et al. EAU Guidelines on RCC. Version 2021. http://uroweb.org/guidelines/compilations-of-all-guidelines/.
2. Gettman MT, Blute ML, Chow GK, et al. Robotic-assisted laparoscopic partial nephrectomy: technique and initial clinical experience with DaVinci robotic system. Urology. 2004;64(5):914–8. https://doi.org/10.1016/j.urology.2004.06.049
3. Wallis CJ, Garbens A, Chopra S, et al. Robotic partial nephrectomy: expanding utilization advancing innovation. J Endourol. 2017;31(4):348–54. https://doi.org/10.1089/end.2016.0639

4. Cignoli D, Fallara G, Larcher A, et al. How to improve outcome in nephron-sparing surgery: the impact of new techniques. Curr Opin Urol. 2021;31(3):255–61. https://doi.org/10.1097/MOU.0000000000000862
5. Buffi NM, Saita A, Lughezzani G, et al. Robot-assisted Partial Nephrectomy for Complex (PADUA Score ≥10) Tumors: techniques and results from a multicenter experience at four high-volume Centers. Eur Urol. 2020;77(1):95–100. https://doi.org/10.1016/j.eururo.2019.03.006
6. Peyronnet B, Seisen T, Oger E, et al. French Comittee of Urologic Oncology (CCAFU). Comparison of 1800 robotic and open partial nephrectomies for renal tumors. Ann Surg Oncol. 2016;23(13):4277–83. https://doi.org/10.1245/s10434-016-5411-0
7. Chang KD, Abdel Raheem A, Kim KH, et al. Functional and oncological outcomes of open, laparoscopic and robot-assisted partial nephrectomy: a multicentre comparative matched-pair analyses with a median of 5 years' follow-up. BJU Int. 2018;122(4):618–26. https://doi.org/10.1111/bju.14250
8. Choi JE, You JH, Kim DK, et al. Comparison of perioperative outcomes between robotic and laparoscopic partial nephrectomy: a systematic review and meta-analysis. Eur Urol. 2015;67(5):891–901. https://doi.org/10.1016/j.eururo.2014.12.028
9. Arora S, Keeley J, Pucheril D, et al. What is the hospital volume threshold to optimize inpatient complication rate after partial nephrectomy? Urol Oncol. 2018;36(7):339.e17-339.e23. https://doi.org/10.1016/j.urolonc.2018.04.009
10. Casale P, Lughezzani G, Buffi N, et al. Evolution of robot-assisted partial nephrectomy: techniques and outcomes from the transatlantic robotic nephron-sparing surgery study group. Eur Urol. 2019;76(2):222–7. https://doi.org/10.1016/j.eururo.2018.11.038
11. Carbonara U, Simone G, Minervini A, et al. Outcomes of robot-assisted partial nephrectomy for completely endophytic renal tumors: a multicenter analysis. Eur J Surg Oncol. 2021;47(5):1179–1186. https://doi.org/10.1016/j.ejso.2020.08.012
12. Beksac AT, Okhawere KE, Elbakry AA, et al. Management of high complexity renal masses in partial nephrectomy: a multicenter analysis. Urol Oncol. 2019;37(7):437–44. https://doi.org/10.1016/j.urolonc.2019.04.019.
13. Amparore D, Pecoraro A, Piramide F, et al. Comparison between minimally-invasive partial and radical nephrectomy for the treatment of clinical T2 renal masses: results of a 10-year study in a tertiary care center. Minerva Urol Nephrol. 2021 Apr 22. https://doi.org/10.23736/S2724-6051.21.04390-1
14. Bertolo R, Autorino R, Simone G, et al. Outcomes of robot-assisted partial nephrectomy for clinical T2 Renal Tumors: a multicenter analysis (ROSULA Collaborative Group). Eur Urol. 2018;74(2):226–32. https://doi.org/10.1016/j.eururo.2018.05.004
15. Yim K, Aron M, Rha KH, et al. Outcomes of robot-assisted partial nephrectomy for clinical T3a renal masses: a multicenter analysis. Eur Urol Focus. 2020;S2405–4569(20):30295–9. https://doi.org/10.1016/j.euf.2020.10.011
16. Larcher A, Wallis CJD, Pavan N, et al. Outcomes of minimally invasive partial nephrectomy among very elderly patients: report from the RESURGE collaborative international database. Cent European J Urol. 2020;73(3):273–9. https://doi.org/10.5173/ceju.2020.0179
17. Porpiglia F, Mari A, Amparore D, et al. RECORD 2 Project. Transperitoneal vs retroperitoneal minimally invasive partial nephrectomy: comparison of perioperative outcomes and functional follow-up in a large multi-institutional cohort (The RECORD 2 Project). Surg Endosc. 2020. https://doi.org/10.1007/s00464-020-07919-4
18. Arora S, Heulitt G, Menon M, et al. Retroperitoneal vs transperitoneal robot-assisted partial nephrectomy: comparison in a multi-institutional setting. Urology. 2018;120:131–7. https://doi.org/10.1016/j.urology.2018.06.026
19. Mittakanti HR, Heulitt G, Li HF, Porter JR. Transperitoneal vs. retroperitoneal robotic partial nephrectomy: a matched-paired analysis. World J Urol. 2020;38(5):1093–99. https://doi.org/10.1007/s00345-019-02903-7
20. Dell'Oglio P, De Naeyer G, Xiangjun L, et al. The impact of surgical strategy in robot-assisted partial nephrectomy: is it beneficial to treat anterior tumours with transperitoneal access and

posterior tumours with retroperitoneal access? Eur Urol Oncol. 2021;4(1):112–6. https://doi.org/10.1016/j.euo.2018.12.010
21. Francavilla S, Abern MR, Dobbs RW, et al. Single-Port robot assisted partial nephrectomy: initial experience and technique with the da Vinci Single-Port platform (IDEAL Phase 1). Minerva Urol Nephrol. 2021. https://doi.org/10.23736/S2724-6051.21.03919-9
22. Greco F, Autorino R, Altieri V, et al. Ischemia techniques in nephron-sparing surgery: a systematic review and meta-analysis of surgical, oncological, and functional outcomes. Eur Urol. 2019;75(3):477–91. https://doi.org/10.1016/j.eururo.2018.10.005.
23. Anderson BG, Potretzke AM, Du K, et al. Comparing off-clamp and on-clamp robot-assisted partial nephrectomy: a prospective randomized trial. Urology. 2019;126:102–9. https://doi.org/10.1016/j.urology.2018.11.053.
24. Porpiglia F, Bertolo R, Amparore D, et al. Evaluation of functional outcomes after laparoscopic partial nephrectomy using renal scintigraphy: clamped vs clampless technique. BJU Int. 2015;115(4):606–12. https://doi.org/10.1111/bju.12834
25. Mari A, Morselli S, Sessa F, et al. Impact of the off-clamp endoscopic robot-assisted simple enucleation (ERASE) of clinical T1 renal tumors on the postoperative renal function: results from a matched-pair comparison. Eur J Surg Oncol. 2018;44(6):853–8. https://doi.org/10.1016/j.ejso.2018.01.093
26. Antonelli A, Cindolo L, Sandri M, et al. Predictors of the transition from off to on clamp approach during ongoing robotic partial nephrectomy: data from the CLOCK randomized clinical trial. J Urol. 2019;202(1):62–8. https://doi.org/10.1097/JU.0000000000000194
27. Gill IS, Eisenberg MS, Aron M, et al. "Zero ischemia" partial nephrectomy: novel laparoscopic and robotic technique. Eur Urol. 2011;59(1):128–34. https://doi.org/10.1016/j.eururo.2010.10.002
28. Delto JC, Chang P, Hyde S, et al. Reducing pseudoaneurysm and urine leak after robotic partial nephrectomy: results using the early unclamping technique. Urology. 2019;132:130–5. https://doi.org/10.1016/j.urology.2019.05.042
29. Desai MM, de Castro Abreu AL, Leslie S, et al. Robotic partial nephrectomy with superselective versus main artery clamping: a retrospective comparison. Eur Urol. 2014;66(4):713–9. https://doi.org/10.1016/j.eururo.2014.01.017
30. Simone G, Gill IS, Mottrie A, et al. Indications, techniques, outcomes, and limitations for minimally ischemic and off-clamp partial nephrectomy: a systematic review of the literature. Eur Urol. 2015;68(4):632–40. https://doi.org/10.1016/j.eururo.2015.04.020
31. Cacciamani GE, Medina LG, Gill TS, et al. Impact of renal hilar control on outcomes of robotic partial nephrectomy: systematic review and cumulative meta-analysis. Eur Urol Focus. 2019;5(4):619–35. https://doi.org/10.1016/j.euf.2018.01.012
32. Bertolo R, Campi R, Mir MC, et al. Systematic review and pooled analysis of the impact of renorrhaphy techniques on renal functional outcome after partial nephrectomy. Eur Urol Oncol. 2019;2(5):572–5. https://doi.org/10.1016/j.euo.2018.11.008
33. Benway BM, Wang AJ, Cabello JM, et al. Robotic partial nephrectomy with sliding-clip renorrhaphy: technique and outcomes. Eur Urol. 2009;55(3):592–9. https://doi.org/10.1016/j.eururo.2008.12.028
34. Bertolo R, Campi R, Klatte T, et al. Suture techniques during laparoscopic and robot-assisted partial nephrectomy: a systematic review and quantitative synthesis of peri-operative outcomes. BJU Int. 2019;123(6):923–46. https://doi.org/10.1111/bju.14537
35. Diana P, Buffi NM, Lughezzani G, et al. The role of intraoperative indocyanine green in robot-assisted partial nephrectomy: results from a large, multi-institutional series. Eur Urol. 2020;78(5):743–9. https://doi.org/10.1016/j.eururo.2020.05.040
36. Porpiglia F, Fiori C, Checcucci E, et al. Hyperaccuracy three-dimensional reconstruction is able to maximize the efficacy of selective clamping during robot-assisted partial nephrectomy for complex renal masses. Eur Urol. 2018;74(5):651–60. https://doi.org/10.1016/j.eururo.2017.12.027.
37. Porpiglia F, Checcucci E, Amparore D, et al. Three-dimensional augmented reality robot-assisted partial nephrectomy in case of complex tumours (PADUA ≥10): a new intraoperative

tool overcoming the ultrasound guidance. Eur Urol. 2020;78(2):229–38. https://doi.org/10.1016/j.eururo.2019.11.024
38. Amparore D, Pecoraro A, Checcucci E, et al. Three-dimensional virtual models' assistance during minimally invasive partial nephrectomy minimizes the impairment of kidney function. Eur Urol Oncol. 2021;S2588–9311(21):00075–4. https://doi.org/10.1016/j.euo.2021.04.001
39. Carbonara U, Eun D, Derweesh I, et al. Retroperitoneal versus transeperitoneal robot-assisted partial nephrectomy for postero-lateral renal masses: an international multicenter analysis. World J Urol. 2021. https://doi.org/10.1007/s00345-021-03741-2
40. Minervini A, Carini M, Uzzo RG, et al. Standardized reporting of resection technique during nephron-sparing surgery: the surface-intermediate-base margin score. Eur Urol. 2014;66(5):803–5. https://doi.org/10.1016/j.eururo.2014.06.002
41. Minervini A, Campi R, Di Maida F, et al. Tumor-parenchyma interface and long-term oncologic outcomes after robotic tumor enucleation for sporadic renal cell carcinoma. Urol Oncol. 2018;36(12):527.e1-527.e11. https://doi.org/10.1016/j.urolonc.2018.08.014
42. Minervini A, Campi R, Lane BR, et al. Impact of resection technique on perioperative outcomes and surgical margins after partial nephrectomy for localized renal masses: a prospective multicenter study. J Urol. 2020;203(3):496–504. https://doi.org/10.1097/JU.0000000000000591

Pushing the Boundaries in Robot—Assisted Partial Nephrectomy for Renal Cancer

Charles Van Praet, Pieter De Backer, Riccardo Campi, Pietro Piazza, Alessio Pecoraro, Alexandre Mottrie, Andrea Minervini, and Karel Decaestecker

Renal cell carcinoma (RCC) incidence increases worldwide and it is highest in developed countries. Due to expanded use of routine imaging for many disorders, nowadays RCC is usually diagnosed as an incidentaloma on abdominal imaging. This has also caused a disease stage migration with average tumour size at diagnosis decreasing over the years [16].

C. Van Praet (✉) · P. De Backer · K. Decaestecker
Department of Urology, ERN eUROGEN Accredited Centre, Ghent University Hospital, Ghent, Belgium
e-mail: charles.vanpraet@uzgent.be

P. De Backer
e-mail: pieter.debacker@uzgent.be

K. Decaestecker
e-mail: karel.decaestecker@uzgent.be

P. De Backer · A. Mottrie
OLV Robotic Surgery Institute (ORSI), Melle, Belgium

R. Campi · A. Pecoraro
Unit of Urological Robotic Surgery and Renal Transplantation, Careggi Hospital, University of Florence, Florence, Italy

R. Campi · A. Minervini
Department of Experimental and Clinical Medicine, University of Florence, Florence, Italy
e-mail: andrea.minervini@unifi.it

R. Campi
European Association of Urology (EAU) Young Academic Urologists (YAU) Renal Cancer Working Group, Arnhem, Netherlands

P. Piazza
Division of Urology, IRCCS Azienda Ospedaliero-Universitaria di Bologna, Bologna, Italy

ORSI Academy, Melle, Belgium

© The Author(s), under exclusive license to Springer Nature Switzerland AG 2022
S. S. Goonewardene et al. (eds.), *Robotic Surgery for Renal Cancer*, Management of Urology, https://doi.org/10.1007/978-3-031-11000-9_6

Therefore, urologists are focusing on strategies to minimize the impact of therapy in terms of overall morbidity and renal function, while maintaining optimal oncological outcome. Minimal-invasive surgery is increasingly adopted to reduce short-term morbidity and allow earlier convalescence. Cancer-specific survival of T1-2 N0M0 RCC is excellent, with cancer specific survival exceeding 92% while chronic kidney disease (CKD) is associated with poor survival [34]. This led to nephron-sparing surgery (NSS) being increasingly performed instead of radical nephrectomy to optimize long-term renal function. European Association of Urology (EAU) guidelines indicate a partial nephrectomy (PN) is indicated for all T1 tumours and it should be considered for T2 tumours, especially in patients with a solitary kidney, bilateral tumours or CKD [35]. A lot of tertiary referral centres in developed countries are currently performing robot-assisted partial nephrectomy (RAPN) as the standard therapy for most of their patients with localized RCC.

A "traditional" RAPN includes the following surgical steps:

1. Development of pneumoperitoneum, placement of trocars and robot docking.
2. Reflecting of the ascending colon and duodenum and mobilization of the liver for right-sided tumours; reflecting of the descending colon and mobilization of pancreas tail and spleen for left-sided tumours.
3. Dissection of the renal hilum with identification of the renal artery (and possibly extra branches).
4. Dissection of the tumour and surrounding renal capsule.
5. Renal artery clamping (warm ischemia).
6. Tumour resection.
7. Renorraphy: classically a separate inner and outer renorraphy.
8. Unclamping and control of hemostasis.
9. Closure of Gerota's fascia, specimen extraction and closure of the abdominal wounds.

Increased experience with robotic surgery, technological improvements, and better awareness of RCC's biological behavior are allowing even more advanced RCC cases to be safely treated with RAPN. As this is an evolving field, this chapter highlights some of these contemporary evolutions. We will focus on preoperative planning using 3D models, different techniques for hilar control and different tumour resection strategies.

A. Minervini
Unit of Oncologic Minimally-Invasive Urology and Andrology, Careggi Hospital, Florence, Italy

A. Mottrie
Department of Urology, OLV Hospital, Aalst, Belgium

6.1 Pre-operative Planning with 3D Models

An accurate surgical planning for renal cancer surgery is mandatory in order to achieve the best surgical outcomes. A comprehensive evaluation of kidney tumours is non-trivial, as tumour size, location and the relationship to the collecting system and the vascular system have to be taken into account. In order to facilitate this process, several nephrometry scores have been implemented in clinical practice over the last ten years, of which PADUA and RENAL are the most widely used [21, 33]. All current nephrometry scores have been developed, validated and calculated using bidimensional imaging. As a consequence, the surgeon is required to create a three-dimensional mental image starting by the observation of two-dimensional images in the three spatial axes (axial, coronal and sagittal), with suboptimal results [50]. Especially when dealing with complex kidney tumours, where bidimensional imaging has been suggested to provide inadequate assessment [59].

Thanks to its ability to overcome some limitations of established imaging techniques [14], the use of 3D technology has widely spread in the urological community since its first use in 2012 [65]. Moreover, 3D reconstructions have been proven to have a stronger correlation with excised renal tumour, in terms of both morphology and volume, when compared with conventional imaging [67].

Available studies on the usefulness of 3D reconstruction report on rather small patient series, which remains a bottleneck in acquiring clear evidence. One key aspect several authors investigated, is the impact on indication shift from radical to partial nephrectomy using 3D models, both virtual and printed. Wake et al. reported a change of 30–50% after visualization of a 3D printed kidney model by the surgeon [68]. Bertolo et al., evaluated the role of 3D planning in highly complex renal tumours, either regarding the size of the tumour or other anatomical characteristics. Of the urologists involved, and regardless of their experience, 25% changed their indication after reviewing the 3D model in favor of PN [9].

In order to overcome the limits of conventional imaging in nephrometry scoring, Porpiglia et al. suggested the use of 3D reconstruction for the assessment of nephrometry scores [49]. Using three-dimensional models, all cases experienced a significant change in the score assigned to renal sinus involvement, urinary collecting system invasion and exophytic rate, while up to 50% of the cases had a downgrade in the PADUA and RENAL risk group. In summary, current evidence suggest that 3D models provide a more accurate overall perspective on renal cancer surgical planning, broadening the indication for nephron sparing surgery. Moreover, these findings may imply a shift in current research trends, moving the focus from "which is the most accurate nephrometry score" to "which is the best imaging tool for tumour complexity evaluation".

While 3D models can help provide anatomical insights and broaden the candidate selection for nephron sparing surgery, other studies have shown that use of 3D models may also lead to reduced operative time, estimated blood loss, clamping time and length of hospital stay [38, 58].

Also the arterial clamping strategy is shown to be altered, resulting in a higher rates of selective and super-selective clamping without increasing intraoperative and postoperative complications [11, 56]. Concerning clinical outcomes of the use of 3D models in renal surgery, the largest retrospective analysis of 3D guided RAPN to date shows significantly higher trifecta achievement rate, lower perioperative transfusion rates and a shorter length of stay [38]. As such, 3D models are expected to further impact intra-, and post-operative outcomes.

6.2 Hilum Control

In a "traditional" PN, renal artery clamping is a standard step just before tumour resection in order to achieve a bloodless resection field. This has many advantages: it allows precise tumour resection without perforation of the tumour (pseudo)capsule, allows minimal resection of normal renal parenchyma and minimizes blood loss. Although prolonged ischemia is a risk factor for acute kidney injury and CKD, the most important determinants of postoperative kidney function are the pre-operative kidney function and the remaining vascularized renal parenchyma [63]. Recent insights learned the human kidney is more tolerable to prolonged ischemia and the concept of 20 to 30 min of "safe ischemia time" is being challenged in patients with bilateral healthy kidneys. Nevertheless, renal ischemia is one of the factors that is surgically modifiable and therefore a lot of effort has been put in developing strategies to minimize healthy renal parenchyma ischemia: off-clamp resection, early unclamping, superselective clamping or establishment of cold ischemia.

6.2.1 Off-Clamp Resection

In an off-clamp resection, the renal hilum is never clamped and all renal parenchyma (and the tumour) remain vascularized during the procedure. For safety, the renal artery is isolated, so it can be clamped in case of excessive bleeding.

Retrospective observational studies comparing on- and off-clamp RAPN demonstrated conflicting results, probably due to selection bias [30, 54]. A meta-analysis in 2019 reported higher blood loss for off-clamp RAPN (mean difference + 47 mL), but similar transfusion rates, complications, and positive surgical margins. Renal function was superior for the off-clamp group both in the short-term change in estimated glomerular filtration rate (GFR; mean difference 7%) and long term (mean difference 4%) [13]. However, the quality of such evidence is very low.

Therefore, two randomized controlled trials (RCTs) analyzed the effect of renal artery clamping versus off-clamp PN on renal function. The recent CLOCK trial randomized 324 patients from several Italian centres with bilateral kidneys, normal kidney function (GFR >60) and a solitary kidney tumour with a RENAL score ≤ 10 to receive either an on-clamp or an off-clamp RAPN [5]. In the "off-clamp" group 43% of patients were crossed over to on-clamp because of excessive bleeding (34%) or because the surgeon desired ischemia 'due to high complexity of the tumour' (9%). No significant differences were seen in terms of estimated blood loss, transfusion rates and postoperative complications [4]. Warm ischemia time (WIT) was limited (median 14 min, interquartile range [IQR] 11–18). No significant difference in postoperative kidney function at 6 months was seen (median -6.2 ml/min [IQR -18 – 0.5] on-clamp versus −5.1 ml/min [IQR -14 – 0.1] off-clamp), nor at 12, 18 and 24 months, both in the intention-to-treat analysis and the per protocol analysis [5].

Similarly, Anderson et al. randomized 71 patients in a single-surgeon RCT between on- and off-clamp RAPN and found no significant difference in 3-month postoperative GFR [3].

It seems that in most patients considered for RAPN, on- or off-clamp strategies have limited impact on clinical outcome. However, this might not be the case for patients with a solitary kidney, pre-existing CKD or more complex tumours with expected longer ischemia time.

6.2.2 Early Unclamping

In early unclamping, perfusion is restored not after double-layer renorraphy but already after internal renorraphy [6]. Some observational series demonstrated a reduction in WIT with a median 5.6 min in RAPN [48]. A meta-analysis of a handful observational series on laparoscopic and robotic PN calculated an increase in mean blood loss of only 37 mL after early unclamping with no difference in transfusion rates or complications [14]. One study assessed postoperative renal function and found no significant difference [48]. When possible, early unclamping is safe, diminishes WIT and provides the surgeon with feedback on hemostasis after internal renorraphy.

6.2.3 Superselective Clamping = "zero Ischemia"

Selective arterial clamping can avoid unnecessary ischemia to healthy renal parenchyma on one side while minimizing the risk of complications such as bleeding on the other side. In superselective clamping (sometimes referred to as the "zero-ischemia" technique), only the tumour-feeding renal vessels are temporarily clamped, to further minimize ischemic damage to healthy tissue and approximate the off-clamp situation. In this technique dating back to 2011 [23], tertiary or higher order branches of the renal artery are dissected. However, the main enigma here remains how to determine up front which vessels need to be dissected/clamped and if this dissection is worth the accruing risks of bleeding and increased operative time. Gill et al. who originally proposed this technique have been using 3D models since 2012 to facilitate this decision [24]. Near-infrared imaging and indocyanine green (ICG) administration was also used in later studies to determine if the clamping was successful at the kidney surface level before starting resection. This showed that a purely cognitive clamping-position estimation does not always establish an avascular resection [12]. Indeed, the clamping strategy is solely based on the surgeon's assessment of which vessels are perfusing the tumour. In lateral rim tumours for instance, vessels are not always connected to the tumour region due to limits in CT imaging resolution. Thus, perfusion needs to be roughly estimated by a 3D 'cognitive region fusion' of nearby vessels.

The first simulation of perfusion regions in 3D renders can be traced back to 2018 [52]. However, no details on the perfusion algorithm or validation are provided and different perfusion zones are separated by straight planes. Each vessel is estimated to perfuse the same perfusion volume with a subsequent linear percentage split (Fig. 6.1).

Figure 6.1a shows how parenchymal percentages can be estimated. Figure 6.1b shows this on a specific case. Figure 6.1c A planar cut is made to estimate which part we need to clamp. Figure 6.1d Looking at this cut, we would estimate the healthy parenchyma which is being clamped to be around 42% (16.6% + 16.6% + 8.3%). It is clear that precise estimation of ischemic volumes is unlikely. Ischemic volumes appear non-physiologic and benefits of a certain clamping strategy are hard to estimate.

More recently, newer perfusion algorithms are demonstrated and validated, based on mathematical models which include several patient-specific arterial features [19]. These models automatically predict ischemic parenchyma and tumour volume percentages and as such objectively inform the surgeon of the risk/benefit ratio in clamping extra vessels (Fig. 6.2).

Figure 6.2: Nearest neighbors approach taking into account arterial path and 3th generation vessels. Fig A. Virtual Model. Fig B–D: Virtual Clamping with ischemic zones indicated in green. Fig B. Clamping of artery headed towards lower pole—anterior view. In this specific case, clamping the inferior artery theoretically

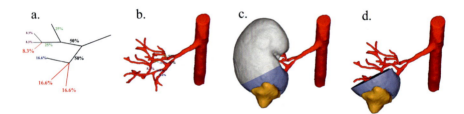

Fig. 6.1 Cognitive estimation of clamped renal volume for partial clamping

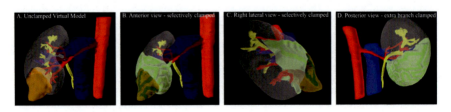

Fig. 6.2 3D perfusion model

results in 77% tumour ischemia and 16% healthy parenchyma clamping. Anterior view looks to be indicating a fully ischemic tumour. Fig C. However, right lateral view reveals the tumour is most likely also perfused by a posterior branch. Fig D. Posterior view when clamping this extra branch, just outside the parenchyma, result in 100% ischemic tumour, however with 36% additional healthy ischemic volume. This approach allows for a more informed clamping strategy.

As tumours are not seldom perfused by several branches, this type of perfusion model lets the surgeon balance off the benefit of encountering a small hemorrhage in certain areas compared to clamping a larger volume of healthy parenchyma. It also informs the surgeon where such a hemorrhage is to be expected or where bloodless enucleation can be started.

6.2.4 Cold Ischemia

In patients were long ischemia times (>30 min) are expected, cold ischemia may limit renal parenchyma damage. Several techniques exist to cool the kidney. In open PN, ice slush can be placed around the kidney. However, in minimal-invasive surgery this is more complex and therefore has not been widely adopted. For laparoscopic PN, cold saline surface irrigation [31], retrograde cooling through the ureter [17] and intra-arterial cold perfusion [29] have been performed. There are no studies comparing these different cooling techniques in terms of kidney temperature and postoperative renal function in minimal invasive surgery. In 1980 Marberger et al. analyzed 95 patient who underwent hypothermic nephrolithotomy. Sixty-three kidneys were cooled by transarterial cold perfusion and 39 were cooled by topical ice slush. Postoperative kidney function decreased less in the perfused group (−19.4% at 2 weeks; −7.9% at 6 months) than in the topical group (−30.3% at 2 weeks; −29.8% at 6 months) [36]. Possibly, intra-arterial cold perfusion delivers a more homogeneous renal parenchyma cooling compared to topical cooling.

A recent systematic review and meta-analysis found no significant difference between cold and warm ischemia in terms of blood loss, surgical margins and postoperative drop in kidney function following PN. However, the number of included studies and patients was low, as was the level of evidence (Oxford level of evidence 4) [25].

Practical considerations and lack of an 'optimal' cooling technique hampered the adoption of cold ischemia in RAPN thus far. It remains an option, however, before autotransplantation and bench surgery or even radical nephrectomy in patients with solitary kidney or CKD with very complex tumours.

In summary, two systematic reviews and meta-analyses in 2019 demonstrated that no ischemia technique (off-clamp, on-clamp, superselective clamping or cold ischemia) is superior over the other in patients with bilateral healthy kidneys. A surgeon must balance between acceptable ischemia time, limited ischemia zone and operative risk and duration, while maintaining maximal oncological control. Additional prudence is required in patients with solitary kidneys or CKD. 3D models can aid in choosing the best strategy.

6.3 Tumour Resection Strategy

Resection strategies and techniques for PN are still object of great interest and debate among urological surgeons and researchers. In fact, the most recent EAU and American Urology Association (AUA) guidelines recommend PN as the gold-standard treatment for patients with localized T1 renal tumours [35], making the technique for tumour excision of great value to achieve the goals of oncologic efficacy, maximal renal function preservation and perioperative safety.

The debate over the merits and potential limitations of different resection strategies and techniques for RAPN has been reinforced by several recent studies. In particular, as the amount of functional parenchymal mass preserved during PN has been shown to be one of the strongest modifiable predictors of functional recovery after surgery (provided that extended warm ischemia time is avoided) [37], some authors have argued that tumour enucleation (TE) may have distinct benefits over "standard" PN (i.e. enucleoresection) without compromising oncologic safety [26]. Among these, TE may allow surgeons to excise the tumour with optimal visualization of its contours (resecting only a microscopic amount of healthy renal tissue [40] and thus reducing the risk of positive surgical margins), while keeping the risk of damages to the urinary collecting system and/or renal sinus to a minimum, especially in case of anatomically complex, hilar renal masses [26]. Importantly, TE may also sponsor a "nephron-sparing" renorrhaphy, especially during RAPN. Indeed, nephron-sparing tumour excision (minimal-margin PN or TE), following a relatively avascular dissection plane, facilitates anatomical nephron-sparing renal reconstruction; this concept is of utmost importance for highly complex and/or hilar tumours, with potential additional benefits in terms of renal function preservation and minimization of perioperative complications [10].

For several years the standard surgical technique PN was the excision of a 1-cm peritumoural tissue to achieve negative margins. This surgical strategy was not without risks, considering the amount of vascularized parenchymal volume resected, the potential urinary collecting system injuries, and the higher risk of prolonged warm ischemia time (WIT) [66].

Interestingly, while originally preferred for nephron-sparing surgery in case of hereditary kidney tumours and for imperative indications, TE has gradually been applied in elective settings for both T1a and T1b/T2 tumours by an increasing number of surgeons [41].

From a pathologic standpoint, tumour enucleation takes advantage of the presence of a distinct fibrous pseudocapsule in most renal tumours as well as of the histologic changes at the tumour-parenchyma interface [44]. This directly translates into the "surgical concept" of TE, which relies on the excision of the tumour predominantly by blunt dissection following the natural cleavage plane between the peritumoural pseudocapsule and the renal parenchyma (without removing a visible rim of healthy renal tissue). In this regard, several studies have shown that the incidence of positive surgical margins after TE is consistently very low, making TE at least non-inferior to standard PN in this regard [43].

A recent study found that, in experienced hands, robotic TE allows to excise the tumour with negative surgical margins even in case of pseudocapsula infiltration, by providing a "microscopic" layer of healthy renal tissue beyond the peritumoural pseudocapsula [39], with no recurrences found in the enucleation bed at a long-term follow-up. As such, robotic TE is oncologically safe and has the potential to meet further essential requirements for PN, such as to widen the indications to tumours with the most unfavourable nephrometry scores while maintaining a low complication rate and maximizing the volume of vascularized parenchyma preserved [44] (Figs. 6.3 and 6.4).

The cornerstones of robotic tumour enucleation are shown in detail at: https://surgeryinmotion-school.org/v/563/. Robotic tumour enucleation has been shown not to be a zero-margin technique but rather a microscopic- margin technique, resecting a microscopic (<1 mm) silver of healthy renal margin in most cases [39].

An anatomic resection strategy (enucleative intent) is key to allow the surgeon to clearly appreciate the tumour's contours and excise the tumour with macroscopically negative surgical margins.

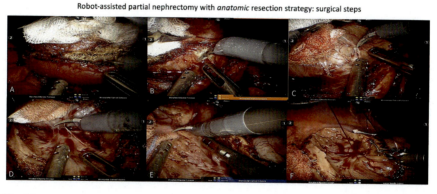

Fig. 6.3 Intraoperative snapshots showing the main steps of robotic tumour enucleation

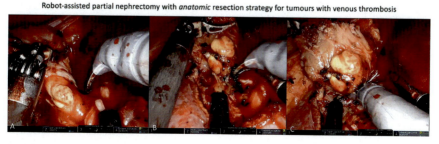

Fig. 6.4 Intraoperative snapshots showing a case of robotic tumour enucleation for a small renal mass with venous thrombosis

Despite the robust evidence confirming the oncologic safety of TE during both open and robotic PN [39, 43], whether TE is ultimately safe for all patients with localized renal tumours who are eligible for nephron-sparing surgery is still debated within the Urology community [26, 42, 64]. In fact, some experts remain sceptic about the real advantages of TE, arguing that TE may lead to insignificant differences in postoperative renal function and complications as compared to standard PN, at the cost of a higher risk of tumour violation (Fig. 6.5).

Figure 6.5: Left side: distinct merits of tumour enucleation from a surgical perspective include the clear visualization of the tumour contours, the possibility to avoid positive surgical margins especially for tumours with no perfectly spherical shape (as in the figure), maximization of the amount of healthy renal parenchyma spared during RAPN and the opportunity for "nephron-sparing" renorrhaphy. Right side: a potential drawback of tumour enucleation is the risk of tumour violation, which increases the risk of true positive surgical margins (residual tumour cells in the enucleation bed).

In a recent review on the key decision-making points in patients with localized renal masses, the authors highlighted how the resection methodology during RAPN should be grounded into a careful consideration of both patients' and tumour's characteristics, and that a wider-margin PN (or even radical nephrectomy) may be safer for in case of tumours with an "infiltrative" tumour growth pattern (in view of a potentially more aggressive histology) [37].

The controversy over the pros and cons of TE versus standard PN is reflected in the historical evolution of EAU Guidelines recommendations. While they originally recommended the removal of a "minimal tumour-free surgical margin" to achieve oncologic efficacy, they subsequently outlined the oncologic efficacy of TE and did not provide further recommendations to guide resection strategies and techniques during open and robotic PN [35]. The same concept can be applied to the AUA Guidelines, which stressed that TE may be more beneficial in patients with familial renal cell carcinoma (RCC), multifocal disease, or severe chronic kidney disease aiming to optimize parenchymal mass preservation [15].

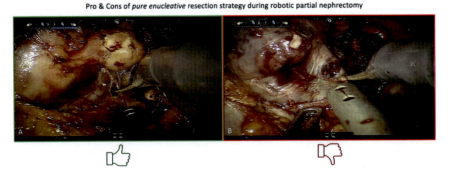

Fig. 6.5 Pros and cons of robotic tumour enucleation for localized renal masses

Unfortunately, the debate over the merits and limitations of different resection techniques has been reinforced over time by the lack of standardized reporting of resection strategies and techniques during PN. Since the initial description of nephron-sparing surgery, a number of technical strategies for excision of the tumour from normal renal parenchyma have been described, including TE, enucleoresection, and wedge resection. Yet, the descriptors of these techniques have been used interchangeably, hindering a meaningful comparison of surgical series until recently. To fill this gap, Minervini and coworkers have proposed in 2014 a standardized reporting system to communicate tumour resection technique in PN series, the Surface-Intermediate-Base (SIB) margin score [45]. This model, based on a visual analysis of the margin of healthy parenchyma scored at the superficial surface, the intermediate surface, and the base of the tumour, was soon validated from a histopathological perspective [40] and tested in a prospective, international multicentre study aiming to assess the impact of resection techniques on PN outcomes [41].

Of note, a more comprehensive model to catch the "whole picture" of tumour excision during RAPN should report not only the final resection technique (according to the SIB scoring system), but also the preoperative surgeon's intent (named "resection strategy") [42]. In fact, tumour excision during PN is a complex surgical task, and the inherent characteristics of the tumour–parenchyma interface allow definition of a constant "anatomic dissection plane" that can always be identified and bluntly developed in close vicinity to the tumour capsule, with or without the removal of a sliver of healthy renal tissue. As such, it is essential to clearly divide the concept of resection strategy (*anatomic vs non-anatomic*) from that of resection technique (*enucleation vs enucleoresection vs resection*, based on the SIB score) (Fig. 6.6).

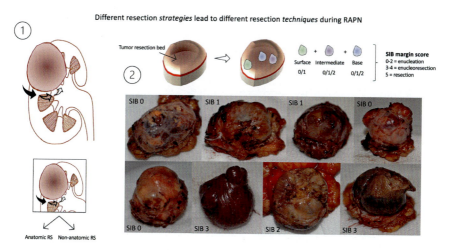

Fig. 6.6 Graphical overview of the integrated model proposed by Minervini and colleagues for standardized reporting of resection strategies and techniques during open and robotic PN [42]

A detailed overview of the SIB scoring system for standardized reporting of PN resection techniques is presented in Fig. 6.6 [45]. A step-by-step tutorial for surgeons on SIB score assignment is available at the link: https://kidney.uroonco.uroweb.org/video/sib-score-tutorial/.

Figure 6.6: (1) Resection strategy (the preoperative surgeon's intent) is classified as *anatomical* or *non-anatomical* according to the surgeon intent to excise the tumour by following the anatomical dissection plane close to the tumour or wider non-anatomical planes, removing a macroscopic layer of healthy renal tissue. (2) In contrast, the resection technique was classified as enucleation (SIB score 0–2), enucleoresection (SIB score 3 or 4) or resection (SIB score 5) according to the SIB score by visual analysis of the specimen performed by the surgeon in the operating room after PN. Details on SIB score assignment are provided in the text as well as in a step-by-step tutorial at this link: https://kidney.uroonco.uroweb.org/video/sib-score-tutorial/.

In this view, the surgeon's preoperative intent during RAPN may be reported in a spectrum ranging from a "pure enucleative" anatomic resection strategy (in this case, the aim is to follow the natural cleavage plane between the tumour and the healthy parenchyma resecting a *microscopic* amount of healthy renal tissue) to a "wedge" non-anatomic resection strategy (in this case, the aim is to excise the tumour with macroscopic margins of healthy renal tissue with no visualization of the anatomic dissection plane). Between these two extremes lie the "minimal-margin" anatomic resection strategy and the "macroscopic-margin" non-anatomic resection strategy [42].

Importantly, a prospective multicentre study has distinctly shown how resection techniques do impact on perioperative and early functional and oncologic outcomes in patients with localized renal masses [41]. In particular, the resection technique, classified after surgery according to the SIB score, was the only significant predictor of positive surgical margins and one of the strongest predictors of Clavien-Dindo grade ≥ 2 surgical complications, postoperative acute kidney injury and Trifecta achievement. This evidence reinforces the clinical relevance of standardized reporting of resection methodology during RAPN.

In summary, the goal of RAPN is complete excision of the tumour with negative margins while maximizing perioperative safety and preservation of vascularized parenchyma. To achieve this goal, individualized tailoring of the excision plane based on intraoperative assessment of the peritumoural tissue planes is needed [55]. To advance this field toward the concept of "precision RAPN", standardized reporting of excision techniques will be key for future studies to understand the impact of resection (and renorrhaphy) strategies and techniques (beyond that of surgeon's experience) on postoperative outcomes after RAPN [10, 18, 41].

6.4 Future Perspectives

6.4.1 3D Model Generation

3D models are typically reconstructed from computed tomography scans using 4 different phases: blanco, early arterial, venous and an excretory phase [11]. MRI scans can technically be used as well, although resolution is often lacking to reconstruct a useful anatomical vascular reconstruction for hilar control. A dedicated software program is to be used to reconstruct these models in a process called 'segmentation' as illustrated in Fig. 6.7.

This means colouring in every artery, vein, ureter, kidney and tumour that is relevant for the final model. Next, these segmentation software packages convert this planar information into a 3D model.

Segmentation software packages are available both open-source for free (e.g. 3DSlicer—http://www.slicer.org) as well as commercially. Segmentation remains a cumbersome, time-consuming, manual task. The advent of artificial intelligence is reducing the time needed for model making by automating the segmentation process. More precisely, so-called deep learning techniques are used to predict a 3D model, which can then be double checked and altered by the physician in the software packages stated above wherever needed [28].

After the generation of such a model, this file can be exported and viewed in several desktop formats. Whenever needed, these files can also be used integrally as input for 3D printing of the anatomy.

6.4.2 Virtual Models and Augmented Reality

When 3D models are viewed in desktop applications or in other purely virtual environments, we refer to them as virtual models. The term augmented reality (AR) refers to the real-time overlaying or superimposition of images captured by the intraoperative field or, more typically, peroperatively, onto a patient's actual endoscopic video [61]. Figure 6.8 shows the difference between both approaches.

The TilePro™ technology enables the surgeon to integrate acquired imaging (3D reconstructions, CT scans, MRI images, ultrasonography) with critical visual information from the operational field. When just the virtual model is imported (Fig. 6.8a), we refer to it as a virtual model. However, a cognitive fusion still needs to take place inside the surgeon's head. On step further (Fig. 6.8b) is to project this 3D model in the operative field. As such, these inputs may 'augment' the limited surgical field and intra-operative perception as associated with laparoscopic

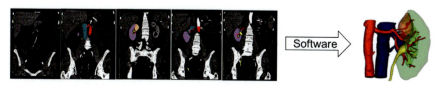

Fig. 6.7 Segmentation is the process where the 3D model maker goes through the entire CT scan using a software package and indicates relevant structures for each slice

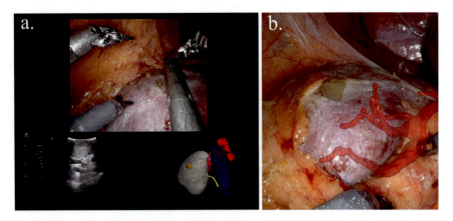

Fig. 6.8 a. Virtual model input using TilePro™, shows a partially endophytic tumour. Ultrasound confirms the location of the tumour. Figure 8.b. Augmented reality setting in which the same 3D model is overlapped to the endoscopic view, also showing the location of the arteries and invisible endophytic part of the tumour. It is to be noted that this is also inputted using the TilePro™ function, as the current systems do not allow to take over the main console view

surgery. In this case, the model needs to be continuously repositioned as to fit the current operative view.

Automation of this process requires image registration, which is the alignment of virtual models with the present intra-operative field. As such, image registration lies at the heart of a successful clinical implementation of AR.

AR image registration can be divided into two main categories: rigid and non-rigid. The former does not account for organ distortion as can be perceived due to repositioning of the body or renal manipulation [57, 60]. For high-precision AR navigation, non-rigid registration is required. However, the dynamic environment of the abdominal cavity makes non-rigid registration incredibly challenging, especially when approaching anatomical structures such as the renal hilum. Several deformation registrations, such as 3D splines [2], non-linear parametric models [51], elastic finite element model (FEM), and biomechanical models [27], can be employed to compensate this necessity.

Most laparoscopic AR navigation systems require so-called manual or semi-automated registration. Manual registration refers to manual alignment of virtual models with endoscopic pictures. Each time the operative view changes, the model must be manually re-aligned using a user interface. Semi-automatic registration necessitates human initial alignment before automatic follow-up. As such, manual and semi-automated registration impair the surgical flow as they require the surgeon or assistant to constantly or intermittently realign the model.

Automatic registration is facilitated by the use of extra sensors in the operative setup. Using electromagnetic or optical tracking sensors to rigidly localize the laparoscope may result in automatic registration. Using fiducials into a kidney silicon model, Teber and Kong et al. demonstrated completely automated augmented reality navigation during laparoscopic PN with great navigation accuracy [32, 62]. However, these tools do not allow the use of a deformable model and because of the intrusive character of the used markers, this approach is not suitable for clinical use [60].

To avoid the use of physical markers, Wild et al. postulated the use of fluorescent dyes, which of course require the procedure to be performed using a laparoscope capable of fluorescence imaging [69].

Further options include the use of stereoscopic laparoscopy to reconstruct the intra-abdominal organ surface to accomplishing registration. In this approach, a live 3D reconstruction is made of the intra-abdominal cavity by using both eyes of a laparoscope with 3D vision, as is the case in robotic surgery. These reconstructions, however, frequently contains insufficient feature points. Furthermore, feature detection may be hampered by several factors, such as texture-poor appearance, specular reflection, and shadows. Moreover, due to the limited endoscopic view (the angle of a laparoscope view is only 70°), only a tiny portion of the organ surface may be rebuilt. It makes automatic registration of an entire 3D anatomical model extremely difficult, necessitating manual initial alignment [8].

Finally, Bernhardt and colleagues proposed a registration algorithm that does not rely on tracking devices or markers. It identifies the location of the endoscopic camera relative to the intra-operative 3D data by incorporating the endoscope tip inside an intra-operative 3D C-arm volume [8]. However, this requires both a setup with a radiographic C-arm inside the operative room as well as the use of a three-axis accelerometer integrated into the endoscopic camera.

Summarizing, to properly incorporate AR in a clinical real-life scenario, some requirements must be fulfilled:

1. Conventional preoperative imaging must be used to easily generate 3D surgical models.
2. The 3D model must be projected onto the live intra-operative anatomy, requiring registration of the model using preferably visual cues and a deformable model.
3. Surgical instruments must be tracked, as well as any mobility of the targeted organs and their surrounding anatomies.

Even if great steps forward have been made in the last few years, we are still just at the beginning of the development of this technology.

6.5 Conclusions

RAPN is no longer a standard 'one technique fits all' procedure, but is continuously evolving towards precision RAPN. A surgeon should encounter every patient with a personalized strategy for hilum control and tumour resection, in order to minimize renal ischemia and maximize the remaining vascularized renal parenchyma. 3D models can aid in pre-operative planning and peroperative guidance, especially in complex cases.

References

1. Abdel Raheem A, Alowidah I, Capitanio U, Montorsi F, Larcher A, Derweesh I, Ghali F, Mottrie A, Mazzone E, G DEN, Campi R, Sessa F, Carini M, Minervini A, Raman JD, Rjepaj CJ, Kriegmair MC, Autorino R, Veccia A, Mir MC, Claps F, Choi YD, Ham WS, Tadifa JP, Santok GD, Furlan M, Simeone C, Bada M, Celia A, Carrion DM, Aguilera Bazan A, Ruiz CB, Malki M, Barber N, Hussain M, Micali S, Puliatti S, Alwahabi A, Alqahtani A, Rumaih A, Ghaith A, Ghoneem AM, Hagras A, Eissa A, Alenzi MJ, Pavan N, Traunero F, Antonelli A, Porcaro AB, Illiano E, Costantini E, Rha KH. Warm ischemia time length during on-clamp partial nephrectomy: dose it really matter? Minerva Urol Nephrol. 2021.
2. Amir-Khalili A, Nosrati M, Peyrat J-M, Hamarneh G, Abugharbieh R. Uncertainty-encoded augmented reality for robot-assisted partial nephrectomy: a phantom study. In: Augmented reality environments for medical imaging and computer-assisted interventions. Springer Berlin Heidelberg; 2013.
3. Anderson BG, Potretzke AM, Du K, Vetter JM, Bergeron K, Paradis AG, Figenshau RS. Comparing off-clamp and on-clamp robot-assisted Partial Nephrectomy: a prospective randomized trial. Urology. 2019;126:102–9.
4. Antonelli A, Cindolo L, Sandri M, Bertolo R, Annino F, Carini M, Celia A, D'orta C, De Concilio B, Furlan M, Giommoni V, Ingrosso M, Mari A, Muto G, Nucciotti R, Porreca A, Primiceri G, Schips L, Sessa F, Simeone C, Veccia A, Minervini A, Group A. Safety of on- vs off-clamp robotic partial nephrectomy: per-protocol analysis from the data of the CLOCK randomized trial. World J U. 2020;38:1101–08.
5. Antonelli A, Cindolo L, Sandri M, Veccia A, Annino F, Bertagna F, Carini M, Celia A, D'orta C, De Concilio B, Furlan M, Giommoni V, Ingrosso M, Mari A, Nucciotti R, Olianti C, Porreca A, Primiceri G, Schips I, Sessa F, Bove P, Simeone C, Minervini A, Group A. Is off-clamp robot-assisted partial nephrectomy beneficial for renal function? Data from the CLOCK trial. BJU Int. 2021.
6. Baumert H, Ballaro A, Shah N, Mansouri D, Zafar N, Molinie V, Neal D. Reducing warm ischaemia time during laparoscopic partial nephrectomy: a prospective comparison of two renal closure techniques. Eur Urol. 2007;52:1164–9.
7. Becker F, van Poppel H, Hakenberg OW, Stief C, Gill I, Guazzoni G, Montorsi F, Russo P, Stockle M. Assessing the impact of ischaemia time during partial nephrectomy. Eur Urol. 2009;56:625–34.
8. Bernhardt S, Nicolau SA, Agnus V, Soler L, Doignon C, Marescaux J. Automatic localization of endoscope in intraoperative CT image: a simple approach to augmented reality guidance in laparoscopic surgery. Med Image Anal. 2016;30:130–43.
9. Bertolo R, Autorino R, Fiori C, Amparore D, Checcucci E, Mottrie A, Porter J, Haber GP, Derweesh I, Porpiglia F. Expanding the indications of robotic partial nephrectomy for highly complex renal tumors: urologists' perception of the impact of hyperaccuracy three-dimensional reconstruction. J Laparoendosc Adv Surg Tech A. 2019a;29:233–9.

10. Bertolo R, Campi R, Klatte T, Kriegmair MC, Mir MC, Ouzaid I, Salagierski M, Bhayani S, Gill I, Kaouk J, Capitanio U, Young Academic Urologists Kidney Cancer Working Group Of The European Urological A. Suture techniques during laparoscopic and robot-assisted partial nephrectomy: a systematic review and quantitative synthesis of peri-operative outcomes. BJU Int. 2019b;123:923–946.
11. Bianchi L, Barbaresi U, Cercenelli L, Bortolani B, Gaudiano C, Chessa F, Angiolini A, Lodi S, Porreca A, Bianchi FM, Casablanca C, Ercolino A, Bertaccini A, Golfieri R, Marcelli E, Schiavina R. The impact of 3D digital reconstruction on the surgical planning of partial nephrectomy: a case-control study. Still time for a novel surgical trend? Clin Genitourin Cancer. 2020;18:e669–78.
12. Borofsky MS, Gill IS, Hemal AK, Marien TP, Jayaratna I, Krane LS, Stifelman MD. Near-infrared fluorescence imaging to facilitate super-selective arterial clamping during zero-ischaemia robotic partial nephrectomy. BJU Int. 2013;111:604–10.
13. Cacciamani GE, Medina LG, Gill TS, Mendelsohn A, Husain F, Bhardwaj L, Artibani W, Sotelo R, Gill IS. Impact of renal hilar control on outcomes of robotic partial nephrectomy: systematic review and cumulative meta-analysis. Eur Urol Focus. 2019;5:619–35.
14. Cacciamani GE, Okhunov Z, Meneses AD, Rodriguez-Socarras ME, Rivas JG, Porpiglia F, Liatsikos E, Veneziano D. Impact of three-dimensional printing in urology: state of the art and future perspectives. A systematic review by ESUT-YAUWP Group. Eur Urol. 2019;76:209–21.
15. Campbell SC, Clark PE, Chang SS, Karam JA, Souter L, Uzzo RG. Renal mass and localized renal cancer: evaluation, management, and follow-Up: AUA guideline: Part I. J Urol. 2021;206:199–208.
16. Cooperberg MR, Mallin K, Ritchey J, Villalta JD, Carroll PR, Kane CJ. Decreasing size at diagnosis of stage 1 renal cell carcinoma: analysis from the National Cancer Data Base, 1993 to 2004. J Urol. 2008;179:2131–5.
17. Crain DS, Spencer CR, Favata MA, Amling CL. Transureteral saline perfusion to obtain renal hypothermia: potential application in laparoscopic partial nephrectomy. JSLS J Soc Laparoendosc Surgeon. 2004;8:217–22.
18. Dagenais J, Bertolo R, Garisto J, Maurice MJ, Mouracade P, Kara O, Chavali J, Li J, Nelson R, Fergany A, Abouassaly R, Kaouk JH. Variability in partial nephrectomy outcomes: does your surgeon matter? Eur Urol. 2019;75:628–34.
19. de Backer P, Vangeneugden J, Van Praet C, Lejoly M, Vermijs S, Vanpeteghem C, Decaestecker K. Robot assisted partial nephrectomy using intra-arterial renal hypothermia for highly complex endophytic or hilar tumors: case series and description of surgical technique. 36th Annual EAU Congress, Virtual Edition, July 8–12. 2021 [Conference presentation].
20. de Backer P, Vermijs S, Van Praet C, Vandenbulcke S, Lejoly M, Vanderschelden S, Debbaut C, Mottrie A, Decaestecker K. Selective arterial clamping in robot assisted partial nephrectomy using 3D nearest distance perfusion zones. American Urology Association Annual Meeting. Las Vegas, USA. 2021. [Conference presentation].
21. Ficarra V, Novara G, Secco S, Macchi V, Porzionato A, de Caro R, Artibani W. Preoperative aspects and dimensions used for an anatomical (PADUA) classification of renal tumours in patients who are candidates for nephron-sparing surgery. Eur Urol. 2009;56:786–93.
22. Gill IS, Abreu SC, Desai MM, Steinberg AP, Ramani AP, Ng C, Banks K, Novick AC, Kaouk JH. Laparoscopic ice slush renal hypothermia for partial nephrectomy: the initial experience. J Urol. 2003;170:52–6.
23. Gill IS, Eisenberg MS, Aron M, Berger A, Ukimura O, Patil MB, Campese V, Thangathurai D, Desai MM. "Zero ischemia" partial nephrectomy: novel laparoscopic and robotic technique. Eur Urol. 2011;59:128–34.
24. Gill IS, Patil MB, Abreu AL, Ng C, Cai J, Berger A, Eisenberg MS, Nakamoto M, Ukimura O, Goh AC, Thangathurai D, Aron M, Desai MM. Zero ischemia anatomical partial nephrectomy: a novel approach. J Urol. 2012;187:807–14.
25. Greco F, Autorino R, Altieri V, Campbell S, Ficarra V, Gill I, Kutikov A, Mottrie A, Mirone V, van Poppel H. Ischemia techniques in nephron-sparing surgery: a systematic review and meta-analysis of surgical, oncological, and functional outcomes. Eur Urol. 2019;75:477–91.

26. Gupta GN, Boris RS, Campbell SC, Zhang Z. Tumor enucleation for sporadic localized kidney cancer: pro and con. J Urol. 2015;194:623–5.
27. Hamarneh G, Amir-Khalili A, Nosrati M, Figueroa I, Kawahara J, Al-Alao O. Towards multimodal image-guided tumour identification in robot-assisted partial nephrectomy. 2nd Middle East Conference on Biomedical Engineering, Doha, Qatar. 2014, p. 159–62.
28. Houshyar R, Glavis-Bloom J, Bui TL, Chahine C, Bardis MD, Ushinsky A, Liu H, Bhatter P, Lebby E, Fujimoto D, Grant W, Tran-Harding K, Landman J, Chow DS, Chang PD. Outcomes of artificial intelligence volumetric assessment of kidneys and renal tumors for preoperative assessment of nephron sparing interventions. J Endourol. 2021.
29. Janetschek G, Abdelmaksoud A, Bagheri F, Al-Zahrani H, Leeb K, Gschwendtner M. Laparoscopic partial nephrectomy in cold ischemia: renal artery perfusion. J Urol. 2004;171:68–71.
30. Kaczmarek BF, Tanagho YS, Hillyer SP, Mullins JK, Diaz M, Trinh QD, Bhayani SB, Allaf ME, Stifelman MD, Kaouk JH, Rogers CG. Off-clamp robot-assisted partial nephrectomy preserves renal function: a multi-institutional propensity score analysis. Eur Urol. 2013;64:988–93.
31. Kijvikai K, Viprakasit DP, Milhoua P, Clark PE, Herrell SD. A simple, effective method to create laparoscopic renal protective hypothermia with cold saline surface irrigation: clinical application and assessment. J Urol. 2010;184:1861–6.
32. Kong SH, Haouchine N, Soares R, Klymchenko A, Andreiuk B, Marques B, Shabat G, Piechaud T, Diana M, Cotin S, Marescaux J. Robust augmented reality registration method for localization of solid organs' tumors using CT-derived virtual biomechanical model and fluorescent fiducials. Surg Endosc. 2017;31:2863–71.
33. Kutikov A, Uzzo RG. The R.E.N.A.L. nephrometry score: a comprehensive standardized system for quantitating renal tumor size, location and depth. J Urol. 2009;182:844–53.
34. Leibovich BC, Lohse CM, Cheville JC, Zaid HB, Boorjian SA, Frank I, Thompson RH, Parker WP. Predicting oncologic outcomes in renal cell carcinoma after surgery. Eur Urol. 2018;73:772–80.
35. Ljungberg B, Albiges L, Bedke J, Bex A, Capitanio U, Giles RH, Hora M, Klatte T, Lam T, Marconi L, Powles T, Volpe A. EAU guidelines on renal cell carcinoma; 2021.
36. Marberger M, Eisenberger F. Regional hypothermia of the kidney: surface or transarterial perfusion cooling? A functional study. J Urol. 1980;124:179–83.
37. Marconi L, Desai MM, Ficarra V, Porpiglia F, van Poppel H. Renal preservation and partial nephrectomy: patient and surgical factors. Eur Urol Focus. 2016;2:589–600.
38. Michiels C, Khene ZE, Prudhomme T, Boulenger De Hauteclocque A, Cornelis FH, Percot M, Simeon H, Dupitout L, Bensadoun H, Capon G, Alezra E, Estrade V, Bladou F, Robert G, Ferriere JM, Grenier N, Doumerc N, Bensalah K, Bernhard JC. 3D-Image guided robotic-assisted partial nephrectomy: a multi-institutional propensity score-matched analysis (UroCCR study 51). World J Urol. 2021.
39. Minervini A, Campi R, Di Maida F, Mari A, Montagnani I, Tellini R, Tuccio A, Siena G, Vittori G, Lapini A, Raspollini MR, Carini M. Tumor-parenchyma interface and long-term oncologic outcomes after robotic tumor enucleation for sporadic renal cell carcinoma. Urologic Oncol. 2018;36:527 e1–527 e11.
40. Minervini A, Campi R, Kutikov A, Montagnani I, Sessa F, Serni S, Raspollini MR, Carini M. Histopathological validation of the surface-intermediate-base margin score for standardized reporting of resection technique during nephron sparing surgery. J Urol. 2015;194:916–22.
41. Minervini A, Campi R, Lane BR, de Cobelli O, Sanguedolce F, Hatzichristodoulou G, Antonelli A, Noyes S, Mari A, Rodriguez-Faba O, Keeley FX, Langenhuijsen J, Musi G, Klatte T, Roscigno M, Akdogan B, Furlan M, Karakoyunlu N, Marszalek M, Capitanio U, Volpe A, Brookman-May S, Gschwend JE, Smaldone MC, Uzzo RG, Carini M, Kutikov A. Impact of resection technique on perioperative outcomes and surgical margins after partial nephrectomy for localized renal masses: a prospective multicenter study. J Urol. 2020;203:496–504.
42. Minervini A, Campi R, Serni S, Carini M, Satkunasivam R, Tsai S, Syan S, et al. Robotic unclamped "Minimal-margin" partial nephrectomy: ongoing refinement of the anatomic zero-ischemia concept. Eur Urol 2015;68:705–12. Eur Urol 2016;70:e47–50.

43. Minervini A, Campi R, Sessa F, Derweesh I, Kaouk JH, Mari A, Rha KH, Sessa M, Volpe A, Carini M, Uzzo RG. Positive surgical margins and local recurrence after simple enucleation and standard partial nephrectomy for malignant renal tumors: systematic review of the literature and meta-analysis of prevalence. Minerva urologica e nefrologica = Italian J Urol Nephrol. 2017; 69:523–38.
44. Minervini A, Carini M. Tumor enucleation is appropriate during partial nephrectomy. Eur Urol Focus. 2019;5:923–4.
45. Minervini A, Carini M, Uzzo RG, Campi R, Smaldone MC, Kutikov A. Standardized reporting of resection technique during nephron-sparing surgery: the surface-intermediate-base margin score. Eur Urol. 2014;66:803–5.
46. Nahar B, Bhat A, Parekh DJ. Does every minute of renal ischemia still count in 2019? Unlocking the chains of a flawed thought process over five decades. Eur Urol Focus. 2019;5:939–42.
47. Parekh DJ, Weinberg JM, Ercole B, Torkko KC, Hilton W, Bennett M, Devarajan P, Venkatachalam MA. Tolerance of the human kidney to isolated controlled ischemia. J Am Soc Nephrol. 2013;24:506–17.
48. Peyronnet B, Baumert H, Mathieu R, Masson-Lecomte A, Grassano Y, Roumiguie M, Massoud W, Abd El Fattah V, Bruyere F, Droupy S, De La Taille A, Doumerc N, Bernhard JC, Vaessen C, Roupret M, Bensalah K. Early unclamping technique during robot-assisted laparoscopic partial nephrectomy can minimise warm ischaemia without increasing morbidity. BJU Int. 2014;114:741–7.
49. Porpiglia F, Amparore D, Checcucci E, Manfredi M, Stura I, Migliaretti G, Autorino R, Ficarra V, Fiori C. Three-dimensional virtual imaging of renal tumours: a new tool to improve the accuracy of nephrometry scores. BJU Int. 2019;124:945–54.
50. Porpiglia F, Bertolo R, Checcucci E, Amparore D, Autorino R, Dasgupta P, Wiklund P, Tewari A, Liatsikos E, Fiori C, Group ER. Development and validation of 3D printed virtual models for robot-assisted radical prostatectomy and partial nephrectomy: urologists' and patients' perception. World J Urol. 2018a;36:201–207
51. Porpiglia F, Checcucci E, Amparore D, Piramide F, Volpi G, Granato S, Verri P, Manfredi M, Bellin A, Piazzolla P, Autorino R, Morra I, Fiori C, Mottrie A. Three-dimensional augmented reality robot-assisted partial nephrectomy in case of complex tumours (PADUA >/=10): a new intraoperative tool overcoming the ultrasound guidance. Eur Urol. 2020;78:229–38.
52. Porpiglia F, Fiori C, Checcucci E, Amparore D, Bertolo R. Hyperaccuracy three-dimensional reconstruction is able to maximize the efficacy of selective clamping during robot-assisted partial nephrectomy for complex renal masses. Eur Urol. 2018;74:651–60.
53. Ramirez D, Caputo PA, Krishnan J, Zargar H, Kaouk JH. Robot-assisted partial nephrectomy with intracorporeal renal hypothermia using ice slush: step-by-step technique and matched comparison with warm ischaemia. BJU Int. 2016;117:531–6.
54. Rosen DC, Paulucci DJ, Abaza R, Eun DD, Bhandari A, Hemal AK, Badani KK. Is off clamp always beneficial during robotic partial nephrectomy? A propensity score-matched comparison of clamp technique in patients with two kidneys. J Endourol. 2017;31:1176–82.
55. Satkunasivam R, Tsai S, Syan S, Bernhard JC, De Castro Abreu AL, Chopra S, Berger AK, Lee D, Hung AJ, Cai J, Desai MM, Gill IS. Robotic unclamped "minimal-margin" partial nephrectomy: ongoing refinement of the anatomic zero-ischemia concept. Eur Urol. 2015;68:705–12
56. Schiavina R, Bianchi L, Chessa F, Barbaresi U, Cercenelli L, Lodi S, Gaudiano C, Bortolani B, Angiolini A, Bianchi FM, Ercolino A, Casablanca C, Molinaroli E, Porreca A, Golfieri R, Diciotti S, Marcelli E, Brunocilla E. Augmented reality to guide selective clamping and tumor dissection during robot-assisted partial nephrectomy: a preliminary experience. Clin Genitourin Cancer. 2021;19:e149–55.
57. Schneider C, Nguan C, Longpre M, Rohling R, Salcudean S. Motion of the kidney between preoperative and intraoperative positioning. IEEE Trans Biomed Eng. 2013;60:1619–27.
58. Shirk JD, Thiel DD, Wallen EM, Linehan JM, White WM, Badani KK, Porter JR. Effect of 3-dimensional virtual reality models for surgical planning of robotic-assisted partial nephrectomy on surgical outcomes: a randomized clinical trial. JAMA Netw Open. 2019;2: e1911598.

59. Silberstein JL, Maddox MM, Dorsey P, Feibus A, Thomas R, Lee BR. Physical models of renal malignancies using standard cross-sectional imaging and 3-dimensional printers: a pilot study. Urology. 2014;84:268–72.
60. Su LM, Vagvolgyi BP, Agarwal R, Reiley CE, Taylor RH, Hager GD. Augmented reality during robot-assisted laparoscopic partial nephrectomy: toward real-time 3D-CT to stereoscopic video registration. Urology. 2009;73:896–900.
61. Tang SL, Kwoh CK, Teo MY, Sing NW, Ling KV. Augmented reality systems for medical applications. IEEE Eng Med Biol Mag Q Mag Eng Med Biol Soc. 1998;17:49–58.
62. Teber D, Guven S, Simpfendorfer T, Baumhauer M, Guven EO, Yencilek F, Gozen AS, Rassweiler J. Augmented reality: a new tool to improve surgical accuracy during laparoscopic partial nephrectomy? Preliminary in vitro and in vivo results. Eur Urol. 2009;56:332–8.
63. Thompson RH, Lane BR, Lohse CM, Leibovich BC, Fergany A, Frank I, Gill IS, Blute ML, Campbell SC. Renal function after partial nephrectomy: effect of warm ischemia relative to quantity and quality of preserved kidney. Urology. 2012;79:356–60.
64. Tsivian M, Packiam VT, Thompson RH. Tumor enucleation is appropriate during partial nephrectomy: against. Eur Urol Focus. 2019;5:925–6.
65. Ukimura O, Nakamoto M, Gill IS. Three-dimensional reconstruction of renovascular-tumor anatomy to facilitate zero-ischemia partial nephrectomy. Eur Urol. 2012;61:211–7.
66. Vermooten V. Indications for conservative surgery in certain renal tumors: a study based on the growth pattern of the cell carcinoma. J Urol. 1950;64:200–8.
67. von Rundstedt FC, Scovell JM, Agrawal S, Zaneveld J, Link RE. Utility of patient-specific silicone renal models for planning and rehearsal of complex tumour resections prior to robot-assisted laparoscopic partial nephrectomy. BJU Int. 2017;119:598–604.
68. Wake N, Rude T, Kang SK, Stifelman MD, Borin JF, Sodickson DK, Huang WC, Chandarana H. 3D printed renal cancer models derived from MRI data: application in pre-surgical planning. Abdom radiol (New York). 2017;42:1501–9.
69. Wild E, Teber D, Schmid D, Simpfendorfer T, Muller M, Baranski AC, Kenngott H, Kopka K, Maier-Hein L. Robust augmented reality guidance with fluorescent markers in laparoscopic surgery. Int J Comput Assist Radiol Surg. 2016;11:899–907.

Perioperative Surgical Complications in Robotic Partial Nephrectomy

7

Riccardo Tellini, Giovanni Enrico Cacciamani, Michele Marchioni, Andrea Minervini, and Andrea Mari

7.1 Introduction

Partial nephrectomy (PN) is the mainstay of treatment for localized renal tumors amenable of surgical excision [1, 9]. PN provides a better preservation of renal function, when compared to radical nephrectomy (RN) [35], which translates in a reduced risk of chronic kidney disease and cardiovascular morbidity and mortality [2, 10]. As for other surgical procedures, minimally invasive approaches have been proposed also for PN procedures. Firstly described in 2004 by Gettman et al. [16], robot-assisted PN (RAPN) has increasingly gained popularity and spread among urologists and nowadays robotic approach is predominant in PN procedures in US and Europe [6, 36]. Indeed, the undeniable advantages of robotic platform including the magnified tridimensional vision, the Endowrist technology and elimination of hand tremor enable an accurate dissection and precise reconstruction, thus allowing to obtain a low rate of positive surgical margins and minimizing the injury to surrounding healthy renal parenchyma, while keeping warm ischemia

R. Tellini (✉) · A. Minervini · A. Mari
Department of Experimental and Clinical Medicine, University of Florence - Unit of Oncologic Minimally-Invasive Urology and Andrology, Careggi Hospital, Florence, Italy
e-mail: riccatello@gmail.com

G. E. Cacciamani
University of Southern California Institute of Urology & Catherine and Joseph Aresty Department of Urology, Keck School of Medicine, University of Southern California, Los Angeles, CA, USA

M. Marchioni
Department of Medical, Oral and Biotechnological Sciences, Laboratory of Biostatistics, University "G. D'Annunzio" Chieti-Pescara, Chieti, Italy

Department of Urology, SS Annunziata Hospital, "G. D'Annunzio" University of Chieti, Chieti, Italy

© The Author(s), under exclusive license to Springer Nature Switzerland AG 2022
S. S. Goonewardene et al. (eds.), *Robotic Surgery for Renal Cancer*, Management of Urology, https://doi.org/10.1007/978-3-031-11000-9_7

times at safe levels. As a fact, current series report more favorable rates of "optimal" perioperative outcomes (i.e., trifecta [17]) after RAPN as compared to open and laparoscopic PN [19, 25, 44].

Moreover, robotic approach allows for a perfect integration of newer technologies in order to further improve perioperative outcomes including augmented reality and intraoperative Indocyanine green [14, 30].

However, despite the aforementioned advantages, PN, regardless of the surgical approach, is often a complex procedure and rate of complications, as well as their potential severity, are not negligible.

Aim of this chapter is to describe and report incidence, predictors and features of both intra- and post-operative complications during robotic PN as well as their specific management.

7.2 Definition and Rates

The first issue regarding perioperative complications of RAPN is the need of shared criteria for defining, reporting and grading the complications. In this context, Cacciamani et al. found that current literature lacks of standardized definition of intraoperative complication (IC) after RAPN and no improvement in reporting and grading of ICs over time was observed while an improvement in outcome reporting in terms of mortality rates and causes of death, definition of complications, severity grade and risk factors was reported for postoperative complications after RAPN [7, 8].

Therefore, we strongly recommend the adoption of standard guidelines and definition for reporting and grading complications. In this regard, the European Association of Urology (EAU) starting from 2012 published an ad hoc guideline about reporting and grading of complications after urologic surgical procedures [27].

In general, IC can be defined as any medical or surgical complication occurring between induction of anesthesia and patient awakening that could cause a potential injury and requiring unplanned medical or surgical maneuvers, while postoperative complications can be defined as any postoperative event caused by surgery, altering the normal postoperative course and/or delaying discharge [26].

The rates of intra- and post-operative complications after RAPN as reported in relevant contemporary series are reported in Table 7.1. As aforementioned, rate and description of intra-operative complication during RAPN is often not reported in current series and conversion rate (to open approach/radical nephrectomy) is low (0.3–2%). Post-operative complications rate ranges from 5.1 to 24.3% among current series with major (Clavien score >2) complications occurring in percentages varying between 0.7 and 10.2%.

Table 7.2 provides a summary of each surgical complication and its management according to the time to onset.

Table 7.1 Summary of the most important studies reporting surgical complications after robotic partial nephrectomy

Author, Year	Patients (n.)	Intraoperative complications, n (%)	Postoperative complications, n (%)	Major (CL >2) postoperative complications, n (%)	Notes
Tanagho, 2013 [37]	886	23 (2.6%)	139 (15.6%)	32 (3.6%)	R.E.N.A.L. score predicts RAPN complications rate
Moskowitz, 2017 [28]	1139	NR	130 (11.3%)	42 (3.7%)	1 (0.09%) Clavien V complication
Mari, 2016 [23]	117	1 (0.9%)	6 (5.1%)	1 (0.9%)	Robotic approach together with comorbidities is independently associated with a lower rate of postoperative complications
Veeratterapillay, 2017 [42]	250	NR	41 (16.4%)	15 (6%)	5 (2%) conversions to open/radical nephrectomy
Bertolo, 2018 [4]	298	16 (5.4%)	62 (21%)	15 (5%)	*Clinical T2 tumors* 1 (0.3%) conversion to radical nephrectomy
Connor, 2019 [12]	395	NR	22 (5.6%)	10 (2.5%)	Incidence of post-operative pseudo-aneurysms was 2.3%, while urinary leak rate was 0.25%
Khene, 2019 [20]	1342	NR	326 (24.3%)	137 (10.2%)	Male gender, tumor complexity and comorbidity were predictors of major complications

(continued)

Table 7.1 (continued)

Author, Year	Patients (n.)	Intraoperative complications, n (%)	Postoperative complications, n (%)	Major (CL >2) postoperative complications, n (%)	Notes
Mari, 2019 [24]	981	NR	79 (8.0%)	7 (0.7%)	3 (0.3%) conversions to open approach
Rosen, 2019 [33]	1770	NR	205 (11.6%)	60 (3.4%)	Obesity did not correlate with an increased complication rate
Diana, 2020 [13]	536	NR	66 (12.3%)	19 (3.5%)	8 (1.5%) conversions to open/radical nephrectomy
Carbonara, 2021 [11]	447	7 (1.6%)	101 (22.6%)	3 (0.67%)	No differences in terms of peri-operative complication between trans- and retro-peritoneal approach

Table 7.2 Summary of the types of surgical complications in robotic partial nephrectomy according to their onset, clinical management of each complication and grading

Intraoperative complications

Description	Management	Grading*
Bleeding	– *Dependent on site of bleeding and entity* – Sutures/Clips/Electrocautery/Hemostatic agents, as appropriate – Intraoperative transfusion may also be required – Conversion to open approach may be required – Radical Nephrectomy (in case of persistent bleeding)	1/2 1/2 3 4A
Vascular injury	– Sutures/Clips/Electrocautery/Hemostatic agents, as appropriate – Intraoperative transfusion may also be required, in case of significant bleeding – Radical Nephrectomy (in case of massive renal vessels injury or massive bleeding)	1/2 1/2 4A
Intraoperative tumor violation (ITV)	– Wider and deeper resection (in case of minor ITV) – Radical Nephrectomy and removal of any macroscopic tumor fragment	1/2/3 4A
Bowel injury	– Suture of laceration (in case of small laceration) – Segmental resection (in case of larger laceration)	1/2 4A
Spleen injury	– Electrocautery/Hemostatic agents – Splenectomy (unstoppable bleeding)	1/2 4A
Liver injury	– Electrocautery/Hemostatic agents – Segmental hepatectomy (unstoppable bleeding/severe injury)	1/2 4A
Pleural injury/ Pneumothorax	– Immediate repair of defect – Possible positioning of chest drain	1/2 1/2
Ureteral/pelvic injury	– Immediate repair of defect and ureteral catheter placement	1/2

(continued)

Table 7.2 (continued)

Postoperative complications		
Description	Management	Grading[#]
Bleeding	– *Dependent on site of bleeding and entity* – Conservative approach (hematocrit and vital parameters monitoring) – Blood transfusion may also be required – Selective Angioembolization – Surgical Exploration (± radical nephrectomy)	1 2 3a 3b/4
RAP / AVF	– Selective Angioembolization	3a
Urinary leak	– Ureteral stent placement and/or percutaneous nephrostomy tube placement	3a/3b

[*] According to Intraoperative Adverse Incident Classification (EAUiaiC) by the European Association of Urology ad hoc Complications Guidelines Panel [5]
[#] According to Clavien-Dindo classification of surgical complications [15]

7.3 Pre-operative Prevention of Complications

The preoperative prevention of complications is essentially based on an accurate imaging and meticulous surgical planning. For these purposes, an abdominal CT scan focused on kidney, tumor and vascular anatomy is indispensable. Arterial, parenchymal, venous and excretory phases are generated for a precise evaluation. If available, a 3D reconstruction of the tumor, intra-renal arterial tree and kidney, and 3D–printed models can facilitate better understanding of the anatomy [21, 29].

Several kidney-, patients- and tumor-related features need a careful evaluation for appropriate surgical planning. Regarding the patient features, particular attention must be turned to body mass index (BMI), previous abdominal surgery and perinephric fat measurements and adhesiveness [22] that could influence port placement as well as surgical access (trans- vs retro-peritoneal).

A clear knowledge of renal vascular anatomy (including number of arteries and veins, relation between the tumor, renal artery and renal vein) could guide the clamping strategy and avoid vascular injuries, while a detailed comprehension of tumor features and its boundaries could prevent tumor violation and forecast potential complications. In this light, nephrometry scores such as R.E.N.A.L, PADUA and Contact Surface Area (CSA) are useful composite tools incorporating the most relevant features [i.e., tumor size, clinical stage, location (anterior, posterior, lateral), relation to polar lines (upper, mid or lower pole), endophytic/exophytic ratio, proximity to the hilum, closeness to collecting system]. All these scores have been validated in several series and were found to predict various perioperative outcomes including post-operative complications [40].

In addition, several clinical nomograms have been proposed and validated for the prediction of overall [24] and major [20] complications following PN.

7.4 Intraoperative Complications

7.4.1 Intraoperative Adverse Events Leading to Bleeding

Unexpected intraoperative bleeding probably represents the most frequent and potentially more severe intraoperative complication during RAPN. Bleeding mainly originates from the PN resection bed, renal hilar vessels or from inferior vena cava (IVC) or aorta. Obviously, management of bleeding is dependent on its location. As aforementioned, an accurate understanding of patient's vascular anatomy is mandatory to prevent and forecast potential complications. Importantly, extensive medial mobilization of the colon/duodenum to expose the kidney, identification of the renal artery and vein and their tributaries is paramount. Dissection towards to the hilum is performed from distally to proximal. The renal vein and renal artery should be carefully isolated and vessel loops should be applied. In these phases, prudent dissection of the tissue in layers and avoid excessive traction on vascular structures is advised. In case of bleeding due to vascular injury, the surgeon needs to rapidly identify the source of bleeding. In these situations, a temporarily increase of the pneumoperitoneum pressure of 2–3 mmHg, basing on the baseline values of pneumoperitoneum and on the anesthesiologist evaluation, could help in reducing bleeding and identifying its origin. The role of bed-assistant is crucial providing adequate suction and irrigation as well as feedback on patient's condition; moreover, the bed-assistant should be ready to place additional ports as well as change instruments as appropriate. The use of mini-lap gauzes (5 × 5 cm or 7 × 5 cm) to compress the bleeding site and remove blood clots is usually helpful. After identification of the bleeding source, it should be controlled by applying clips or suturing, as appropriate. The type of bleeding generally depends on the source of bleeding (arterial or venous) and the dimension of the vessel injured. The vessel injured, either arterial or venous, could be closed with a metal clip or with a hem-o-lok. Indeed, the surgeon should carefully balance the consequences and the risk–benefit related to the closure of each clipped vessel. In case of damage of a significant venous vessel such as the renal vein or one of its segmentary branches, the surgeon should try to manage the bleeding closing the defect with a monofilament 3.0 suture. The vein could be closed with a clamp upstream and downstream depending on the grade of bleeding. Generally, the venous bleeding is higher on the right renal vein due to the downstream blood reflux from the inferior vena cava. The main artery should be clamped before the renal vein to avoid upstream bleeding from the kidney. The surgical management of arterial injury is more complex due to the higher intensity of bleeding. The closure of the arterial vessel is adopted as last chance only, while the closure of the arterial defect with single sutures or a running suture is often difficult. In case of a clinically significant arterial bleeding from the renal artery or the aorta, the apposition of a patch could be necessary to close the defect without reducing the diameter of the vessel. The intervention of vascular surgeon may be required. Despite an experienced robotic surgeon could theoretically manage any of these accidents robotically, in case of massive bleeding and/or hemodynamic instability or failure to identify the source of bleeding, a prompt open conversion should be considered.

Intraoperative bleeding is a potentially significant clinical complication in the tumor resection phase or renorraphy during partial nephrectomy. In these cases, the surgeon could consider performing a precise electrocautery of any bleeding points when possible or using adsorbable clips on single major bleeding vessel on tumor resection bed or placing additional deeper stiches. Otherwise, different hemostatic matrix sealants could be applied with adequate compression (over a gauze) of the bleeding site.

Finally, in case of uncontrolled bleeding compromising clear vision of the surgical field during the resection phase, some strategies could be attempted:

- In case of initial clampless approach, consider clamping the renal artery that should have been previously identified and isolated;
- If the renal artery has already been clamped, it should be re-checked for uneffective clamp placement (e.g., in case of inadequate isolation the vessel from perivascular tissue). Moreover, it should be verified that clamp has been placed

on the main renal artery and not on a secondary branch. Similarly, the presence of multiple renal arteries should be excluded. Indeed, the preventive use of green indocyanine before renal clamping and tumor resection could be of great help for the surgeon [40].
- In case of persistent bleeding despite these precautions, the surgeon should consider clamping also the renal vein, especially in case of right-sided endophytic and/or hilar masses due to the possibility of relevant blood backflow coming from the inferior vena cava.
- In case of uncontrollable/life-threatening bleeding, radical nephrectomy is advisable.

Some surgical tips to prevent bleeding from resection bed include an effective closure of the medullary defect starting from the inner layer taking care to include any visible source of bleeding (e.g., horizontal mattress suture technique). Moreover, the closure of cortical defect should be considered to improve the hemostatic action of renorraphy; in this scenario, the "sliding-clip" technique is a quick and effective strategy for renal defect closure in most cases [3].

7.4.2 Intraoperative Tumor Violation (ITV)

Since renal tumors are often frail, with a discontinuous, thin or absent pseudocapsule or with necrotic component, ITV may occur during PN and it should be cautiously avoided. The occurrence of ITV could increase the risk of positive surgical margins (PSM) or lead to tumor spillage that, especially in case of pneumoperitoneum, may jeopardize oncologic outcomes [38].

ITV during RAPN can be prevented by cautious handle of the tumor avoiding excessive traction on it and direct grasping of its surface. It can be helpful avoiding a complete de-fatting of the exophytic portion of the lesion to take advantage this peritumoral fatty tissue for the manipulation/traction of the tumor during the resection. Lastly, intraoperative ultrasound (US) may be used to precisely identify tumor shape, depth and margins, especially for endophytic masses, allowing the definition of surgical landmarks. In case of minor ITV, an immediate acknowledgement allows a conservative management including a prompt suction of any spilled tumoral material and a wider and deeper resection. In a case of major tumor violation leading to massive tumor spillage or impossibility to obtain a clear resection plane, a radical nephrectomy may be necessary, followed by an accurate inspection of the renal fossa and surrounding organs with removal of any tumor fragments. In all cases of ITV, the procedure should be completed as soon as possible, and the specimen should be placed in an endocatch bag immediately averting any further tumor seeding.

7.4.3 Visceral Injuries

Bowel injury rarely occurs with a incidence rate around 0.25% [34]. This complication could happen during the trocar placement or during the manipulation of the bowel.

It is very important a prompt identification of the bowel injury to manage intraoperatively this complication and to avoid postoperative complications due to bowel perforation. In these cases, the injury can be extremely difficult to identify and could be difficulty managed with a minimally invasive approach.

Trocar placing should be performed with a visual control of the access of trocars. Furthermore, manipulation of the bowel during surgery should be performed with atraumatic instruments or better avoiding a direct contact with the bowel and manipulating only the mesenteric.

Small lacerations in the bowel (without spillage of bowel content into the abdomen) can be sutured if immediately identified during surgery. Serosal injuries should be repaired as it may result in a damaged bowel wall as a result of absent anatomical support of the serosal layer with or without a localized area of ischaemia: this condition may determine intestinal leakage or fistula formation.

Larger, full-thickness lacerations or those diagnosed postoperatively may require resection and a general surgeon intervention. A particular attention should be taken to avoid damage to the duodenum in case of right-sided tumors.

Splenic injuries during RAPN occur in around 0.08% of cases [34] and their treatment depend on their severity. Electrocautery and hemostatic agents are usually used to control bleeding; however, if the bleeding does not stop, a splenectomy can be required.

Hepatic injury is typically related to a thermal injury or laceration from retraction. In general, thermal injuries do not require any intervention. Hepatic lacerations can determinate relevant bleeding and should be initially addressed with electrocautery and application of hemostatic agents. Larger lacerations with uncontrolled bleeding or damage to the biliary system (including a laceration of the gallbladder) should involve an hepatic surgeon.

Injury to the pancreas represents a rare occurrence (in case of left-sided tumors) and capsular injuries can be closed primarily. However, pancreatic leaks may require a partial pancreatectomy and patients require close postoperative monitoring for pancreatitis. In these cases, an abdominal drainage is usually required to monitor post-operative pancreatic juices drain.

7.4.4 Thoracic Complications

Pleural injuries and pneumothorax can occur during port placement or during the dissection.

Sometimes, right-sided pneumothorax happens due to the grasper used to retract the liver.

If it grasps the diaphragm, it can determinate diaphragmatic injuries that lead to a CO_2 leakage into the thorax due to high pressure pneumoperitoneum.

Management of a pleural lesion and a pneumothorax includes an immediate report to the anesthesiologist that can regulate airway pressure and flows to help the surgeon to better repair the lesion. Generally, a reduction of the pneumoperitoneum induce a retraction of the diaphragm toward the abdomen that could help during these complications. In case of small defects and immediate repair, no other actions are usually required. In case of larger defects and a pneumothorax causing hemodynamic instability or respiratory compromise, an immediate chest drain placement will be required to ensure resolution. Serial postoperative chest x-rays are necessary to exclude eventual failures or persisting pneumothorax. In these cases, the consultation of a thoracic surgeon is preferable.

7.5 Postoperative Complications

7.5.1 Postoperative Bleeding

Immediate or early postoperative bleeding is a relatively frequent and potentially life-threatening complication after RAPN. Treatment of post-operative bleeding ranges from a conservative management to blood transfusions administration till emergency surgical exploration according to patient conditions and extent of blood loss. Hemodynamic instability, decreasing hematocrit, low/absent urine output and abdominal distention and pain may represent signs and symptoms of post-operative hemorrhage and require an immediate recognition and intervention. The presence of a bloody drain output makes hemorrhage evident and measurable. Usually, the source of bleeding is the resection bed, however, it can originate from other areas including renal vessels, adrenal, lumbar veins, epigastric vessels or port sites.

Once hemorrhage is suspected, hemodynamic stabilization and fluid resuscitation, if necessary, represent the priorities. The execution of a CT renal angiography often allows a correct identification of the active bleeding site and enable its selective angioembolization (Fig. 7.1), whose efficacy as primary treatment is high. Blood transfusions are often required in case of sever acute anemia and/or hemodynamic instability.

In case hemodynamic instability persists or in case of failure to identify the bleeding site or to perform an effective angioembolization, surgical exploration is required. Usually, open exploratory laparotomy is needed for clot evacuation and bleeding control. If the bleeding is from the PN resection bed and cannot be properly controlled, completion nephrectomy may be required.

Late (>14 post-operative days) post-operative bleeding is likely due to renal artery pseudo-aneurysms (RAP) or arteriovenous fistula (AVF) [34]. These complications have been reported in up to 2.3% of patients after RAPN [12]. RAP derive from intraoperative arterial trauma resulting in communication with the extravascular space or formation of a fistula with the collecting system [18]. Patients typically present with symptoms of hematuria and/or flank pain. AVF occur less frequently

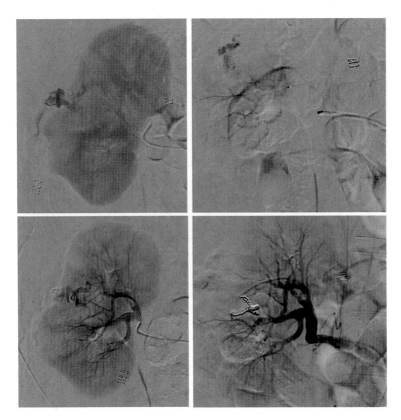

Fig. 7.1 Renal angiography showing a bleeding from the resection bed after RAPN. Superselective embolization of bleeding branch with microcoils enabled immediate cessation of bleeding. Post embolization angiogram showed no further bleeding from the resection bed while preserving vascular supply in the surrounding areas

than renal artery pseudo-aneurysms [18]. Most AVF are asymptomatic but can also present with symptoms of pain, hematuria, hypertension, or high-output cardiac failure. Selective angio-embolization is an effective treatment for AVF and RAP in approximately 95% of cases [18].

7.5.2 Urinary Leak

Urinary leak (UL) is a rare complication after RAPN with a reported incidence of 0.5–4% in contemporary series [34]. UL is associated with larger, endophytic tumors that are centrally located or near the renal collecting system. The Renal Pelvic Score is the best predictor of UL among nephrometry scores [39, 41]. Routine intraoperative ureteral catheterization does not reduce the probability of postoperative UL and therefore is not routinely recommended [43]. Symptoms and signs of a urine leak include increased drain output, fever, abdominal pain, and peritonitis. The time at presentation is variable, with a median of 13 days [31]. In case of evident urinary collecting system entry during the resection, a careful closure of the defect during the renorraphy is mandatory; in case of large defects, a ureteral catheter could be placed endoscopically (and left in place for 2–5 days) to favorite healing and permit a urine drainage in a "low-pressure" system. Similarly, in case of ureteral damage in any stage of the procedure, a primary repair should be performed and a JJ ureteral stent should be placed. Usually, the placement of an abdominal drain is strongly recommended in these situations to monitor post-operative UL and its evolution.

In case of post-operative UL and/or urinoma, the creation of a "low-pressure" excretory system is paramount and can be achieved with ureteral stent placement and/or nephrostomy tube placement and urethral catheterization. Percutaneous nephrostomy in these patients can be difficult, as typically, the renal pelvis is not dilated due to the urine leak [34].

7.5.3 Acute Kidney Injury

Acute Kidney Injury (AKI) after RAPN is a relatively frequent event and several features including female gender, age, baseline estimated glomerular filtration rate, pedicle clamping and tumor complexity were found to be predictors of its occurrence [2]. AKI occurs as a result of acute tubular necrosis secondary to global renal ischemia. Methods to reduce renal ischemia include decreasing warm ischemia time (WIT) and reducing the effects of decreased renal perfusion by early unclamping of the artery [34]. Traditionally, WIT should not exceed 25 min and prolonged WIT has been shown to negatively impact post-operative renal function. In case of expected longer WIT, cold ischemia techniques should be taken into consideration in the preoperative setting One method for reducing the effects of ischemia is cooling the kidney with ice; this should be considered if the anticipated ischemic time is >25 min [32].

Treatment of postoperative AKI includes reducing further insult to the kidney by ensuring adequate hydration, avoiding hypotension, and avoiding nephrotoxic agents. Dialysis is usually unnecessary in patients without severe pre-operative renal function impairment.

7.6 Conclusions

Perioperative complications after RAPN are often underreported and there is lack adoption of standardized criteria for their reporting and grading. Most frequent intraoperative complications are bleeding from tumor resection bed or abdominal arterial or venous vessels, tumor violation, visceral lesions. Most frequent post-operative complications are hemorrhagic, urinary leakage and acute kidney injury. Despite the robot-assisted approach seems to be associated with a significantly lower rate of postoperative complications compared to the open approach, RAPN remains a complex major surgery that can determine intraoperative and postoperative complications. Any robotic surgeon should be aware of all the adverse events that could happen during or after RAPN and know how to better manage these events intraoperatively avoiding whenever possible a conversion to open surgery.

References

1. Albiges L, et al. European association of urology guidelines on renal cell carcinoma: The 2019 Update 2019. https://doi.org/10.1016/j.eururo.2019.02.011.
2. Antonelli A, et al. Role of clinical and surgical factors for the prediction of immediate, early and late functional results, and its relationship with cardiovascular outcome after partial nephrectomy: results from the prospective multicenter RECORd 1 Project. J Urol. 2018;199(4). https://doi.org/10.1016/j.juro.2017.11.065.
3. Benway BM, et al. Robotic partial nephrectomy with sliding-clip renorrhaphy: technique and outcomes. Eur Urol (Switzerland). 2009;55(3):592–99. https://doi.org/10.1016/j.eururo.2008.12.028.
4. Bertolo R, et al. Outcomes of robot-assisted partial nephrectomy for clinical T2 renal tumors: a multicenter analysis (ROSULA Collaborative Group). Eur Urol (Switzerland). 2009;74(2):226–32. https://doi.org/10.1016/j.eururo.2018.05.004.
5. Biyani CS, et al. Intraoperative adverse incident classification (EAUiaiC) by the European association of urology ad hoc complications guidelines panel. Eur Urol. 2020;77(5):601–10. https://doi.org/10.1016/j.eururo.2019.11.015.
6. Bravi CA, et al. Perioperative outcomes of open, laparoscopic, and robotic partial nephrectomy: a prospective multicenter observational study (The RECORd 2 Project). Eur Urol Focus (Netherlands). 2021;7(2):390–96. https://doi.org/10.1016/j.euf.2019.10.013.
7. Cacciamani GE, Medina LG, et al. Impact of implementation of standardized criteria in the assessment of complication reporting after robotic partial nephrectomy: a systematic review. Eur Urol Focus (Netherlands). 2020;6(3):513–17. https://doi.org/10.1016/j.euf.2018.12.004.
8. Cacciamani GE, Tafuri A, et al. Quality assessment of intraoperative adverse event reporting during 29 227 robotic partial nephrectomies: a systematic review and cumulative analysis. Eur Urol Oncol (Netherlands). 2020;3(6):780–83. https://doi.org/10.1016/j.euo.2020.04.003.
9. Cadeddu JA, et al. American Urological Association (AUA) Renal mass and localized renal cancer: aua guideline american urological association (AUA) Renal Mass and Localized Renal Cancer. Am Urol Assoc 2017;1–49. http://auanet.org/guidelines/renal-mass-and-locali zed-renal-cancer-new-(2017).
10. Capitanio U, et al. Hypertension and cardiovascular morbidity following surgery for kidney cancer. Eur Urol Oncol (Netherlands). 2020;3(2):209–15. https://doi.org/10.1016/j.euo.2019.02.006.
11. Carbonara U, et al. Retroperitoneal versus transeptitoneal robot-assisted partial nephrectomy for postero-lateral renal masses: an international multicenter analysis. World J Urol (Germany). 2021. https://doi.org/10.1007/s00345-021-03741-2.
12. Connor J, et al. Postoperative complications after robotic partial nephrectomy. J Endourol (United States). 2020;34(1):42–7. https://doi.org/10.1089/end.2019.0434.
13. Diana P, Lughezzani G, et al. Multi-institutional retrospective validation and comparison of the simplified PADUA REnal nephrometry system for the prediction of surgical success of robot-assisted partial nephrectomy. Eur Urol Focus (Netherlands). 2020. https://doi.org/10.1016/j.euf.2020.11.003.
14. Diana P, Buffi NM, et al. The role of intraoperative indocyanine green in robot-assisted partial nephrectomy: results from a large, multi-institutional series. Eur Urol. 2020;78(5):743–9. https://doi.org/10.1016/j.eururo.2020.05.040.

15. Dindo D, Demartines N, Clavien P-A. Classification of surgical complications: a new proposal with evaluation in a cohort of 6336 patients and results of a survey. Ann Surg. 2004;205–13. https://doi.org/10.1097/01.sla.0000133083.54934.ae.
16. Gettman MT, et al. Robotic-assisted laparoscopic partial nephrectomy: technique and initial clinical experience with DaVinci robotic system. Urology (United States). 2004;64(5):914–18. https://doi.org/10.1016/j.urology.2004.06.049.
17. Hung AJ, et al. "Trifecta" in partial nephrectomy. J Urol (United States). 2013;189(1):36–42. https://doi.org/10.1016/j.juro.2012.09.042.
18. Hyams ES, et al. Iatrogenic vascular lesions after minimally invasive partial nephrectomy: a multi-institutional study of clinical and renal functional outcomes. Urology (United States). 2011;78(4):820–26. https://doi.org/10.1016/j.urology.2011.04.063.
19. Khalifeh A, et al. Comparative outcomes and assessment of trifecta in 500 robotic and laparoscopic partial nephrectomy cases: a single surgeon experience. J Urol (United States). 2013;189(4):1236–42. https://doi.org/10.1016/j.juro.2012.10.021.
20. Khene Z-E, et al. A preoperative nomogram to predict major complications after robot assisted partial nephrectomy (UroCCR-57 study). Urol Oncol Seminars Original Investigat. 2019;37(9):577.e1-577.e7. https://doi.org/10.1016/j.urolonc.2019.05.007.
21. Kyung YS, et al. Application of 3-D printed kidney model in partial nephrectomy for predicting surgical outcomes: a feasibility study. Clin Genitourin Cancer. 2019;17(5):e878–84. https://doi.org/10.1016/j.clgc.2019.05.024.
22. Di Maida F, et al. Clinical predictors and significance of adherent perinephric fat assessed with Mayo Adhesive Probability (MAP) score and Perinephric Fat Surface Density (PnFSD) at the time of partial nephrectomy for localized renal mass. A single high-volume referral ce. Minerva urologica e nefrologica = Italian J Urol Nephrol (Italy). 2020. https://doi.org/10.23736/S0393-2249.20.03698-X.
23. Mari A, et al. Predictive factors of overall and major postoperative complications after partial nephrectomy : results from a multicenter prospective study (The RECORd 1 project). Eur J Surgical Oncol (Elsevier Ltd.). 2016. https://doi.org/10.1016/j.ejso.2016.10.016.
24. Mari A, et al. Nomogram for predicting the likelihood of postoperative surgical complications in patients treated with partial nephrectomy: a prospective multicentre observational study (the RECORd 2 project). BJU Int. 2019. https://doi.org/10.1111/bju.14680.
25. Mari A, et al. Perioperative and mid-term oncological and functional outcomes after partial nephrectomy for complex (PADUA Score $\geq$10) renal tumors: a prospective multicenter observational study (the RECORD2 Project). Eur Urol Focus (Netherlands). 2020. https://doi.org/10.1016/j.euf.2020.07.004.
26. Minervini A, et al. The occurrence of intraoperative complications during partial nephrectomy and their impact on postoperative outcome: results from the RECORd1 project. Minerva urologica e nefrologica = Italian J Urol Nephrol (Italy). 2019;71(1):47–54. https://doi.org/10.23736/S0393-2249.18.03202-2.
27. Mitropoulos D, et al. Reporting and grading of complications after urologic surgical procedures: an ad hoc EAU guidelines panel assessment and recommendations. Eur Urol (Switzerland). 2012;61(2):341–49. https://doi.org/10.1016/j.eururo.2011.10.033.
28. Moskowitz EJ, et al. Predictors of medical and surgical complications after robot-assisted partial nephrectomy: an analysis of 1139 patients in a multi-institutional kidney cancer database. J Endourol (United States). 2017;31(3):223–8. https://doi.org/10.1089/end.2016.0217.
29. Porpiglia F, et al. Development and validation of 3D printed virtual models for robot-assisted radical prostatectomy and partial nephrectomy: urologists' and patients' perception. World J Urol. 2018;36(2):201–7. https://doi.org/10.1007/s00345-017-2126-1.
30. Porpiglia F, et al. Three-dimensional augmented reality robot-assisted partial nephrectomy in case of complex tumours (PADUA$\geq$;10): a new intraoperative tool overcoming the ultrasound guidance. Eur Urol (Elsevier). 2020;78(2):229–38. https://doi.org/10.1016/j.eururo.2019.11.024.

31. Potretzke AM, et al. Urinary fistula after robot-assisted partial nephrectomy: a multicentre analysis of 1791 patients. BJU Int (England). 2016;117(1):131–7. https://doi.org/10.1111/bju.13249.
32. Rogers CG, et al. Robotic partial nephrectomy with cold ischemia and on-clamp tumor extraction: recapitulating the open approach. Eur Urol. 2013;63(3):573–8. https://doi.org/10.1016/j.eururo.2012.11.029.
33. Rosen DC, et al. The impact of obesity in patients undergoing robotic partial nephrectomy. J Endourol (United States). 2019;33(6):431–7. https://doi.org/10.1089/end.2019.0018.
34. Ryan J, et al. A systematic management algorithm for perioperative complications after robotic assisted partial nephrectomy. Can Urological Associat J = Journal de l'Association des urologues du Canada (Canadian Medical Association). 2019;13(11):E371–E376.https://doi.org/10.5489/cuaj.5750
35. Scosyrev E, et al. Renal function after nephron-sparing surgery versus radical nephrectomy: results from EORTC Randomized Trial 30904. Eur Urol (European Association of Urology). 2013;1–6. https://doi.org/10.1016/j.eururo.2013.06.044.
36. Shah PH, et al. The temporal association of robotic surgical diffusion with overtreatment of the small renal mass. J Urol (United States). 2018;200(5):981–8. https://doi.org/10.1016/j.juro.2018.05.081.
37. Tanagho YS, et al. Perioperative complications of robot-assisted partial nephrectomy: analysis of 886 patients at 5 United States centers. Urology (United States). 2013;81(3):573–9. https://doi.org/10.1016/j.urology.2012.10.067.
38. Tellini R, et al. Positive surgical margins predict progression-free survival after nephron-sparing surgery for renal cell carcinoma: results from a single center cohort of 459 cases with a minimum follow-up of 5 years. Clinic Genitour Cancer (Elsevier). 2019;17(1):e26–31. https://doi.org/10.1016/j.clgc.2018.08.004.
39. Tomaszewski JJ, et al. Renal pelvic anatomy is associated with incidence, grade, and need for intervention for urine leak following partial nephrectomy. Eur Urol (Switzerland). 2014;66(5):949–55. https://doi.org/10.1016/j.eururo.2013.10.009.
40. Veccia A, Antonelli A, Hampton LJ, et al. Near-infrared fluorescence imaging with indocyanine green in robot-assisted partial nephrectomy: pooled analysis of comparative studies. Eur Urol Focus (Netherlands). 2020;6(3):505–12. https://doi.org/10.1016/j.euf.2019.03.005.
41. Veccia A, Antonelli A, Uzzo RG, et al. Predictive value of nephrometry scores in nephron-sparing surgery: a systematic review and meta-analysis. Eur Urol focus (Netherlands). 2020;6(3):490–504. https://doi.org/10.1016/j.euf.2019.11.004.
42. Veeratterapillay R, et al. Early surgical outcomes and oncological results of robot-assisted partial nephrectomy: a multicentre study. BJU Int (England). 2017;120(4):550–5. https://doi.org/10.1111/bju.13743.
43. Zargar H, et al. Urine leak in minimally invasive partial nephrectomy: analysis of risk factors and role of intraoperative ureteral catheterization. Int braz j urol : Official J Brazil Soc Urol (Brazil). 2014;40(6):763–71. https://doi.org/10.1590/S1677-5538.IBJU.2014.06.07.
44. Zargar H, et al. Trifecta and optimal perioperative outcomes of robotic and laparoscopic partial nephrectomy in surgical treatment of small renal masses: a multi-institutional study. BJU Int (John Wiley & Sons Ltd.). 2015;116(3):407–14. https://doi.org/10.1111/bju.12933.

Renal Robotic Surgery for Lefties: Left-Handedness in Upper Tract Robotic Surgery

Mylle Toon, Challacombe Ben, Uvin Pieter, and Mottrie Alexandre

8.1 Introduction

Handedness or chirality, is a characteristic of a person defined by the unequal distribution of fine motor skills in both hands. Although right-handedness predominates, an estimated 9.3–18.1% of the global population are left-handed. Recent publications show an increase in the reported rate of left-handedness [8]. A contributing factor may be the easing of cultural pressure against this sinistrality. For centuries, left handers have endured discrimination in a world designed for right hand preference. Literally, 'right' means 'correct' and 'sinister' means 'left' or 'omnious'. Left-handedness is still considered an exception and a physical deviation. It may however be a potential advantage as left-handers are more likely to be better users of their non-dominant hand and many are effectively ambidextrous. This allows more flexibility in complex surgical tasks and the potential to change to the better positioned but non-dominant hand.

M. Toon (✉)
University Hospital of Ghent, Corneel Heymanslaan 10, 9000 Gent, Belgium
e-mail: toon.mylle@ugent.be

C. Ben
Guy's Hospital, Guy's and St Thomas' Trust (GSTT), London, UK
e-mail: benchallacombe@doctors.org.uk

U. Pieter
AZ Sint-Jan, Ruddershove 10, 8000 Brugge, Belgium
e-mail: Pieter.uvin@azsintjan.be

M. Alexandre
O.L.V. Clinic, Moorselbaan 164, 9300 Aalst, Belgium

Every day, left-handed individuals experience difficulties with tools designed for the right-handed persons [4]. These problems extend to instruments as simple as scissors and many other within the operating room. Surgical residents report anxiety about their left-handedness, inconveniences during assisting, and lack of mentorship [9] For some right-handed senior surgeons, tutoring a left-handed trainee is an uphill task [1]. The default option is to train the left handed surgeon to perform the operation in a right handed manner but this is disadvantageous to the leftie. Surgeons and surgical trainees have indicated that difficulties arise in both open and minimally invasive surgery [6].

With a growing rate of left-handedness, there is a need to adapt and expand our surgical training and practice. For the moment, few teaching materials and even less technical reports are available for left-handed surgeons. A more personal approach, adapted for the dominant hand is needed. With a vast majority of laparoscopic and robotic surgeons being right-handed, proper guidelines for left-handed surgeons are in short supply.

The goal of this chapter is to provide tips and tricks to left-handed surgeons. As it rethinks the different possibilities in instrument usage within upper tract robotic surgery, it could be of interest to every upper tract surgeon. To our knowledge, no similar chapter has been written before. This chapter fills a gap that exists in current literature and is therefore based on experience and expert opinions.

8.2 Upper Tract Robotic Surgery

The introduction of the Da Vinci Robotic Surgical System by Intuitive has brought urological surgery into a new era. The engineering feat comes with multiple advances in 'minimally invasive surgery', such as seven degrees of freedom, 3-dimensional view, tremor filtration and better instrument precision. The system allows the surgeon to operate in an ergonomic non-sterile manner and -theoretically- at a distant location [2].

The robotic system of Da Vinci got designed to allow as much degrees of freedom as possible. Not only provides the robotic system a better range of motion than a surgeon's wrist and fingers, recent studies showed that it also can minimize the innate chirality of the surgeon. Novel studies are needed to further distinguish how big the elimination of the chirality is [2, 7]

A second advantage of the Xi system is the possibility of port hopping with the endoscope. Allowing the surgeon to switch positions in the middle of the operation, new possibilities arise. When using the Xi system correctly, being a leftie should not have any impact. Left-handed surgeons can use various unique tips and tricks to use their left-handedness in their advantage. We made them a summary of those tips and tricks.

8.2.1 Instruments

According to a statement Intuitive made for this chapter, all da Vinci Instruments are meant to be used for left-handed and right-handed surgeons. Concerning the da Vinci Instruments with curved tip design (Maryland Bipolar Forceps, Monopolar Curved Scissors, Curved Bipolar Dissector), the designers consider task and approach to tissue regardless of the dominant hand of the surgeon. The curve of the instrument tip can be rotated tip-up or tip-down with the instrument's roll capability to the surgeon's preference by rolling the hand controller. This will move the instrument tip in the direction most comfortable to the surgeon. Intuitive tests the usability of the instrument with both left-handed and right-handed surgeons by evaluations with engineers who observe user interaction to confirm if the device is safe and intuitive to the user. Currently, anno 2021, Intuitive does not sell instruments for left-handed or right-handed surgeons. All the instruments can be used by both.

8.2.2 Renal Robotic Surgery: Positioning and Port Placement

The positioning of the patient during renal robotic surgery is identical as in the right-handed procedure. Secure the patient in a modified lateral position with a 45° angle. Make sure the patient is fitted at the lateral edge of the operative table and the ipsilateral arm is as low as possible to maximize the range motion of the different arms of the robotic system.

Placement of the ports is different with changing handedness. First, the Hasson technique is used to place the assisting port. After pneumoperitoneum is achieved, a first look intra-abdominally must be undertaken to be sure the peritoneum is free of injuries and adhesions. The four remaining ports will be placed in a straight line at the lateral border of the rectus abdominus muscle. For left-handed surgeons, optimal port placement is displayed at Figs. 8.1 and 8.2. At the start of the procedure, scissors will be placed at the most cranial port. The endoscopic camera will be placed at the second most cranial port. In ports number 3 and 4, respectively a ProGrasp and needle holder (or fenestrated bipolar) can be placed.

Note that right-handedness surgery on the right kidney often requires an additional 5 mm port. With the help of this additional port a liver retractor is put in place. With left-handed surgeons, there is no need for a retractor or an extra entry. Using the pitch degree of the robotic instrument in port 4, ProGrasp, the surgeon can easily push aside the liver, gaining view and necessary workspace.

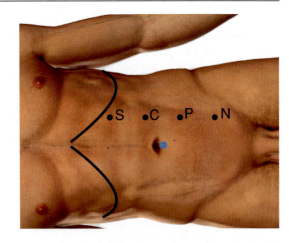

Fig. 8.1 Port placement at start of procedure Da Vinci Xi, left kidney surgery (left-handed). **C**: Camera / **N**: Needle holder / **S**: Bipolar scissors / **P**: Prograsp / Blue dot: Assisting Port

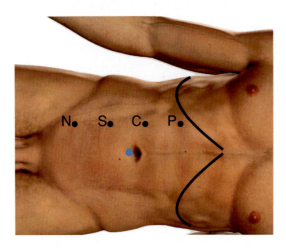

Fig. 8.2 Port placement at start of procedure Da Vinci Xi, right kidney surgery (left-handed). **C**: Camera / **N**: Needle holder / **S**: Bipolar scissors / **P**: Prograsp / Blue dot: Assisting Port

8.2.3 Port hopping During (Partial) Nephrectomy

During a (partial) nephrectomy, the Xi Da Vinci system allows us to easily switch the camera and the different instruments. Port hopping can provide a better view of the kidney tumor, can facilitate manipulation of the kidney and offers a safe access to cranial, caudal or posterior tumors. Repositioning of the ports displayed on Figs. 8.3 and 8.4 grants the needle holder to grasp adjacent kidney tissue. Now the kidney can be moved around freely around the pedicle.

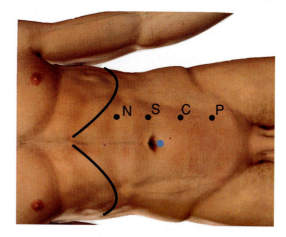

Fig. 8.3 Port hopping during ischemia time Da Vinci Xi, left kidney surgery (left-handed). **C**: Camera / **N**: Needle holder / **S**: Bipolar scissors / **P**: Prograsp / Blue dot: Assisting Port

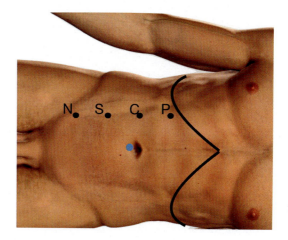

Fig. 8.4 Port hopping during ischemia time Da Vinci Xi, right kidney surgery (left-handed). **C**: Camera / **N**: Needle holder / **S**: Bipolar scissors / **P**: Prograsp / Blue dot: Assisting Port

8.2.4 Nephro-Ureterectomy

During the nephrectomy with or without lymphadenectomy, the left-handed console surgeon may use the same setup and starting position as mentioned before (Figs. 8.1 and 8.2).

After the completion of the first portion, ureterectomy may be performed with a different port position. A brief undocking may be helpful for targeting the pelvis. The boom is now rotated and the required angle differences are met. Position the camera port more caudally so the downwards dissection of the ureter can be achieved up to the ureterovesical junction. After the excision of the bladder cuff is finalized, the specimen can be placed in a laparoscopic bag and removed. Repair of cystotomy is performed using either of both hands to suture.

Fig. 8.5 Setup during upper tract surgery in the pelvic region. Da Vinci Xi. Left-handed assisting port. **C**: Camera / **N**: Needle holder / **S**: Bipolar scissors / **P**: Prograsp / Blue dot: Assisting Port

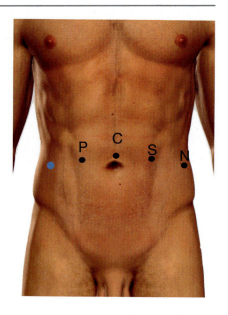

8.2.5 Cystoureterostomy/Ureterovesical Junction Surgery

Setup for distal ureteral repair and upper tract surgery limited to the pelvis region is similar to other pelvic surgery. Place the ports in a standard 'prostatectomy' fashion. Place the 12 mm assistant trocar at the right side if the assistant is left-handed. Favorable placement for left-handed surgeons of the other ports is shown at Fig. 8.5.

Our camera is placed at the umbilical port, between the monopolar scissors at the left and the Prograsp at the right side. At the left lateral port, a needle holder is the preferred choice. With this layout, the surgeon is capable of showing all tissues with the both lateral instruments while operating with the left hand. The endoscope is placed next to the bipolar scissors so that the instruments are as lateral as possible.

8.3 Assisting Upper Tract Robotic Surgery

The success of robot assisted procedures depend on a successful team. However, the literature focuses on the performance of the console surgeons, one study showed that the experience of the bedside assistant is of almost equal interest, shortening the total operation time [3]. Our believe is that adaptation to the right- or left-handedness of the assistant can be helpful, further studies are necessary to review the impact of trocar adjustment.

In case of the upper tract surgery, adaptation of the assisting port can be useful. For a left-handed assistant, the port has to be more cranial or caudal if the targeted region is respectively the right and left kidney. An illustration is added to gain a

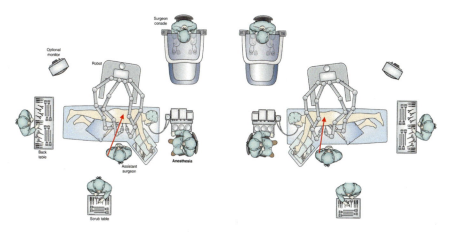

Fig. 8.6 Adaptation of the assisting port following handedness of bedside assistant [5]

better insight in the situation (Fig. 8.6). The scrub table is placed at the right side of the left-handed assistant, so to secure a smooth and elegant transition when changing instruments or loading clip appliers.

8.4 Epilogue

Experienced surgeons often develop their own individualized technique, rather than using the theoretically optimal technique for their dominant hand. When trying the "optimal" technique, it doesn't always meet the expectations but to apply a different technique or setup, one must leave behind standardized routines, which is not a comfortable process. Every possible setup mentioned above can be adapted to individual preferences. The correct technique, based on the dominant hand, should be educated from the start of training. Therefore, not only literature on specific procedure guidelines is necessary, training should always include the difference between right and left-handedness and their practical consequences. They used to say that left-handers were the only people in their right minds but, it may be that sinister surgeons actually are in a good place for upper tract robotic surgery.

References

1. Adusumilli PS, Kell C, Chang JH, Tuorto S, Leitman IM. Left-handed surgeons: are they left out? Curr Surg. 2004;61:587–91.
2. Badalato GM, Shapiro E, Rothberg MB, Bergman A, Roychoudhury A, Korets R, Patel T, Badani KK. The da vinci robot system eliminates multispecialty surgical trainees' hand dominance in open and robotic surgical settings. JSLS J Soc Laparoendosc Surg. 2014;18(e2014):00399.

3. Cimen HI, Atik YT, Altinova S, Adsan O, Balbay MD. Does the experience of the bedside assistant effect the results of robotic surgeons in the learning curve of robot assisted radical prostatectomy? Int Braz J Urol. 2019;45:54–60.
4. FLATT, A. E. Is being left-handed a handicap? The short and useless answer is "yes and no." Proc (Bayl Univ Med Cent). 2008;21:304–7.
5. Leveillee RJ, Ashouri K. Robot-assisted pyeloplasty. In: SU L-M, editor. Atlas of robotic urologic surgery. Cham: Springer International Publishing; 2017. p. 148.
6. LIESKE B. The left handed surgical trainee. BMJ. 2008;337:a2883.
7. Mucksavage P, Kerbl DC, Lee JY. The da Vinci(®) Surgical system overcomes innate hand dominance. J Endourol. 2011;25:1385–8.
8. Papadatou-Pastou M, Ntolka E, Schmitz J, Martin M, Munafò MR, Ocklenburg S, Paracchini S. Human handedness: a meta-analysis. Psychol Bull. 2020;146:481–524.
9. Tchantchaleishvili V, Myers PO. Left-handedness–a handicap for training in surgery? J Surg Educ. 2010;67:233–6.

Training with New Robots and How to Transition from One System to the Next in Renal Cancer Surgery

Kenneth Chen, Kae Jack Tay, John Shyi Peng Yuen, and Nathan Lawrentschuk

9.1 Introduction

The introduction of robotics into the field of minimally invasive surgery marked a significant milestone in the evolution of surgery. The formidable combination of precision, flexibility and control helped overcome many technical challenges, particularly for operations within confined spaces. Since its inception at the turn of the millennium, robotic-assistance has pervaded a range of surgical operations across various subspecialties with Urologists being early adopters of the technology.

The da Vinci surgical system (Intuitive Surgical, Sunnyvale, CA, USA) was unveiled in 1999 and received U.S. Food and Drug Administration (FDA) approval in 2000 for human use [21]. For nearly 20 years, it has been the standard for robot-assisted surgery. A strong patent filing including ownership of intellectual

K. Chen (✉) · K. J. Tay · J. S. P. Yuen
Department of Urology, Singapore General Hospital, Singapore, Singapore
e-mail: Kenneth.chen@singhealth.com.sg

K. J. Tay
e-mail: tay.kae.jack@singhealth.com.sg

J. S. P. Yuen
e-mail: john.yuen.s.p@singhealth.com.sg

K. Chen · N. Lawrentschuk
Division of Cancer Surgery, Peter MacCallum Cancer Centre, Melbourne, Australia
e-mail: lawrentschuk@gmail.com

N. Lawrentschuk
Department of Surgery, University of Melbourne, Royal Melbourne Hospital, Melbourne, Australia

EJ Whitten Prostate Cancer Research Centre, Epworth Healthcare, Melbourne, Australia

© The Author(s), under exclusive license to Springer Nature Switzerland AG 2022
S. S. Goonewardene et al. (eds.), *Robotic Surgery for Renal Cancer*, Management of Urology, https://doi.org/10.1007/978-3-031-11000-9_9

property on multiple component technology, constant modifications, updated regulatory approvals, an established global network of training centres, distributors and technical support have all allowed da Vinci to maintain its dominance in the field.

Competition is the essential catalyst for growth in any field. As patents last a maximum duration of 20 years, the expiry of the original patent portfolio held by Intuitive has primed its competitors and caused quite a stir of excitement in the industry. This has resulted in many companies investing in their own research and development in the last decade and the current emergence of various new robotic platforms (Table 9.1). However, with a history of such strong presence from a single robotic system, what challenges lie ahead for the generations of robotic surgeons trained on da Vinci when they transition to the next system?

9.2   Console Concept and Display Technology

Intuitive Surgical has constructed an iconic closed console with the da Vinci system which has advantages in reducing distractions and increasing surgeon's focus, as well as providing a more immersive experience. However, the lack of awareness of the surgical environment may compromise communication with the rest of the surgical and anaesthetic team. While the concept of open consoles is refreshing, the design has its shortcomings which are mainly related to a difference in the ergonomics and operative vision. Indeed, the console design is inherently intertwined with the style of visual optics presented to the surgeon (Fig. 9.1).

The advancements in visual optics systems paved the way for realistic 3-dimensional view of the operative field, a main attraction of robot-assisted surgery. True stereopsis capture of the operative field is essential for the composition of a high definition stereoptic image for the operating surgeon. A 3D operating system comprises 2 main components: image capture and projection system. With the traditional rod-lens laparoscope, image capture of the operative field is transmitted externally to a video camera which then sends the image as electrical signals to an image processor. This has been supplanted by "chip on the tip" technology where miniature camera chips convert the image to electrical signals at the tip of the laparoscope and externalizes the signals to the image processor. Single channel systems use refraction to split a single image to provide 2 perspectives, while dual channel systems provide 2 separate point of views and hence, offers a true binocular vision of the operative field [29]. Projection systems on the other hand help deliver a 3D visual field to the surgeon. There are two main 3D vision systems. Da Vinci offers the fixed screen 3D stereoscopic design where stereoptic vision is achieved with separate image captures from 2 camera heads on the endoscope delivered respectively to each eye within the console. This negates the need for cumbersome active shuttering glasses that are required in active shuttering projection, which is a different technique where alternate left and right views are displayed at high frequency on a single flat display screen and polarized glasses

9 Training with New Robots and How to Transition from One System …

Table 9.1 Current approved robotic systems and characteristics

Robotic system	Year of approval	Approval authority	Surgeon console	Display system	Patient cart	Master controller	Haptic feedback	Camera diameter (mm)	Instrument profile/DOF	Dedicated training simulator
da Vinci Xi	2014	FDA	Closed	Fixed screen	Single	Finger loops	No	8	8 mm/7°	da Vinci® Skills Simulator™, SimNow® by da Vinci®
Senhance	2017	FDA	Open	3D polarized glasses	Multiple	Laparoscopic handles	Yes	10	10 mm/7° 5 mm/6° 3 mm/6°	NA
Revo-I	2017	KMFDS	Closed	Fixed screen	Single	Finger loops	Yes	10	7.4 mm/7°	Revo-Sim
Da Vinci SP	2018	FDA	Closed	Fixed screen	Single	Finger loops	No	12 × 10	6 mm/7°	NA
Versius	2019	CE Mark	Open	3D polarized glasses	Multiple	Joystick	Yes	10	5 mm/7°	Versius trainer
Avatera	2019	CE Mark	Semi-closed	Fixed screen	Single	Finger loops	Yes	10	5 mm/7° (single use)	Avatera VR simulator
Hinotori	2020	JMHLW	Semi-closed	Fixed screen	Single	Finger loops	No	NA	NA	hi-Sim™

DOF, degrees of freedom; FDA, U.S. Food and Drug Administration; SP, Single-Port; 3D, three dimensional; KMFDS, Korean Ministry of Food and Drug Safety; NA, no available data; JMHLW, Japanese Ministry of Health, Labor and Welfare; TM, trademark

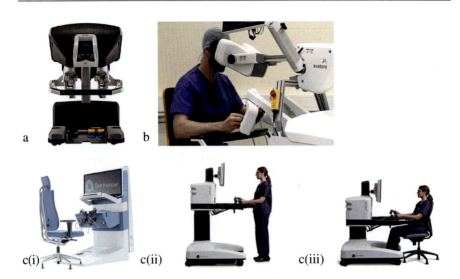

Fig. 9.1 Different concept of console. **a** Closed console and fixed screen 3D stereoscopic system of da Vinci [7]. **b** Semi-closed console of Avatera [2]. **c** Open console and 3D polarized display of (i) Senhance (*The Senhance Surgical System*) (ii) Versius, standing position (iii) Versius, sitting position (*Versius For Surgeons—CMR Surgical*)

help ensure each eye receives the corresponding image. This form of 3D polarized display is utilized in robotic systems with open consoles offered by Senhance (TransEnterix Surgical Inc., Morrisville, NC, USA), Versius (Cambridge Medical Robotics Ltd., Cambridge, UK) and Hugo (Medtronic Inc, Minnesota, USA) (not commercially available as of article).

There is abundance of evidence on the advantages of 3D vs 2D vision in operative time and errors, reduced motion, and all other comparative markers for surgical performance [34]. Even with the leap into 3D visualization, there are significant differences between the two modes of 3D view mentioned above. In transitioning between robots, users have to be cognizant of these fundamental differences in the acquisition of surgical field stereopsis between fixed (closed) console viewing and open consoles mandating use of polarized shuttering glasses. In particular, the latter may suffer from issues of user discomfort with the additional weight of polarizing glasses, decreased brightness resulting from filtering of polarized glasses and more importantly, a lower horizontal resolution compared to the 3D stereoscopic system which boasts a higher fidelity image. In addition, with open sided eye units, the user may not be entirely excluded from surrounding visual stimuli which may cause headaches and neurovestibular disturbances arising from sensory conflicts from visual input and body position.

9.3 Ergonomics

The robotic console is essentially a bustling center of human–computer interactions. There is a constant flow of visual information to the surgeon, who then effects a change in vision or tissue control via master controllers on the console. With this understanding, we can appreciate the importance of the interplay between master–slave motion alignment, hand–eye coordination, ergonomics of the console and its direct impact on surgeon comfort and sense of surgical immersion [9]. A main tenet in the design of the robotic console is ensuring the optimal balance between the concepts of ergonomics and master–slave motion alignment.

With the closed consoles such as da Vinci and Revo-I, the surgeon's head is fixed as is the eye-to-screen relationship (Fig. 9.1). While there are advantages as mentioned above in reducing surrounding sensory distractions, remaining in this constant posture has been shown to strain the cervical spine [31]. While open consoles such as Versius and Senhance allow free movement, they do not necessarily mitigate the musculoskeletal strain on the surgeon. Some systems which allow eye-tracking such as Senhance may introduce similar problems with strain on neck if the display and eye alignment is not optimal. Studies show that eye fatigue is contributed by operator-display distance and the viewing angle of the operator [16, 17]. Research has also shown that a downward gaze at the display is more likely to cause cervical strain on the surgeon, an observation reported for the da Vinci's console as well [3, 11, 35]. In addition, the allowance of a more casual sitting posture without resting points may also hold potential for poor posturing of the surgeon. A unique feature of Versius is that the open console offers both standing and sitting configurations for the robotic surgeon, allowing more flexibility and potentially more comfort as well (Fig. 9.1). These posture related nuances are considered important for the transitioning surgeon especially in crossing from a closed console to an open concept. The awareness of these issues should prompt a proper induction course that emphasizes on proper posturing to optimize ergonomics as an early step in the training on a new system. The conversation on ergonomics extends beyond the relationship of the surgeon's posture with the robotic console into the type of master controllers.

9.4 Master Controllers

The design of the master controllers on the robotic console is of paramount importance and a comfortable manipulator enhances surgical precision and surgeon experience. Current robotic platforms employ 2 main types of grips—the pinch or the power grip (Fig. 9.2). There are inherent differences between the two. The pinch grip is optimal for precise movement but increases the tension and fatigue of small muscles of the hand [23, 32]. In contrast, the power grip offers less muscle tension but lacks precision, with movements effected from large group muscles of the arm while finger movements are restricted due to their commitment to gripping a handle. Jeong and Tadano [18] investigated the design of a combined-grip-handle

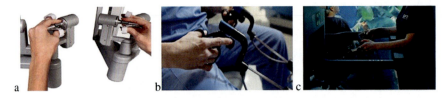

Fig. 9.2 Different types of grips for master controllers. **a** pinch grip in da Vinci [7]. **b** Power grip in Senhance [37]. **c** power grip (joystick) in Versius [38]

in master–slave configuration and showed better performance on the positioning operation and provided a possibility to perform precise work at lower scale factors.

With the above in mind, a surgeon could possibly experience the biggest change in terms of transitioning between a pinch grip and a handle grip controller. This may form the biggest hurdle to cross. The pinch movements are more naturalistic and approximate fine open surgery with forceps and hand-held diathermy. While laparoscopic surgeons would have more affinity for the handle grip controllers as they resemble laparoscopic equipment. Given the generations of robotic surgeons that have been trained on da Vinci's pinch grip controllers, the adopter of the handle grip controller will have a larger learning curve to mount and possibly a different skillset to pick up.

9.5 Haptic Feedback

One of the vexations of robotic surgical systems is the glaring lack of haptic feedback. The absence of this safety feature coupled with the capability of robotic arms to exert significant amount of force over a small area explains the inherent increased risk of tissue damage and surgical mishaps [10, 20, 30]. It is not surprising therefore that newer robots endeavor to provide a solution in this space.

There has been much research done in the field of haptics in the past decade [5, 8, 26, 39] particularly in the area of kinesthetic force feedback (KFF) [4, 6, 33], which involves activation of receptors in the muscles to create awareness of the position and movement of the human musculoskeletal system. However, focusing on one aspect oversimplifies the human sense of touch, which also encompasses tactile feedback through activation of mechanoreceptors in the skin [33]. It has been shown that a multi-modal haptic feedback system that includes synergistic simultaneous activation of various receptors is most optimal for approximating natural human touch and performance [1]. The da Vinci has yet to offer haptic feedback and users presently rely on visual cues such as tissue deformation and blanching for gauging tissue tension, which is not a foolproof method and unnecessary damage can still occur with misappropriation of force. Significant advancement has been made with Senhance and Versius which offers haptic feedback in the console handles however, this is at present still a single modality feedback and has yet to be shown to translate into better surgical and clinical outcomes. Nonetheless, this is an exciting feature that will require transiting da Vinci users to be recalibrated and accustomed to. Having said so, this added feature is likely be more facilitative than disruptive and may even reduce the learning curve of robotic surgery now that surgeons no longer have to rely solely on visual cues for tissue tension.

9.6 Learning Pedagogy and Training from Industry

Beyond the race for technological and design supremacy, emerging robotic platforms also need to devote equal attention to understanding the science of learning. At the end of the day, a new system will require a period of training to surmount the steepest part of the learning curve. And this is where the industry can play a bigger role. Indeed, one may argue that how well a robotic surgeon adopts a new system is only dependent on how well he is trained for it.

Training a new user for a robotic system can be undertaken in 2 stages. Firstly, a dry lab simulator training is essential in acclimatizing the user to the different concept, design and functionality of the system. Emerging robotic surgical systems can differ in so many aspects as touched on earlier in this chapter and a new user will need time to develop muscle memory and a mindset change to achieve a minimum level of proficiency before operating on actual patients. Simulation-based learning has changed the way we learn and the old adage of "see one, do one, teach one" often used for surgical trainees can no longer stand up to the rigor of medical standards today. There is strong evidence today for simulation-based training [22, 25, 40] for robotic surgeons and we can certainly draw lessons from the success of da Vinci Skills Simulator (dVSS; Intuitive Surgical Inc., Sunnyvale, California, USA) in providing structured skills training for robot novices [13, 19]. New robotic platforms should endeavor to provide a high face, content and construct validity simulator to allow new users to surmount the early part of the learning curve in a safe and controlled environment with the mastery of basic skillsets. For kidney surgery in particular, the commercially available Mimic dV-Trainer (MdVT, Mimic Technologies, Seattle, Wash., USA) offers an augmented simulation of partial nephrectomy that provides 3-dimensional videos of robotic partial nephrectomy, superimposed virtually to help learners with surgical skills and renal anatomy at each step of the operation. It boasts a high construct validity in all domains of the Global Evaluative Assessment of Robotic Skills (GEARS) and in one study that included in vivo experiment, showed a high GEARS correlation of transferability of skills from the virtual simulator compared to live tissue operation [14]. On top of that, the dV-Trainer® also offers meaningful personalized tracking of progress with the help of Mimics's MScore® (Mimic Technologies, Inc, Seattle, USA) which utilizes data from expert robotic surgeons to provide benchmarking and objective assessment (Fig. 9.3).

Once that initial proficiency has been established with skills-based simulators, new users can move on to operation-based training in the wet lab or on actual

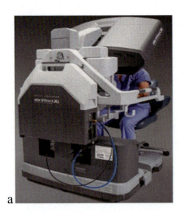 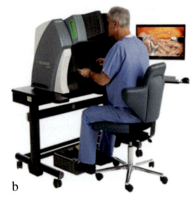

Fig. 9.3 Different virtual reality robotic simulators. **a** da Vinci skills simulator [15]. **b** dV-Trainer® [28]

patients. Many systematic reviews have been done on the learning curves for robotic surgery and all have identified substantial differences in the length of learning curves, largely arising from lack of consensus amongst studies on the metrics and outcomes as well as terminologies needed to construct the learning curve [27, 36]. Similar to the modular training established for robotic prostatectomies [24], it is imperative that more research be done on establishing and validating structured training pathways and assessment metrics for kidney surgery. Progress has been made recently in this area in validating automated performance metrics during robotic-assisted partial nephrectomy [12] for 7 segmented steps of the surgery: colon mobilization, identification and dissection of ureter, tumour exposure, hilar dissection, scoring of margins with intra-operative ultrasound, tumor excision and renorrhaphy. Such data helps establish formal metrics of assessment for training and should be implemented in all training curriculum for robotic kidney surgery.

9.7 Summary

The training of new generations of robotic surgeons is an important agenda, however let us not forget that in the past 2 decades of the 'da Vinci' era, a substantial number of robotic surgeons have come through the robotic system and have been honed to be the experts they are today. What does it mean for a surgeon of mastery level on one robotic platform when he has to transition to another robotic platform? And will his performance on a new robotic platform be commensurate with his experience on da Vinci? Would there necessarily be a shorter learning curve for him? These are important considerations as we see an explosion of new robotic platforms in the market.

Transferability of skillsets between robotic platforms is not well studied as there has only been one dominant robotic system up to now. Dissecting robotic surgical skills and evaluating which skillsets have favorable pedagogical characteristics such as high transferability and a milder learning curve between different robotic platforms could provide more insight into transitioning robotic surgeons. This may shape the design and focus of future robotic systems if they were to be well received by the community of robotic surgeons. Emerging platforms should reach out to current robotic surgeons to understand their needs and facilitate early learning with simulators.

The future of robotic surgical landscape is one that is highly variable. With different systems emerging, new robotic users face hopes of a more intuitive and user-friendly interface while existing robotic surgeons may face more challenges in transitioning between different platforms. More questions will arise not just on clinical efficacy and outcomes of new robotic systems, but on training as well as accreditation of robotic surgeons and the economic impact of this evolution. One thing may remain certain and that is with more competition, comes progress. With more emerging robotic platforms, robotic surgery looks set to be further refined and enhanced in the next decades.

References

1. Abiri A, Pensa J, Tao A, Ma J, Juo YY, Askari SJ, Bisley J, Rosen J, Dutson EP, Grundfest WS. Multi-modal haptic feedback for grip force reduction in robotic surgery. Sci Rep. 2019;9(1):5016.
2. Avatera System. https://www.avatera.eu/en/avatera-system/#c3151. Accessed 8 Aug 2021.
3. Bauer W, Wittig T. Influence of screen and copy holder positions on head posture, muscle activity and user judgement. Appl Ergon. 1998;29(3):185–92.
4. Benali-Khoudja M, Hafez M, Alexandre J-M, Kheddar A. Tactile Interfaces: a state-of-the-art survey. Inform Syst Res—ISR. 2004.
5. Bethea BT, Okamura AM, Kitagawa M, Fitton TP, Cattaneo SM, Gott VL, Baumgartner WA, Yuh DD. Application of haptic feedback to robotic surgery. J Laparoendosc Adv Surg Tech A. 2004;14(3):191–5.
6. Bholat OS, Haluck RS, Murray WB, Gorman PJ, Krummel TM. Tactile feedback is present during minimally invasive surgery. J Am Coll Surg. 1999;189(4):349–55.
7. Da Vinci systems and simulation—Press Resources. 2017. https://www.intuitive.com/en-us/about-us/press/press-resources. Accessed 8 Aug 2021.
8. Demi B, Ortmaier T, Seibold U. The touch and feel in minimally invasive surgery. In: IEEE international workshop on haptic audio visual environments and their applications, 1 October 2005, 6 pp.
9. Du Z, Wang W, Yan Z, Dong W. Variable admittance control based on fuzzy reinforcement learning for minimally invasive surgery manipulator. Sensors (Basel). 2017;17(4).
10. Enayati N, De Momi E, Ferrigno G. Haptics in robot-assisted surgery: challenges and benefits. IEEE Rev Biomed Eng. 2016;9:49–65.
11. Fries Svensson H, Svensson OK. The influence of the viewing angle on neck-load during work with video display units. J Rehabil Med. 2001;33(3):133–6.
12. Ghodoussipour S, Reddy SS, Ma R, Huang D, Nguyen J, Hung AJ. An objective assessment of performance during robotic partial nephrectomy: validation and correlation of automated performance metrics with intraoperative outcomes. J Urol. 2021;205(5):1294–302.
13. Hertz AM, George EI, Vaccaro CM, Brand TC. Head-to-head comparison of three virtual-reality robotic surgery simulators. JSLS. 2018;22(1).

14. Hung AJ, Shah SH, Dalag L, Shin D, Gill IS. Development and validation of a novel robotic procedure specific simulation platform: partial nephrectomy. J Urol. 2015;194(2):520–6.
15. Intuitive Surgical, I. 'da Vinci Xi skills simulator manual'. https://manuals.intuitivesurgical.com/c/document_library/get_file?uuid=75bf45ec-9595-0b19-4ff3-c2cf0a90be89&groupId=73750789. Accessed 8 Aug 2021.
16. Jaschinski W, Heuer H, Kylian H. Preferred position of visual displays relative to the eyes: a field study of visual strain and individual differences. Ergonomics. 1998;41(7):1034–49.
17. Jaschinski-Kruza W. Eyestrain in VDU users: viewing distance and the resting position of ocular muscles. Hum Fact. 1991;33(1):69–83.
18. Jeong S, Tadano K. Manipulation of a master manipulator with a combined-grip-handle of pinch and power grips. Int J Med Robot. 2020;16(2): e2065.
19. Kelly DC, Margules AC, Kundavaram CR, Narins H, Gomella LG, Trabulsi EJ, Lallas CD. Face, content, and construct validation of the da Vinci skills simulator. Urology. 2012;79(5):1068–72.
20. Kirkpatrick K. Surgical robots deliver care more precisely. Commun ACM. 2014;(8):14–6.
21. Koukourikis P, Rha KH. Robotic surgical systems in urology: what is currently available? Investig Clin Urol. 2021;62(1):14–22.
22. Kumar A, Smith R, Patel VR. Current status of robotic simulators in acquisition of robotic surgical skills. Curr Opin Urol. 2015;25(2):168–74.
23. Lee MR, Lee GI. Does a robotic surgery approach offer optimal ergonomics to gynecologic surgeons?: a comprehensive ergonomics survey study in gynecologic robotic surgery. J Gynecol Oncol. 2017;28(5):e70.
24. Lovegrove C, Novara G, Mottrie A, Guru KA, Brown M, Challacombe B, Popert R, Raza J, Van der Poel H, Peabody J, Dasgupta P, Ahmed K. Structured and modular training pathway for robot-assisted radical prostatectomy (RARP): validation of the RARP assessment score and learning curve assessment. Eur Urol. 2016;69(3):526–35.
25. MacCraith E, Forde JC, Davis NF. Robotic simulation training for urological trainees: a comprehensive review on cost, merits and challenges. J Robot Surg. 2019;13(3):371–7.
26. Martell J, Elmer T, Gopalsami N, Park YS. Visual measurement of suture strain for robotic surgery. Comput Math Methods Med. 2011;2011:879086.
27. Mazzon G, Sridhar A, Busuttil G, Thompson J, Nathan S, Briggs T, Kelly J, Shaw G. Learning curves for robotic surgery: a review of the recent literature. Curr Urol Rep. 2017;18(11):89.
28. Mimic Technologies, I. Mimic marketing brochure. Accessed 8 Aug 2021.
29. Mitchell TN, Robertson J, Nagy AG, Lomax A. Three-dimensional endoscopic imaging for minimal access surgery. J R Coll Surg Edinb. 1993;38(5):285–92.
30. Nayyar R, Gupta NP. Critical appraisal of technical problems with robotic urological surgery. BJU Int. 2010;105(12):1710–3.
31. Niemeyer G, Nowlin W, Guthart G. Alignment of master and slave in a minimally invasive surgical apparatus. 2002.
32. Santos-Carreras L, Hagen M, Gassert R, Bleuler H. Survey on surgical instrument handle design: ergonomics and acceptance. Surg Innov. 2012;19(1):50–9.
33. Schostek S, Schurr MO, Buess GF. Review on aspects of artificial tactile feedback in laparoscopic surgery. Med Eng Phys. 2009;31(8):887–98.
34. Schwab K, Smith R, Brown V, Whyte M, Jourdan I. Evolution of stereoscopic imaging in surgery and recent advances. World J Gastrointest Endosc. 2017;9(8):368–77.
35. Seghers J, Jochem A, Spaepen A. Posture, muscle activity and muscle fatigue in prolonged VDT work at different screen height settings. Ergonomics. 2003;46(7):714–30.
36. Soomro NA, Hashimoto DA, Porteous AJ, Ridley CJA, Marsh WJ, Ditto R, Roy S. Systematic review of learning curves in robot-assisted surgery. BJS Open. 2020;4(1):27–44.
37. The Senhance Surgical System. https://www.senhance.com/us/digital-laparoscopy. Accessed 8 Aug 2021.
38. Versius For Surgeons—CMR Surgical. https://cmrsurgical.com/versius/surgeon. Accessed 8 Aug 2021.

39. Wagner CR, Stylopoulos N, Jackson PG, Howe RD. The benefit of force feedback in surgery: examination of blunt dissection. Presence. 2007;16(3):252–62.
40. Walliczek-Dworschak U, Mandapathil M, Förtsch A, Teymoortash A, Dworschak P, Werner JA, Güldner C. Structured training on the da Vinci skills simulator leads to improvement in technical performance of robotic novices. Clin Otolaryngol. 2017;42(1):71–80.

New Robots and How this has Changed Operative Technique in Renal Cancer Surgery

Christopher Soliman, Marc A. Furrer, and Nathan Lawrentschuk

10.1 Introduction

Since the 1990s, laparoscopic surgery has undergone unprecedented change and expansion. The benefit and attraction of minimally invasive surgery to both patients and surgeons alike forced this growth and a necessity to perform more and more complex operations laparoscopically [1, 2]. Predictably, a threshold was reached, and surgical advancement plateaued. In response, robotic surgery was introduced, and since then its evolution has transformed minimally invasive surgery (MIS) worldwide [3]. This bourgeoning field of robotics has redefined the gold standard of surgical care for many staple uro-oncological procedures. The introduction of the da Vinci Surgical System in 2000 changed the face of modern MIS [4].

Distinct advantages of the robotic approach, compared to laparoscopic surgery, include a surgeon-controlled camera, three-dimensional high-definition magnified surgical vision, and EndoWrist enhanced manoeuvrability with seven degrees of freedom and 90° articulation [5]. Moreover, providing natural movements consequently enhances dexterity and dissection, precise coordination of hands and eyes, filtration of physiological tremor, and motion scaling [6] which allows for precise tissue dissection and suturing [7, 8]. These advantages enable surgeons to perform more complex MIS procedures and extend the feasibility, and therefore benefits, of MIS to more specialists by reducing the learning curve [9, 10]. Consequently, robotic surgery continues to be rapidly adopted in renal and prostate surgery worldwide [11].

C. Soliman (✉) · M. A. Furrer · N. Lawrentschuk
Department of Urology, The University of Melbourne, The Royal Melbourne Hospital, Parkville, VIC, Australia
e-mail: chrissol1312@gmail.com

10.2 Background

10.2.1 The Origin of Robotic Surgery and Intuitive Surgical

Although Intuitive Surgical, Inc. was founded in 1995, the current Da Vinci platform is an amalgamation of research and innovation that originated prior in the late 1980s at the non-profit Stanford Research Institute (SRI) International. Through combined efforts, Phil Green and Richard Satava pioneered the prototype robotic surgical system. During its evolution, the "telepresence surgery system" caught the attention of the Defence Advanced Research Projects Agency (DARPA), whose focus under the Advanced Biomedical Technologies (ABMT) program was directed toward improving emergency surgical care to combat casualties [12, 13]. The incorporation of telepresence into medical forward advanced surgical treatment (MEDFAST), in conjunction with key technologies from IBM and MIT, would revolutionise the idea of specialised remote operating and was a landmark inspiration for John Freund, Frederick Moll, and Rob Younge to collectively form Intuitive Surgical, Inc. [12–14].

After several prototypes, the landmark da Vinci Surgical System was created in 1999, and by 2000 it was approved by the U.S. Food and Drug Administration (FDA) for use in general laparoscopic surgery. In 2001, the FDA approved use of the system for prostate surgery; and since then has revolutionised Uro-oncological surgical procedures and completely changed operative techniques in renal cancer surgery [15].

Shortly before its public release, Intuitive Surgical was sued for patent infringement by Computer Motion, Inc. Computer Motion had already released the ZEUS Robotic Surgical System (ZRSS), which was approved in Europe although not yet so by the FDA. After generating uncertainty for several years and stifling each company's growth, Intuitive Surgical and Computer Motion agreed to merge in 2003, and the ZEUS system was subsequently phased out in favour of the da Vinci system [12, 13] (see Fig. 10.1).

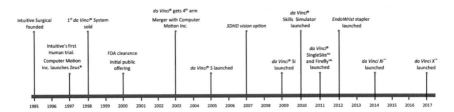

Fig. 10.1 Timeline of selected company milestones [14]

10.3 The Da Vinci Robotic Surgical System

Since the initial public release of the da Vinci Surgical System in 2000, four further generations of da Vinci systems have been introduced to the market: the da Vinci S platform, da Vinci Si platform, da Vinci Xi platform, and da Vinci X platform (see Fig. 10.2). Each generation platform has distinct technological upgrades to optimise surgical techniques and performance. In addition, with each design, the Intuitive market has expanded with rapid succession of innovation from instruments and accessories to systems and services, heralding with it global dissemination, acceptance, and integration of robotic-assisted surgery. At present, 5989 da Vinci systems are in use across 67 different countries, performing over 8.5 million procedures through 2020 [16].

At its foundation, compared to prototypes and the ZEUS platform, the original 'Classic' da Vinci Surgical System displayed significant enhancements. The robotic system was composed of 3 components—a surgeon console, a patient cart, and a vision cart. All robotic arms originated from a single patient cart, alleviating the need to mount individual arms to the operating table, while providing a solution for optimal table position. The surgeons console provided an innovative three-dimensional visual display with the trademark binocular visualisation which allowed greater optical accommodation and focus, resulting in improved concentration, and reducing surgical fatigue. Additionally, complimentary EndoWrist instrumentation with seven degrees of freedom and two degrees of axial rotation combined with intuitive motion and superior ergonomics culminated in advanced surgical precision. The Classic platform patient cart was originally composed of one endoscope port and two instruments. However, before long, in 2003 a fourth arm was added to overcome exposure limitations. The fourth arm allowed the surgeon greater control of retraction, improved exposure of the surgical field, and reduced dependence on surgical assistance [17].

By 2006, Intuitive Surgical introduced their first generational upgrade in the form on the da Vinci S platform. The new platform offered modest improvements in the form of high-definition (HD) camera vision with an interactive touch display and a more streamlined set-up. In 2009, not satisfied with the previous model, the da Vinci Si platform was released, offering a dual console to optimise collaborative operating and training. Additionally, the incorporation of TilePro software modernised the imaging system, allowing real-time fluorescence imaging with Firefly technology. The Si would become one of the most worldwide distributed platforms for Intuitive since creation. Although remarkable in its time, the Si system had distinct structural limitations. A single, large, vertical column exoskeleton meant that reachable workspace was highly dependent on the orientation of the cart and, combined with bulky robotic arms, frequent external clashing was highly troublesome. Furthermore, multi-quadrant surgery required complete repositioning of the patient cart and redocking of the robotic arms intraoperatively, increasing overall surgical and anaesthetic time.

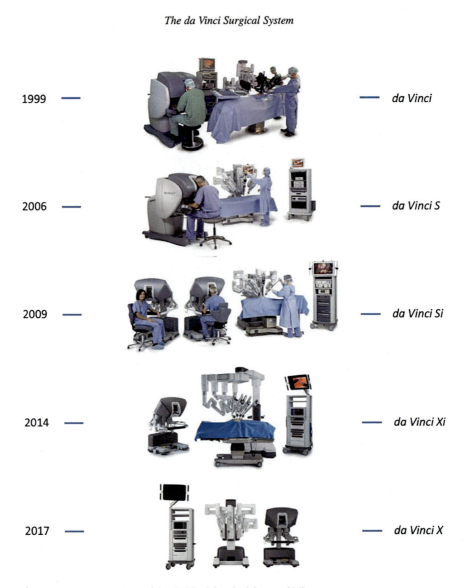

Fig. 10.2 Five generations of the da Vinci Surgical System [14]

It wouldn't be until 5 years later that Intuitive Surgical developed the da Vinci Xi system, which currently still resides today as the flagship platform and most capable system yet. In 2014, the Xi model reinvented the concept of the patient cart design with tremendous mobility, flexibility, and versatility. It introduced new, advanced instrumentation, vision, cart design, table motion and setup automation which almost completely resolved patient cart and arm limitations in previous prototypes. The Xi's boom-mounted architectural design allows complete rotational all-quadrant access with docking from any angle. This remodelled gantry positions instrument arms directly over operating table, making positioning of the cart base largely independent from workspace orientation, providing overall greater internal range of motion, improving patient access, and minimising external collisions. Additionally, the redesigned flex joints permit robotic arms to be slimmer and compact, unlike earlier da Vinci system generations which required widely spaced external arms to maximise working space. Furthermore, docking of the Xi is streamlined and semi-automated, simple targeting of the surgical field with the endoscope disposes the robotic arms effortlessly into optimal position with appropriate patient clearance. In conjunction with significant upgrades to the patient cart, the surgeon console was modernised with ergonomic refinement, precision control, and improved visualisation technology. Endoscope size was reduced to an 8 mm from previous models, making it less bulky, while providing higher resolution three-dimensional high-definition view, brighter and more immersive images, and longer scope length. Additionally, the Xi 30° camera could be inverted from the surgeon console without bedside assistance. The four now identical robotic arms allowed for versatility and positioning of any instrument in any port at any given time. Moreover, integrated FireFly fluorescence imaging technology, with the administration of indocyanine green, allowed for real-time intraoperative decision-making (e.g., tissue perfusion). Finally, additional instruments were made available (e.g., robotic suction, irrigation, and clip application) and current energy device performance were amplified (e.g., Vessel Sealer Extend) [18, 19].

Most recently, in 2017, Intuitive Surgical released the da Vinci X Surgical System in an expansion bid to provide a financial economical solution to global customers in which cost was a limiting factor. This lower-fee platform offered several key innovative developments taken from the da Vinci Xi system. Although the patient cart is structurally more similar to the Si platform, and despite the lack of a gantry, it boasts a 1.5× greater workspace field than the Si—as compared to 3× greater workspace of the Xi (see Fig. 10.3). This enables the X to provide a more optimised, quadrant-focused surgery (e.g., prostatectomy, partial nephrectomy) and allows the use of finer surgical instruments. Furthermore, the X uses the same vision cart, surgeon console, many of the same advanced instruments and accessories as the Xi, thus providing customers with an upgrade pathway should they desire [14].

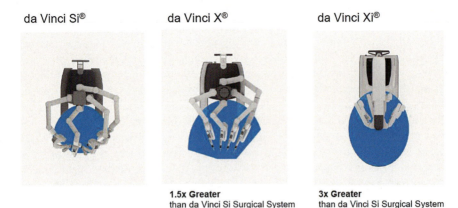

Fig. 10.3 Worspace comparison between the three latest da Vinci Surgical System generations. *Credit* Intuitive Surgical, Inc.

10.4 New Robots in Renal Cancer Surgery

Robot-assisted procedures have become a staple in renal surgery, gaining robust clinical status reflected by the current literature. However, the focus and favour of robotic renal surgery lies in technically demanding procedures (i.e., complex and partial nephrectomy, nephroureterectomy, with or without vena cava thrombus, complex transplant surgery, and difficult anatomy as in patients with obesity or adhesions) rather than simple uncomplicated nephrectomies. As described above, the latest generations of leading surgical robots (i.e., da Vinci Xi Surgical System) offer countless mechanical advantages to aid these technical demands, such as (1) three-dimensional high-definition stereoscopic vision, (2) fine-motor tissue manipulation with higher quality instrumentation, (3) ability to perform multi-quadrant surgical procedures (i.e., nephroureterectomy) without the need to re-dock the patient console and thus reduce operative time, (4) easily accessible and integrated FireFly fluorescence imaging technology to assess perfusion and assist with tumour resection [19]. These advancements have been clearly shown to accelerate the learning curve for non-laparoscopic surgeons [20].

Laparoscopic approaches are limited by the challenges of tumour dissection and intracorporal suturing, and in non-robotic institutions open surgery, which carries a longer hospital stay and increased estimated blood loss, may be the only alternative [21]. At present, cost, longer set-up time, and longer overall operative time remain the greatest criticisms for robotic surgery. The role of routine robotic-assisted radical nephrectomy (RARN) is still debatable, primarily due these disparagements of cost and time, versus laparoscopic nephrectomy (LN) [22]. In contrast, a review of 150 nephrectomies revealed that costs of RARN are comparable to LN when a robot is already present [23]. Furthermore, a retrospective single centre review demonstrated that costs of disposable instruments used in LN were comparable to the disposables used in RARN, concluding that robotic surgery for nephrectomy

10 New Robots and How this has Changed Operative …

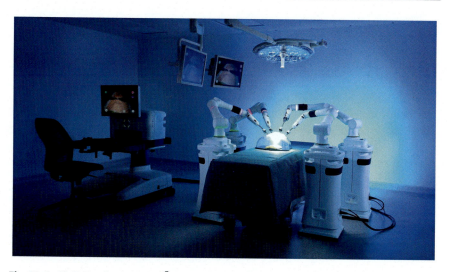

Fig. 10.4 CMR Surgical's Versius® surgical Robotic System. *Credit* CMR surgical

does not always correlate with greater costs [24]. Whether or not these studies are currently widely applicable is unclear; however, if issues of cost are somewhat mitigated in future, then robotic surgery for renal cancer will undeniably become the baseline gold standard approach.

In addition, the Versius Surgical Robotic System (CMR Surgical, Cambridge, UK) is a new tele-operated robotic surgical system designed to assist surgeons in performing MIS and overcome some of the challenges associated with available surgical robots mentioned above (see Fig. 10.4). The Versius System mimics the articulation of the human arm, and with V-wrist technology, the wristed instrument tip provides seven degrees of freedom inside the patient, allowing for even greater surgical access. Instruments and visualisation arms are attached to their own discrete wheeled cart to form a compact and mobile bedside unit. The surgeon interacts with the system via the "game controller" handgrip and visual feedback from the surgeon console. The consoles head-up display relays the three-dimensional video from the endoscopic camera together with a display overlay. Its open design allows surgeons to sit or stand for optimal ergonomics, ensures patient accessibility at all times, and permits easier communication between the surgeon and the team, facilitating training and teaching. The operating room team accesses controls and feedback on the visualisation bedside unit and up to three instrument bedside units, while viewing a two-dimensional version of the endoscope feed and display overlay on an auxiliary display. The systems modular design increases its potential for flexible use, as the bedside units are small enough to be used in a standard operating room and can easily be moved within a single operating room or between operating rooms. The safety and effectiveness of the system in renal cancer surgery have been demonstrated in a feasibility study of 24 procedures successfully completed in cadavers [25].

The main clinical advantages of the robot, compared to a laparoscopic approach, remain the shorter learning curve and more efficient renorrhaphy. Rapid suturing shortens ischemia time associated with renal artery clamping and crucially maximises preservation of renal parenchyma. Hence, the robotic approach sanctions operations of larger and more complex renal masses, especially in the presence of a solitary kidney [26–28].

Notably, refinement and development of the da Vinci systems have facilitated optimisation of robotic arm positioning, allowing for a more flexible port placement in renal surgery. This positioning permits multi-quadrant surgery with a wider range of motion of the robotic instruments, while preventing clashing and making several surgical steps such as bowel mobilisation easier. These advantages become even more evident in complex renal cancer surgery (e.g., when performing retroperitoneal lymph node dissection for upper tract urothelial cancer, or more complex surgeries such as cava thrombectomy or renal transplants).

With regards to port placement for renal surgery, the da Vinci X and Xi systems allow for a straight line ('in-line') placement of the ports rather than a L-shaped line. In comparison, the S and Si systems narrow range of port placement configurations may make access to the bedside difficult or uncomfortable. Furthermore, the newer da Vinci generation allows for camera targeting, camera hopping, better spatial awareness, and therefore more flexibility to expose the operative field.

Below is a review of the current literature evidence for comparing clinical outcomes of robot-assisted RN and PN versus open and laparoscopic techniques.

10.5 Current Evidence

10.5.1 Radical Nephrectomy (RN)—Robotic Versus Laparoscopic Approach

Data from a large retrospective cohort study on robot-assisted RN (RARN) versus laparoscopic RN (LRN) revealed that RARN was not associated with increased risk of any or major complications; but, had longer operative times and higher hospital costs as compared to LRN [29]. While a systematic review on RARN versus LRN showed no substantial differences in local recurrence rates, or all-cause cancer-specific mortality [30]. The improved dexterity of the robotic nephroureterectomy has clear benefit compared to the laparoscopic approach by improving distal ureteric dissection, excision of bladder cuff and bladder closure. However, the advantages of the robotic approach for nephrectomy, compared to the laparoscopic procedure, are not evident from a pure surgical perspective. This is because the extirpative procedure is technically less challenging. Despite the lack of proven benefit for robotic compared to laparoscopic radical nephrectomy, use of the robot has increased over the last decade. This trend primarily results from the surgeon endeavour to gain experience in hilar dissection during radical nephrectomy to complement the learning curve for partial nephrectomies. Additionally, these skills are essential before adopting more complex renal surgery such as donor nephrectomies or radical nephrectomy with inferior vena cava thrombectomy.

10.5.2 Partial Nephrectomy (PN)—Robotic Versus Open Approach

Data from a prospective, single-surgeon study which compared peri-operative outcomes of robot-assisted PN versus open PN reported lower estimated blood loss and shorter hospital stay in the RAPN group. Complications, operative time, warm ischaemia time, variation in creatinine levels and positive margins were similar in both groups [31]. While a multicentre French prospective database compared outcomes of 1800 patients who underwent RAPN and OPN, and found that the RAPN cohort had lower morbidity with less transfusions, less major complications, less overall complications, and a much shorter hospital stay [32].

10.5.3 Partial Nephrectomy (PN)—Robotic Versus Laparoscopic Approach

Data from a retrospective propensity-score-matched study, comparing RAPN, LPN and OPN demonstrated similar rates of local recurrence, distant metastasis, and cancer-related death rates after 5-year median follow-up [33]. While a meta-analysis compared peri-operative outcomes of RAPN versus LPN, and found that the RARP arm had significantly lower rate of conversion to open surgery and to radical surgery, shorter warm ischaemia time, smaller change in eGFR postoperatively, and shorter length of hospital stay. No significant differences were observed between the two groups regarding complications, change of serum creatinine post-operatively, operative time, estimated blood loss and positive surgical margins [34].

10.5.4 Surgical Volume, Positive Margins and RAPN

Data from a retrospective US study of 18,724 patients which the evaluated prognostic impact of hospital volume on outcomes post-RAPN revealed that undergoing higher-volume hospitals may have better peri-operative outcomes (conversion to open and length of hospital stay) and lower positive surgical margin rates [35]. While a French study of 1222 RAPN patients showed that hospital volume was the main predictive factor of the trifecta achievement (warm ischaemia time < 25 min, no complications, and a negative surgical margins) [36].

10.6 Future Challenges

Of course, future challenges remain. Improved identification of key anatomic structures remains paramount for a successful outcome. This can be facilitated by technological advancements offered by robotics such as Indocyanine green (ICG) [administered intravenously or through an extracorporeal access point (i.e., percutaneous nephrostomy or indwelling catheter)] to identify vascular perfusion [37].

The next very challenging step in robotic surgery, which is facilitated by refinement of da Vinci systems, will be the standardised implementation of radical nephrectomy with inferior vena cava thrombectomy. In highly specialised centres this operation has been performed up to a level III thrombus [38]. Given the large incision required for the open approach the robotic management is assumed to significantly reduce morbidity, length of hospital stay and hence, economic burden.

Further procedures which are assumed to be adopted robotically include renal transplant surgeries. The evolution of this technique is in progress. Importantly, not only kidney transplantation but also donor nephrectomy, which require optimal operative conditions, can be performed safely. Evidence in the literature show that robotic kidney transplantation is feasible, reducing complications while maintaining the functional results achieved by the open approach [39].

It is expected that both urologic surgeons and robotic systems will steadily continue to advance as experience evolves. Consequently, technically challenging robotic procedures will likely be reserved for tertiary referral centres, whereas lower-volume and less experienced centres will perform common and less complex procedures.

10.7 Conclusion

The current robotic era has already shown huge impact in the field of Uro-oncology and renal cancer surgery. It's worldwide dissemination and integration has made it clear that robotic surgery will continue to shape and play a significant role in the natural evolution of future minimally invasive surgery. Latest generation da Vinci Surgical Systems, and potentially other innovations such as the Versius Surgical System, have marched forth as the pinnacle of surgical technology, having overcome the intrinsic limitations of laparoscopy years ago, they now provide enticement for experienced surgeons to push the barrier for more and more complex upper tract procedures. Cost remains the rate-limiting factor for these devices, and likely will continue for several years to come; however, similar to any previous innovation or technological advancement, initially thought to be unaffordable, it is possible that further analysis reports will prove cost-effective.

References

1. Rukstalis DB, Chodak GW. Laparoscopic retroperitoneal lymph node dissection in a patient with stage 1 testicular carcinoma. J Urol. 1992;148:1907–9; discussion 1909–1910.
2. Berkman DS, Taneja SS. Laparoscopic partial nephrectomy: technique and outcomes. Curr Urol Rep. 2010;11:1–7.
3. Yates DR, Vaessen C, Roupret M: From Leonardo to da Vinci: the history of robot-assisted surgery in urology. BJU Int. 2011;108:1708–13; discussion 1714.
4. McGuinness LA, Prasad Rai B. Robotics in urology. Ann R Coll Surg Engl. 2018;100:38–44.
5. Lanfranco AR, Castellanos AE, Desai JP, Meyers WC. Robotic surgery: a current perspective. Ann Surg. 2004;239:14–21.
6. Hanna T, Imber C. Robotics in HPB surgery. Ann R Coll Surg Engl. 2018;100:31–7.
7. Cwach K, Kavoussi L. Past, present, and future of laparoscopic renal surgery. Investig Clin Urol. 2016;57:S110–3.
8. Babbar P, Hemal AK. Robot-assisted urologic surgery in 2010—advancements and future outlook. Urol Ann. 2011;3:1–7.
9. Pal RP, Koupparis AJ. Expanding the indications of robotic surgery in urology: a systematic review of the literature. Arab J Urol. 2018;16:270–84.
10. Finkelstein J, Eckersberger E, Sadri H, Taneja SS, Lepor H, Djavan B. Open versus laparoscopic versus robot-assisted laparoscopic prostatectomy: the European and US experience. Rev Urol. 2010;12:35–43.
11. Ishii H, Rai BP, Stolzenburg JU, Bose P, Chlosta PL, Somani BK, Nabi G, Qazi HA, Rajbabu K, Kynaston H, et al. Robotic or open radical cystectomy, which is safer? A systematic review and meta-analysis of comparative studies. J Endourol. 2014;28:1215–23.
12. George E, Brand T, LaPorta A, Marescaux J, Satava R. Origins of robotic surgery: from Skepticism to standard of care. JSLS: J Soc Laparoendosc Surg. 2018;22:e2018.00039.
13. Satava RM. Robotic surgery: from past to future–a personal journey. Surg Clin North Am. 2003;83(1491–1500):xii.
14. Azizian M, Liu M, Khalaji I, Sorger J, Oh D, Daimios S. 3—The da Vinci Surgical System. In: Abedin-Nasab, editor. Handbook of robotic and image-guided surgery. MH: Elsevier;2020. p. 39–55. https://doi.org/10.1016/B978-0-12-814245-5.00003-7.
15. Satava RM. Surgical robotics: the early chronicles: a personal historical perspective. Surg Laparosc Endosc Percutan Tech. 2002;12:6–16.
16. Intuitive History on World Wide Web. https://www.intuitive.com/en-us/about-us/company/history.
17. Takács Á, Nagy D, Rudas I, Haidegger T. Origins of surgical robotics: from space to the operating room. 2016;13:13–30.
18. Damle A, Damle RN, Flahive JM, Schlussel AT, Davids JS, Sturrock PR, Maykel JA, Alavi K. Diffusion of technology: trends in robotic-assisted colorectal surgery. Am J Surg. 2017;214:820–4.
19. Wirth GJ, Hauser J, Caviezel A, Schwartz J, Fleury N, Tran SN, Iselin CE. Roboterassistierte Operationen in der Urologie. Urologe. 2008;47:960–3.
20. Hanzly M, Frederick A, Creighton T, Atwood K, Mehedint D, Kauffman EC, Kim HL, Schwaab T. Learning curves for robot-assisted and laparoscopic partial nephrectomy. J Endourol. 2015;29:297–303.
21. Gill IS, Kavoussi LR, Lane BR, Blute ML, Babineau D, Colombo JR Jr, Frank I, Permpongkosol S, Weight CJ, Kaouk JH, et al. Comparison of 1,800 laparoscopic and open partial nephrectomies for single renal tumors. J Urol. 2007;178:41–6.
22. Yang DY, Monn MF, Bahler CD, Sundaram CP. Does robotic assistance confer an economic benefit during laparoscopic radical nephrectomy? J Urol. 2014;192:671–6.
23. Roos FC, Thomas C, Neisius A, Nestler S, Thüroff JW, Hampel C. Robot-assisted laparoscopic partial nephrectomy: functional and oncological outcomes. Urologe A. 2015;54:213–8.

24. Petros FG, Angell JE, Abaza R. Outcomes of robotic nephrectomy including highest-complexity cases: largest series to date and literature review. Urology. 2015;85:1352–8.
25. Thomas BC, Slack M, Hussain M, Barber N, Pradhan A, Dinneen E, Stewart GD. Preclinical evaluation of the versius surgical system, a new robot-assisted surgical device for use in minimal access renal and prostate surgery. Eur Urol Focus. 2021;7:444–52.
26. Laviana AA, Hu JC. Current controversies and challenges in robotic-assisted, laparoscopic, and open partial nephrectomies. World J Urol. 2014;32:591–6.
27. Gill IS, Kamoi K, Aron M, Desai MM. 800 Laparoscopic partial nephrectomies: a single surgeon series. J Urol. 2010;183:34–41.
28. Leow JJ, Heah NH, Chang SL, Chong YL, Png KS. Outcomes of robotic versus laparoscopic partial nephrectomy: an updated meta-analysis of 4,919 patients. J Urol. 2016;196:1371–7.
29. Jeong IG, Khandwala YS, Kim JH, Han DH, Li S, Wang Y, Chang SL, Chung BI. Association of robotic-assisted vs laparoscopic radical nephrectomy with perioperative outcomes and health care costs, 2003 to 2015. JAMA. 2017;318:1561–8.
30. Asimakopoulos AD, Miano R, Annino F, Micali S, Spera E, Iorio B, Vespasiani G, Gaston R. Robotic radical nephrectomy for renal cell carcinoma: a systematic review. BMC Urol. 2014;14:75.
31. Masson-Lecomte A, Yates DR, Hupertan V, Haertig A, Chartier-Kastler E, Bitker MO, Vaessen C, Rouprêt M. A prospective comparison of the pathologic and surgical outcomes obtained after elective treatment of renal cell carcinoma by open or robot-assisted partial nephrectomy. Urol Oncol. 2013;31:924–9.
32. Peyronnet B, Seisen T, Oger E, Vaessen C, Grassano Y, Benoit T, Carrouget J, Pradère B, Khene Z, Giwerc A, et al. Comparison of 1800 robotic and open partial nephrectomies for renal tumors. Ann Surg Oncol. 2016;23:4277–83.
33. Chang KD, Abdel Raheem A, Kim KH, Oh CK, Park SY, Kim YS, Ham WS, Han WK, Choi YD, Chung BH, et al. Functional and oncological outcomes of open, laparoscopic and robot-assisted partial nephrectomy: a multicentre comparative matched-pair analyses with a median of 5 years' follow-up. BJU Int. 2018;122:618–26.
34. Choi JE, You JH, Kim DK, Rha KH, Lee SH. Comparison of perioperative outcomes between robotic and laparoscopic partial nephrectomy: a systematic review and meta-analysis. Eur Urol. 2015;67:891–901.
35. Xia L, Pulido JE, Chelluri RR, Strother MC, Taylor BL, Raman JD, Guzzo TJ. Hospital volume and outcomes of robot-assisted partial nephrectomy. BJU Int. 2018;121:900–7.
36. Peyronnet B, Tondut L, Bernhard JC, Vaessen C, Doumerc N, Sebe P, Pradere B, Guillonneau B, Khene ZE, Nouhaud FX, et al. Impact of hospital volume and surgeon volume on robot-assisted partial nephrectomy outcomes: a multicentre study. BJU Int. 2018;121:916–22.
37. Diana P, Buffi NM, Lughezzani G, Dell'Oglio P, Mazzone E, Porter J, Mottrie A. The role of intraoperative indocyanine green in robot-assisted partial nephrectomy: results from a large. Multi-inst Ser Eur Urol. 2020;78:743–9.
38. Gill IS, Metcalfe C, Abreu A, Duddalwar V, Chopra S, Cunningham M, Thangathurai D, Ukimura O, Satkunasivam R, Hung A, et al. Robotic level III inferior Vena Cava Tumor Thrombectomy: initial series. J Urol. 2015;194:929–38.
39. Territo A, Mottrie A, Abaza R, Rogers C, Menon M, Bhandari M, Ahlawat R, Breda A. Robotic kidney transplantation: current status and future perspectives. Minerva Urol Nefrol. 2017;69:5–13.

Use of Indocyanine Green (ICG) During Robotic Surgery for Renal Cancer

Geert De Naeyer, Carlo Andrea Bravi, and Alexandre Mottrie

11.1 Introduction

Robotic technology enables the performance of complex urologic surgeries with greater precision, miniaturization of instruments, and smaller incisions than traditional laparoscopic or open approaches. An evolution is image-guided surgery: the principle that optical enhancements can improve visualization of internal anatomical structures or pathological features and can facilitate surgery. Real-time intraoperative identification of malignant versus benign tissue can help surgical outcomes by simultaneously decreasing positive surgical margin and local recurrence rate while preventing over-aggressive resection of vital structures. A particular enhancement in image-guided surgery that has been utilized significantly for both oncologic and non-oncologic surgeries is the Fire-Fly technology using indocyanine green (ICG) for near-infrared fluorescence imaging (NIRF). In contrast to white light, NIRF, with the addition of fluorophores, permits deeper photon penetration, superb optical contrast, less scatter, and a high signal-to-background ratio [7], van den [21]. Optical enhancement using ICG-NIRF has been shown to facilitate surgical performance in both the oncologic and non-oncologic settings. ICG received initial FDA approval in 1959 (NDA 011525). Based on the most

---

G. De Naeyer (✉) · C. A. Bravi · A. Mottrie
Department of Urology, Onze Lieve Vrouw Hospital, Aalst, Belgium
e-mail: geert.de.naeyer@olvz-aalst.be

A. Mottrie
e-mail: alex.mottrie@olvz-aalst.be

ORSI, Academy, Melle, Belgium

C. A. Bravi
Unit of Urology, Division of Experimental Oncology, Urological Research Institute (URI), IRCCS San Raffaele Scientific Institute, Vita-Salute San Raffaele University, Milan, Italy

recent labeling package insert submitted in 2015, the current FDA-approved indications for ICG include determination of cardiac output, hepatic function, and liver blood flow, as well as, ophthalmic angiography.

ICG has been used off-label for urologic surgery since 2006 [19, 20]. Initially described for open partial nephrectomy in the urologic literature, intravenous injection of ICG was utilized to clearly demarcate the vasculature and fluorescence patterns of the tumor in 15 patients [19, 20]. The technology was later developed in a laparoscopic and robotic cohort utilizing the Endoscopic SPY Imaging System [19, 20]. The da Vinci® surgical platform (Intuitive Surgical, Sunnyvale, CA) equipped with Firefly technology (Novadaq Technologies, Mississauga, ON) allows surgeon-controlled utilization of NIRF. The robotic application was first studied in patients with suspected renal cell carcinoma [10]. Subsequently, other urologic organs have been extensively studied including prostate, bladder, and adrenal glands. The urologic oncologic and non-oncologic applications of ICG-NIRF are vast [2, 3, 14]. For oncologic surgery, molecular-guided surgery can facilitate upper, combined upper and lower, and lower tract pathologies as well as lymph node dissection within the retroperitoneum and pelvis. For non-oncologic surgery, specifically reconstructive surgery, ICG-NIRF allows for deeper tissue penetration and real-time perfusion status that can aid in ureteral stricture repair, anastomotic viability, and identification of critical vasculature. Despite its vast applications in urology, dedicated recommendations for the use of ICG are not available in urological guidelines.

11.2 Pharmacodynamics

ICG, a tricarbocyanine, is a water-soluble molecule with a peak spectral absorption at 806 nm and with peak emission fluorescence at 830 nm. ICG is only visualized with near-infrared fluorescence (found on the da Vinci Surgical Systems equipped with Firefly® technology). After intravenous administration, ICG becomes rapidly bound to albumin (95%) and can be near-instantaneously visualized within the vasculature and target organs through a NIR fluorescence camera system. The novel Firefly® system incorporates a NIR fluorescence camera system, namely the SPY Imaging System (Novadaq Inc., Mississaugua, ON, Canada), directly into the da Vinci Si® and Xi® and allows the surgeon to switch between visible light and fluorescence-enhanced views in real time [11].

ICG should be handled in with generalized sterile techniques as with an intravenously administered agent. Common drug interactions that can reduce the peak absorption of ICG include sodium bisulfate found in many heparin products (NDA 011525 Food and Drug Administration Suppl-27 Labeling-Packaging Insert 2021). ICG is classified as a pregnancy category C compound and thus further research in this area is warranted prior to administering ICG in pregnant females (NDA 011525 Food and Drug Administration Suppl-27 Labeling-Packaging Insert 2021). According to the FDA, the usual dose for ICG varies with age with adults receiving a maximum total dose of 5.0 mg and children and infants receiving a maximum

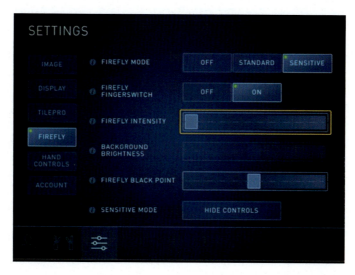

Fig. 11.1 On the da Vinci Xi the Fire-Fly modus can be adjusted selecting "sensitive" modus

total dose of 2.5 mg and 1.25 mg, respectively. The total dose should anyway be <2 mg/kg, and specific dosages are recommended according to the target organ [15]. ICG is removed from circulation exclusively by the liver to bile juice, and, depending on liver performance, is eliminated from the body with a half-life of about 3–4 min.

11.3 Firefly Technology

The technique of fluorescence imaging, the so-called Firefly System®, is integrated into the robotic console, and allows the surgeon to switch to fluorescence mode on using the fingerswitch on the surgical handles after ICG injection. As a result, the surgical field is illuminated with a special infrared light source that is able to see the glowing areas infused with the dye. On the da Vinci® Xi system he Fire-Fly modus can be adjusted selecting "sensitive" modus (Fig. 11.1). This can be done by the surgeon at the console or by anybody at the vision screen cart.

11.4 Side Effects

ICG should not be used in patients with concomitant allergy to iodides and it is considered contraindicated for these patients. Anaphylactic deaths have occurred after administration of ICG during cardiac procedures [4], however, no studies have found any impact of ICG on carcinogenesis, mutagenesis, and impairment of fertility. ICG can be used in patients with chronic kidney disease, since it is not nephrotoxic and is cleaned by hepatic metabolism [16].

11.5 Indications for ICG During Robotic Surgery for Renal Cancer

11.5.1 Vasculature Identification

Renal vascular anatomy can have a lot of variations, and one of the most popular uses of ICG technology, especially during surgery for renal cancer, is vasculature identification [5, 6]. This application may include intra-operative identification of vessels for selective clamping during partial nephrectomy, or the assessment of arterial and/or venous clamping.

11.5.1.1 Identification of the Vessels
The identification of vessels in the renal hilum may be challenging, especially for less experienced surgeons. In these cases, the use of ICG technology might be of help, allowing for a precise description and identification of renal vessels, and providing a helpful guide for surgical dissection.

11.5.1.2 Selective Clamping
ICG may support selective clamping and thereby minimize ischemia time of healthy and non-tumor-bearing renal parenchyma, by improving identification of the renal vascular anatomy and the arterial blood supply to the tumor [9]. Indeed, when a selective clamping is planned or if an incomplete clamp is suspected, due to the possible presence of non-diagnosed ancillary renal arteries, the exclusion of blood supply from the target resection area can be confirmed with ICG.

In addition, ICG technology can be used to check selective blood supply to specific parts of the kidney. From a technical standpoint, after all renal vessels are clamped, the bulldogs are removed one by one to observe which part of the parenchyma is perfused, with the goal to preserve kidney perfusion, especially in patients with solitary kidney or reduced kidney function.

11.5.1.3 Check Adequate Clamping During On-Clamp Partial Nephrectomy
In case of difficult hilar anatomy, and in absence of 3-D reconstruction, the surgeon might be in doubt whether all arteries are identified or isolated, or whether the target area of the kidney will be still perfused after clamping (e.g. lower pole for lower pole tumor). In this situation, ICG can be used to assess whether the area that has to be dissected is still receiving blood supply or not.

11.5.2 Dissection of Tumor Margins

The use of ICG may facilitate the identification of the tumor which appears hypo-fluorescent as opposed to the highly vascularized healthy renal tissue, hence allowing a more accurate dissection and proper preservation of renal parenchyma [1, 12, 17, 19, 20]. This is because renal cell carcinomas lack bilitranslocase, a

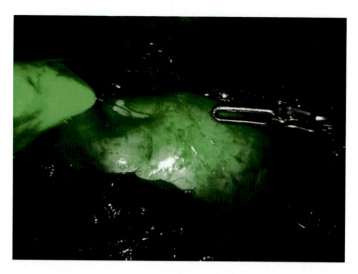

Fig. 11.2 Complete parenchyma reperfusion after renorrhaphy with ICG fluorescence imaging

carrier protein of ICG present in normal proximal tubule cells [8], allowing for clear discrimination between cancer and normal kidney tissues. By contrast, oncocytomas and chromophobe RCC are both known to express bilitranslocase and as such, may appear iso-fluorescent after ICG infusion.

An extension of this application is that, after tumor resection, the surgeon can evaluate the surgical margins and inspect whether there might be macroscopic residuals (R2 resection). Although this use is not validated, ICG technology might be of added value to assess the completeness of resection.

11.5.3 Check Tissue Viability After Renorrhaphy

ICG may also be used to assess the amount of remnant vital renal parenchyma by exploring the integrity of vascularization, which might have been compromised during renorrhaphy. Once the bulldog clamp is removed, and the kidney is re-vascularized, ICG fluorescence can be used to check for tissue perfusion (Fig. 11.2). If there is no ICG uptake on the resection margin, the surgeon can untighten the renorrhaphy in order to restore adequate perfusion.

11.5.4 Other Indications for ICG in Robotic Renal Surgery and New Applications

Other applications of ICG technology in partial and/or radical nephrectomy may include sentinel lymph node dissection during partial and/or radical nephrectomy, or super-selective infusion of ICG during partial nephrectomy for the identification of endophytic tumors. This new technique has been developed recently, and includes a super-selective catheterization of tertiary and quaternary arterial branches supplying the renal tumors [18]. Via a femoral approach, interventional uro-radiologist selectively delivers ICG mark into the tertiary-order arteries feeding the tumor, in order to mark the tumor and minimize any ischemic injury to the surrounding parenchyma. In case of avascular renal masses, the mixture can be delivered in close proximity to the lesion in order to obtain a peripheral ICG-marked rim of healthy parenchyma.

11.6 Conclusions

ICG technology has now emerged as a safe and feasible tool for an enhanced surgical experience. Its introduction in robotic surgery for renal cancer has changed practice, facilitating surgical performance mainly with respect to vascular identification. Given the versatility of ICG technology, other applications are possible but have to be further validated. Although the applications of ICG in renal surgery are promising, the actual clinical benefit for the patient remains to be determined and as such, further investigations are needed to improve the understanding on the impact of ICG.

References

1. Angell JE, Khemees TA, Abaza R. Optimization of near infrared fluorescence tumor localization during robotic partial nephrectomy. JURO. 2013;190(5):1668–73.
2. Bjurlin MA, McClintock TR, Stifelman MD. Near-infrared fluorescence imaging with intraoperative administration of indocyanine green for robotic partial nephrectomy. Curr Urol Rep. 2015;1–7.
3. Cacciamani GE, et al. Best practices in near-infrared fluorescence imaging with indocyanine green (NIRF/ICG)-guided robotic urologic surgery: a systematic review-based expert consensus. World J Urol. 2019;38(4):883–96.
4. Chu W, et al. Anaphylactic shock after intravenous administration of indocyanine green during robotic partial nephrectomy. Urol Case Rep. 2017;12:37–8.
5. Diana P, et al. The role of intraoperative indocyanine green in robot-assisted partial nephrectomy: results from a large, multi-institutional series. Eur Urol. 2020;1–7.
6. Gadus L, et al. Robotic partial nephrectomy with indocyanine green fluorescence navigation. Cont Media Mol Imaging. 2020;1–8.
7. Gioux S, Choi HS, Frangioni JV. Image-guided surgery using invisible near-infrared light: fundamentals of clinical translation. Mol Imaging. 2010;1–31.
8. Golijanin DJ, et al. Bilitranslocase (BTL) is immunolocalised in proximal and distal renal tubules and absent in renal cortical tumors accurately corresponding to intraoperative near infrared fluorescence (NIRF) expression of renal cortical tumors using intravenous indocyanin green (ICG). J Urol. 2008;1.
9. Harke N, et al. Selective clamping under the usage of near-infrared fluorescence imaging with indocyanine green in robot-assisted partial nephrectomy: a single-surgeon matched-pair study. World J Urol. 2014;1–7.
10. Krane LS, Manny TB, Hemal AK. Is near infrared fluorescence imaging using indocyanine green dye useful in robotic partial nephrectomy: a prospective comparative study of 94 patients. Urology. 2012;80(1):110–8.

11. Malthouse T. The future of robotic-assisted partial nephrectomy. 2017;1–9.
12. Manny TB, Krane LS, Hemal AK. Indocyanine green cannot predict malignancy in partial nephrectomy: histopathologic correlation with fluorescence pattern in 100 patients. J Endourol. 2013;1–4.
13. NDA 011525 Food and Drug Administration Suppl-27 Labeling-Packaging Insert, 2021.
14. Pandey A, et al. Usefulness of the indocyanine green (ICG) immunofluorescence in laparoscopic and robotic partial nephrectomy. Arch Esp Urol. 2019;1–6.
15. Pathak RA, Hemal AK. Intraoperative ICG-fluorescence imaging for robotic-assisted urologic surgery: current status and review of literature. Int Urol Nephrol. May 2019;51(5):795–771. https://doi.org/10.1007/s11255-019-02126-0. Epub 2019 Mar 22. PMID: 30903392.
16. Rao AR. Occlusion angiography using intraoperative contrast-enhanced ultrasound scan (CEUS): a novel technique demonstrating segmental renal blood supply to assist zero-ischaemia robot-assisted partial nephrectomy. Eur Urol. 2013;1–7.
17. Sentell KT, Ferroni MC, Abaza R. Near-infrared fluorescence imaging for intraoperative margin assessment during robot-assisted partial nephrectomy. BJU Int. 2020;1–6.
18. Simone G, et al. "Ride the Green Light": indocyanine green–marked off-clamp robotic partial nephrectomy for totally endophytic renal masses. Eur Urol. 2018;1–7.
19. Tobis S. Robot-assisted and laparoscopic partial nephrectomy with near infrared fluorescence imaging. J Endourol. 2012;1–6.
20. Tobis S, et al. Near infrared fluorescence imaging after intravenous indocyanine green: initial clinical experience with open partial nephrectomy for renal cortical tumors. Urology. 2012;79(4):958–64.
21. van den Berg NS. Fluorescence guidance in urologic surgery. Curr Opinion Urol. 2012;1–12.

3D Virtual Models and Augmented Reality for Robot-Assisted Partial Nephrectomy

12

E. Checcucci, P. Verri, G. Cacciamani, S. Pulliatti, M. Taratkin, J. Marenco, J. Gomez Rivas, D. Veneziano, and F. Porpiglia

12.1 Introduction

Nowadays, urological surgery has been changing its prerogatives, heading towards a patient-tailored management, especially when facing malignancies [7]. This new approach aims to obtain an equal balance between oncological safety and functional results. Focusing on renal cancer and the related surgery, the maintenance of functional results covers a crucial role, since renal function is fundamental for the body homeostasis and for potential medical treatment [9, 10, 22]. Because of these

E. Checcucci (✉)
Department of Surgery, Candiolo Cancer Institute, FPO-IRCCS, Candiolo, Turin, Italy
e-mail: checcu.e@hotmail.it

G. Cacciamani · M. Taratkin · J. Marenco · J. G. Rivas · D. Veneziano
Uro-Technology and SoMe Working Group of the Young Academic Urologists (YAU) Working Party of the European Association of Urology (EAU), Arnhem, The Netherlands

E. Checcucci · P. Verri · F. Porpiglia
Division of Urology, Department of Oncology, University of Turin, Turin, Italy

G. Cacciamani
USC Institute of Urology, University of Southern California, Los Angeles, CA, USA

S. Pulliatti
ORSI Academy, Melle, Belgium

Department of Urology, OLV Hospital, Aalst, Belgium

Department of Urology, University of Modena and Reggio Emilia, Modena, Italy

M. Taratkin
Institute for Urology and Reproductive Health, Sechenov University, Moscow, Russia

J. Marenco
Department of Urology, Hospital Instituto Valenciano de Oncología, Valencia, Spain

specific characteristics, the handling of renal lesions with nephron-sparing techniques, even in case of complex tumors, became increasingly popular, also taking advantage of the technological novelties, in particular robotic-surgery [11]. In order to reach optimal oncological and functional results by creating a patient-tailored approach, the performance of image-guided surgery is crucial [5, 8].

Amongst the different technologies available, the three-dimensional (3D) image guided surgery is one of the most attractive ones, with very promising clinical application.

In this chapter we will explore the universe of 3D guided surgery, starting from the realization of the 3D models, to their application in surgical planning and navigation.

12.2 What is a 3D Model?

A 3D-model is a virtual or physical representation of the surface of an object. It can be obtained by using a dedicated software (virtual model) or it may also be physically manufactured (printed model). The operator (i.e., modeller) recreates and transforms an idea (i.e., virtual model) or a real object into a different product, using the available technologies. In the past, the first 3D-modellers were artists: sculptors and painters had the ability to shape different materials into the chosen form, using various instruments, which were the most disparate, translating their ideas (e.g., virtual models) into actual objects (i.e., printed models). The advent of the computer and informatics brought great innovations, which allowed artists and scientists to create and benefit from new techniques, changing the status quo of their respective fields. A modern example is represented by the movie industry, twisted by the advent of 3D-rendering softwares allowing to outline the human presence from the movie-set.

In the medical field, particularly in the surgical environment, the creation of 3D models represents one of the cornerstones of the so called "surgery 4.0" [20].

Each patient is unique, his/her anatomy is at the same time identical and different from the other patients, so it is mandatory to study each case with the aim to offer a tailored and personalized treatment.

It is important to underline that the correct interpretation of the information obtained from the standard preoperative 2D images (e.g., contrast-enhanced CT scan) requires a thorough anatomical knowledge and clinical experience. In addition, the mental transformation from 2 to 3D is not an easy process. Therefore, following this principle and trying to overcome these problems, 3D technology finds its role, progressively becoming an important tool in the daily clinical practice [17].

J. G. Rivas
Department of Urology, Hospital Clinico San Carlos, Madrid, Spain

D. Veneziano
Department of Urology and Renal Transplantation, Bianchi-Melacrino-Morelli Hospital, Reggio Calabria, Italy

12.3 How to Create a 3D Model?

In the framing process of the major part of urological diseases, radiological imaging such as CT or MRI, represents a fundamental step in order to plan the best treatment for each single patient. The main limit of these radiological instruments is represented by the two-dimensionality of the images, which require an accurate anatomical knowledge in order to avoid misinterpretations, in particular when the operator are young urologists with limited experience [23]. In fact, the "building in mind" process a surgeon is required to perform, needs to follow a learning curve, which takes time to be walked. As evident as it can be, 3D reconstructions offer immediate and intuitive information, more easily accessible when compared to 2D CT/MRI images: proportions and relationships between nearby organs are more understandable and the pathology itself (whether malignant or benign) can be displayed and visualized in a different fashion.

The realization of a 3D models starts from the processing of bi-dimensional images. Commonly, almost every DICOM viewers software provide, by default, a 3D reconstruction, thanks to an automatic rendering process. Unfortunatly, the quality is often poor in resolution and the model lacks many details.

Notwithstanding the quality of these models, they can add some information and details when compared to 2D images, thanks to the organs' visualization and the display of the disease's features.

However, surgeons cannot rely on poor quality models before performing a surgical procedure and, in order to realize better reconstructions, a new specialized figure was introduced: the bioengineer. The collaboration between surgeons and engineers has led to the creation of more satisfying models in terms of details and anatomical accuracy.

The interaction and communication between these two parts (doctors and engineers) is fundamental: engineers must understand the surgeon's needs and vice versa, in order to create an accurate computer project.

Practically speaking, the realization of the models starts from the acquisition of bidimensional images. The most useful material is obtained by CT scan (multi-slice is preferred) or MRI images, which can be easily exported in DICOM format.

The image quality is fundamental, since it increases linearly with the precision of the 3D reconstruction; in order to obtain good quality models, the thickness of the single slice should not exceed 5 mm.

First of all, using DICOM images displaying softwares, the object must be analyzed, the most useful images (e.g., arterial or late phase of a CT-scan) must be selected and specific parameters (e.g., image contrast and luminosity) have to be modified and regulated in accordance with the project's needs. This phase is named "preprocessing phase".

Subsequently, a volume rendering is created: the software automatically generates an initial version of the 3D model, using the information included in the image voxels. A voxel is the basic volume unit, the equivalent of a pixel in a 2D system. Thanks to this rendering, the engineer can have an overall idea of the project, identifying the project's critical issues.

Afterwards, a process called "segmentation" is performed thanks to a dedicated software. Segmentation is defined as the isolation of pixels included in regions or objects of interest (ROIs/OOIs), selected on the basis of a subjective similarity criterion (e.g., color). The best method to identify different ROIs/OOIs is called "thresholding", which is based on the selection of a specific range of a defined parameter (e.g., gray scale). After the range has been set, the software can consequently identify all the regions with the chosen characteristics and, subsequently, specific algorithms are generated, and other regions/objects are automatically discarded. This represents a fundamental step for the realization of the 3D models: in some cases, the software is not able to correctly identify and depict the different features and this process needs to be done manually. The experience of the engineer is particularly relevant at this stage, since the reconstruction must be precisely tailored, almost such as a dressmaker would do in a fashion atelier.

Once this process is completed, the project can be exported and saved in.stl (Standard Triangulation Language) format and, when needed, the operator can perform furtherly modify the rendering, using dedicated softwares. Finally, the virtual 3D model is completed (Fig. 12.1).

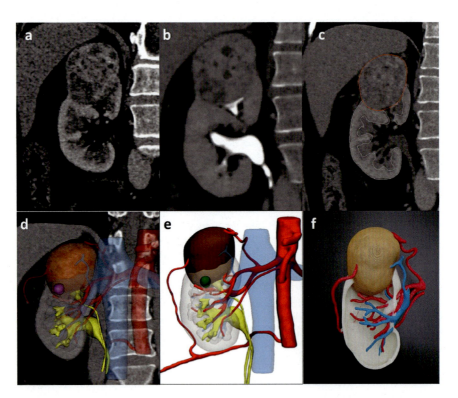

Fig. 12.1 3D model processing: **a** CT scan; **b** c.e. CT scan; **c** segmentation phase aimed to identify the different anatomical structures; **d** 3D model obtained can be overlapped to the CT images; **e** hyper-accurated 3D virtual model; **f** 3D printed model with FDM technology

12 3D Virtual Models and Augmented Reality ...

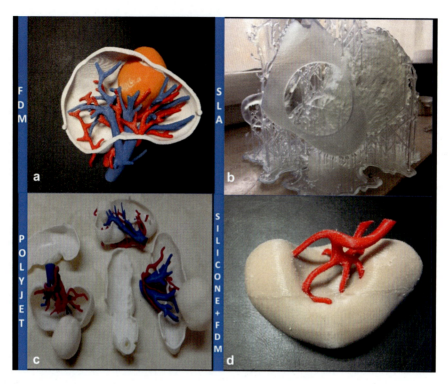

Fig. 12.2 3D printing technologies: **a** Fused Deposition Modeling (FDM); **b** Stereolitography (SLA); **c** Multi-material Plastic Jetting (Polyjet); **d** Silicone mold pouring combined with FDM printing

Once obtained, the model can be uploaded on almost any electronic devices (*see subchapter below*) for its virtual three-dimensional visualization.

Alternatively, using dedicated hardware, it can be printed using different 3D printing technologies, with different characteristics and potential applications [12, 26] (Fig. 12.2).

12.4 How to Review the 3D Models?

There are essentially two different ways to review 3D reconstructions: display them on an electronic device (virtual models) or create a physical object (printed models).

Nowadays, virtual models represent the most appealing tool amongst the two, since they are accessible from any electronic device (e.g., smartphones, tablets, laptops) and offer an intuitive experience. The chance to export.stl files in.pdf format allows to easily send 3D models via email or via dedicated platforms (e.g., MyMedics–Medics Srl©), allowing a joint teamwork between different people in different hospitals.

Table 12.1 Summary of the different display systems for 3D virtual models

	Vision	Environment	Consultation	Clinical application
2D flat screen	2D	Real + Virtual monitor	2D monitor (tablet, smartphone)	Surgical planning
Mixed reality	3D	Virtual + Real	Head mounted display (i.e., Hololens)	Surgical planning and surgical navigation
Virtual reality	3D	Virtual	Immersive head mounted display (i.e., Oculus Rift)	Surgical planning and training
Augmented reality	2D/3D	Virtual + Real	Robotic console	Surgical navigation and training

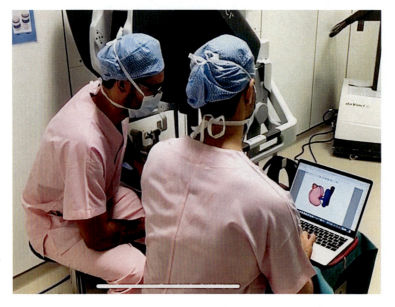

Fig. 12.3 2D flat screen visualization of the 3D models during cognitive robotic partial nephrectomy

3D models can be displayed variably, depending by the surgeon needs and by the hardware's availability (Table 12.1):

- 2D screen (e.g., TV, tablet): the virtual model is displayed on a 2D surface and can be zoomed, tilted, rotated and translated according to the operator's needs, using a touch screen or a joystick/mouse.
- The model can also be variably modified (e.g., transparency, colors), compatibly with the software used. In this setting, the absence of 3D vision represents the main limitation (Fig. 12.3).

12 3D Virtual Models and Augmented Reality ...

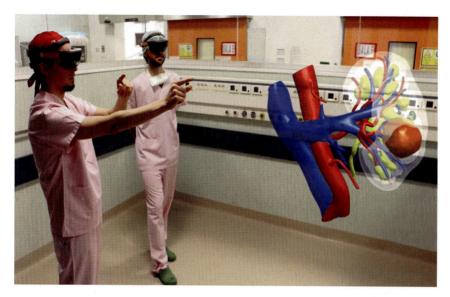

Fig. 12.4 3D mixed reality visualization of the 3D virtual model for preoperative surgical planning

- Mixed Reality (MR): in this setting, the use of dedicated devices (e.g., head mounted displays, such as HoloLens®) allows the superimposition of virtual elements to live images. Thanks to this instruments, three-dimensional virtual images are merged with the real environment. This technique finds its principal application in during preoperative planning, allowing the operator to physically walk around the model and to interact with it through gestures. These devices are usually equipped with broadcasting technology, so that an audience can experience what the operator sees through the lenses, live (Fig. 12.4).
- Virtual reality (VR): this technology allows the operator, using dedicated visors, to interact with a fully virtual environment. In this setting, surgeons are immersed into a totally virtual reality where they have the chance to interoperate, through preset gestures, with the 3D model; it must be emphasized that this technology totally excludes the real environment from the operator's view. VR can alternatively be enjoyed using virtual simulators [e.g., for robotic surgery: dV-Trainer (Mimic, Seattle, WA, USA), da Vinci Skills Simulator (Intuitive Surgical, Sunnyvale, CA, USA)]: these machines serve as training devices for surgeons of different levels of experience, offering the possibility to practice particular tasks (e.g., suturing, moving objects) or entire procedures (e.g., partial nephrectomy, radical prostatectomy) while being immersed in a fully virtual environment. The most realistic devices also offer a haptic feedback, resembling the actual intraoperative scenario.
- Augmented Reality (AR): AR can be defined as the overlay of digitally created content into the user's real-world environment with the aim of enhancing

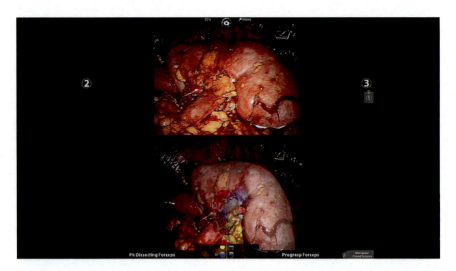

Fig. 12.5 3D augmented reality image was overlapped to in-vivo anatomy during robotic partial nephrectomy

real-word features. This technique finds its perfect application during surgical procedures, since the surgeon can overlap virtual reconstruction to the intraoperative images, adding important information during the surgical procedure (e.g., tumor margins, vascular anatomy) (Fig. 12.5).

In a recently published survey [2], all of the aforementioned methods were analyzed, and surgeons of different experience level were asked to evaluate each modality applied to different fields of interest. The most appealing technology for intraoperative guidance and training for kidney surgery was the AR technology, (58.3 and 40%), whilst during surgical planning and patient counselling, the use of HoloLens device and printed models were rated as the most effective in 60 and 61.8% of the cases, respectively. Another interesting point was that, amongst the interviewers, a poor knowledge of 3D printing costs and production times was identified.

12.5 Applications of 3D Models for Robotic Partial Nephrectomy

12.5.1 Patient Counselling

Patient counselling covers a fundamental role in the reaching of a globally successful medical act, but the communication can sometimes be tricky and challenging, since the surgeon must often face limits given by the patient's scholarship and socio-cultural extraction. Images, on the opposite, represent a straightforward and intuitive tool, easy to understand, with the power to communicate an idea in a blink of an eye.

3D models (whether virtual or printed) offer a precise and comprehensive anatomical representation of both the organ/s and lesion/s in exam, therefore they can be used to provide patients with a more immediate visualization and comprehension of their pathology.

As reported by Porpiglia et al. [11] and Checcucci et al. [16], patients and surgeons find very interesting and useful the use of 3D models, whether virtual or printed. During the 2017 Edition of Techno Urology Meeting (TUM) held in San Luigi Gonzaga Hospital (TO), specific questionnaires were administered to patients and operators. The results were satisfying both from the surgeon's and patient's point of view.

In a work by Atalay et al. [6], the importance of 3D models in the preoperative phase was highlighted: the author, by administering questionnaires to patients, showed how the overall comprehension of the anatomy, disease, treatment and related complications was improved up to 64% when compared to baseline tests. This work proved once again the great communicative power of 3D models.

Despite the higher costs of 3D printed models respect to virtual counterpart, this kind of fruition seems to be the most appreciated by the patients [2].

12.5.2 Surgical Training

Surgical training and simulation probably represent the most attractive field of application of the 3D modelling technology [13, 14] according to epidemiological studies, in fact, in the US more than 400,000 deaths by year due to medical errors have been reported and part of these unfortunate cases are determined by surgical errors [9]. The classic Halstedian model, based on the "see one, do one, teach one" paradigm must be overcome in favor of new and safe approach to learn surgical techniques. Furthermore, in order to standardize the evaluation of trainees, instruments based on virtual exercises were created: in case of robot-assisted surgery, the most known evaluating instrument is represented by the "Global Evaluative Assessment of Robotic Skills (GEARS)" [21]. By assessing six different domains (depth perception, bimanual dexterity, efficiency, autonomy, force sensitivity and robotic control), the experimenters were able to validate this tool, which has also been integrated by several institutions as a part of the curriculum.

Considering robotic-surgery simulators, the most popular and commercially available machines are the da Vinci Skills simulator (dVSS; Intuitive Surgical, Sunnyvale, CA, USA), the Mimic dV-Trainer (Mimic Technologies, Inc, Seattle, WA, USA), the Robotic Surgical Simulator (RoSS; Simulated Surgical Systems, Buffalo, NY, USA), SimSurgery Educational Platform (SEP, SimSurgery, Norway) and RobotiX Mentor (Simbionix USA Inc., Cleveland, OH). The da Vinci Skills simulator is the only platform which is based on the actual Da Vinci surgical console, simulating the use of the actual machinery. Thanks to all the aforementioned platforms, trainees can perform basic surgical skills exercises (e.g., suturing) or entire procedures (e.g., robot-assisted radical prostatectomy, RARP) accordingly to their experience, immersed in a fully virtual 3D environment. The technical differences between the different platforms and their effectiveness during training represent a topic of interest, since it is fundamental for the acquired skills to be actually useful in a real environment. All the platforms are validated, demonstrated to offer an optimal experience for trainees and their use was significantly associated to surgical skills improvement [12].

Portelli et al. published a meta-analysis concerning the impact of virtual training on laparoscopic and robotic surgery, including 24 RCTs (Randomized Controlled Trials). The Authors analyzed different parameters, such as time, path length, instrument and tissue handling and technical skills scoring, including different simulators. The final results proved that the use of virtual training improves efficiency in terms of surgical practice but also increases the quality of the surgical act itself, reducing the error rates and improving tissue handling [29].

12.5.3 Surgical Planning

The most important crossroad in the path of surgeons and, consequently, patients is represented by the treatment indication. When deciding how to approach complex diseases, the surgeon must find the perfect balance between personal experience and international guidelines and recommendations and, when necessary, discussing the case in a multidisciplinary setting, in order to take the best decisions for the patient. In this scenario, 3D reconstructions can be very important, since surgeons can gather together and discuss the clinical case, choosing the best treatment (e.g., minimally invasive vs open surgery) and the most suitable surgical approach, according to the patient's and tumor's characteristics [25].

In their work, Porpiglia et al. realized hyper accuracy three-dimensional (HA3D™) reconstructions, allowing a clear visualization of the vascular anatomy and of the intraparenchymal vessels supplying the tumor. Thanks to this precise instrument and to dedicated algorithms, it was possible to simulate the selective clamping phase during partial nephrectomy and to highlight the corresponding rate of ischemized parenchyma. This instrument revealed to be particularly useful, proving to be effective in avoiding global ischemia of the kidney [27] (Fig. 12.6).

These findings were later confirmed by a RCT demonstrating that patients treated with the aid 3-D models had reduced operative time, estimated blood loss, clamp time, and length of hospital stay [30].

3D virtual models, as previously described, can be visualized as holograms in a mixed reality setting. Antonelli et al. [4] developed a mixed-reality tool using the zSpace workstation, a Windows-based laptop connected to a stereoscopic screen displaying virtual objects. This station was designed specifically for a mixed-reality experience, giving the chance to visualize a simulation environment over

12 3D Virtual Models and Augmented Reality …

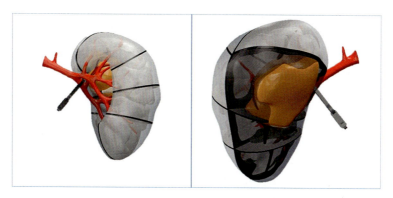

Fig. 12.6 Thanks to the 3D virtual model is possible to visualize the vessels feeding the tumour and respective rate of vascularized parenchyma; then a selective clamping can be planned

the real one. Thanks to this experience, the Authors concluded that mixed reality could improve preoperative planning for partial nephrectomy, since it provides higher quality details when compared to a computer tomography scan.

The mixed realty setting was also evaluated in another work by Checcucci et al., which focused on the high-resolution 3D perception of the organ anatomy offered by this technology and on the possibility to virtually interact with the model. Using HoloLens device, several surgeons had the chance to enjoy 3D reconstructions of complex clinical cases, displayed as 3D models "floating" in space [16]. The interviewed surgeons gave a positive feedback both for surgical planning (scored 8/10) and anatomical accuracy (9/10) on 1–10 Likert Scale. Moreover, the potential role of this technology in surgical planning and in the understanding of surgical complexity was highlighted. The impact of this technology on the decision making process was furtherly investigated by asking surgeons about the best surgical approach for each analysed clinical case: after a firsthand experience with HoloLens and MR, 64.4% and 44.4% of the surgeons changed their clamping and resection approach, respectively—ompared to CT image visualization only—in favour of a more selective one.

12.6 Surgical Navigation

Considering the increasing number of works published, only few and exploratory clinical studies have focused on the application of AR during partial nephrectomy [19].

In 2009 Su et al. [32] developed a markerless intraoperatory tracking system based on preoperatory CT images, performing an AR real-time stereo-endoscopic robot-assisted nephron sparing procedure. After calibrating the system intraoperatively, the 3D-to-3D registration was performed, and an error between the superimposed images and the real surgical field of only 1 mm was recorded.

An alternative technique was developed by Nostrati et al. [24] for the localization of visible and hidden structures, during endoscopic procedures. During a challenging robotic nephron-sparing procedures, thanks to their specifically developed method, the intraoperative accuracy of the surgical act was improved by 45% compared to standard techniques. In this specific case, the procedure was helped by the vascular pulsation cues registered using dedicated instruments [1].

In 2018, Wake et al. published an article, describing the step-by-step creation of 3D printed and AR kidney models with Unity® software, used during robotic nephron sparing surgery. These models were successively deployed to Microsoft's HoloLens® system. 3D models and AR were used preoperatively and intraoperatively to assist the surgeon. Conclusions assessed that the use of AR 3D models is safe, feasible and that it has an impact on the surgeon's decision-making process, without significant changes in the procedure's outcome [3].

In 2017 Singla et al. [31] created an AR guidance system applied during robotic nephron-sparing procedures' simulations, using ultrasonography for lesion tracking during. The registered error was around 1 mm, and the authors could consequently assess that the tested system could significantly reduce the excised volume of peritumoral healthy tissue during surgery (30.6 vs. 17.5 cm^3).

A pioneering experience was published by Porpiglia et al. [27, 28]. The Authors merged hyper-accuracy models (HA3D™) with the DaVinci software using Tile-Pro® and tested their use during partial nephrectomy. Concerning selective ischemia, AR guidance proved to be as valid as the cognitive guidance while offering the surgeon the chance to stay constantly focused on the surgical field, avoiding distraction errors. This preliminary experience implied the use of rigid 3D virtual models, unsuitable to simulate intraoperative tissue deformations. For this reason, the same group, collaborating with the engineers of *Politecnico* of Turin, consequently developed a dedicated software, introducing elastic AR. This system proved to be particularly useful during the identification and resection of hidden, endophytic tumors, especially when they were located in the posterior face of the kidney. During the procedure, in order to prove the 3D-overlapping accuracy, endoscopic ultrasonography was used, showing a perfect match between the virtual model and the lesion. Moreover, the AR images allowed to visualize intraparenchymal structures, such as vessels and calyxes, invisible with the aid of ultrasound only [28] (Fig. 12.7).

However, at current times, AR still remains a newborn and emerging technology with consequent limitations that need to be overcome [15]. The major limitation is represented by the manual overlapping process, performed by an expert assistant who needs to help the operator during the procedure. To overcome this limit, two main strategies have been theorized. The first one implies the identification of endoscopic landmarks, which can be consequently detected by the AR system [4, 24]. The second strategy, more challenging and expensive, involves a markerless approach.

Again, the group directed by professor Porpiglia, firstly start to explore this innovative approach [3] Thanks to a constant collaboration with the engineers, they created an algorithm-based computer vision dedicated software, with the objective

12 3D Virtual Models and Augmented Reality ...

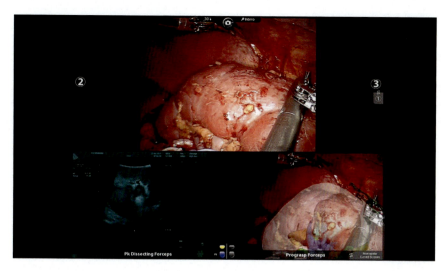

Fig. 12.7 3D augmented reality images perfectly correspond to the real time ultrasound ones

to automatize 3D virtual and endoscopic images co-registration. In particular, by leveraging the enhanced vision provided by indocyanine green (ICG), the software allowed a precise intraoperative kidney identification and a consequent automatic overlap of the 3D mesh with live intraoperative images was successfully performed (Fig. 12.8). In a pilot study, ten patients were enrolled: in all the cases, the automatic tracking was successful, allowing to perform an enucleoresection of the lesion without damaging the pseudocapsule and avoiding the occurrence of positive surgical margins.

Notwithstanding these encouraging findings, this approach was not devoid of limitations: in fact, when the kidney is rotated in order to approach posterior lesions, the shape of the organ changes dramatically, and the software is therefore unable to overlap the images. To overcome this problem, it will probably be essential the development of artificial intelligence with deep learning algorithms [18, 19], which will train the software to recognize the kidney's features and texture, reaching a more precise and stable automatic tracking during the whole procedure.

12.7 Conclusions

In an even more tailored surgery era, the image guided surgery plays a fundamental role especially during complex procedures such as partial nephrectomy. Nowadays, a paradigm shift is happening thanks to the advent of 3D models. The possibility to visualize the patient's specific anatomy three-dimensionally offers an unprecedent comprehension of the surgical complexity with a subsequent more patient-specific surgical planning. Moreover, by using augmented reality systems, these virtual 3D reconstructions can be the virtual eyes of the surgeon guiding him during the entire procedure.

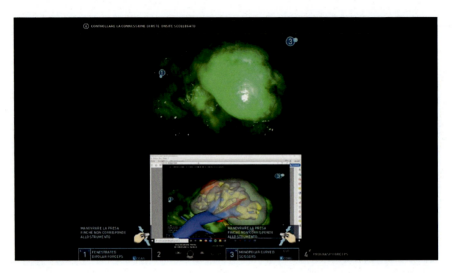

Fig. 12.8 Thanks the enhanced vision provided by indocyanine green (ICG) the computer-vision based software was able to recognize the kidney shape and automatically anchor the 3D virtual images of the kidney

References

1. Amir-Khalili A, et al. Auto localization and segmentation of occluded vessels in robot-assisted partial nephrectomy. In: Lecture notes in computer science (including subseries Lecture notes in artificial intelligence and Lecture notes in bioinformatics). Springer;2014. p. 407–14. https://doi.org/10.1007/978-3-319-10404-1_51.
2. Amparore D, et al. 3D imaging technologies in minimally-invasive kidney and prostate cancer surgery: which is the urologists' perception? Minerva Urol Nephrol. 2021. https://doi.org/10.23736/S2724-6051.21.04131-X.
3. Amparore D, Checcucci E, Piazzolla P, Piramide F, De Cillis S, Piana A, Verri P, Manfredi M, Fiori C, Vezzetti E, Porpiglia F. Indocyanine Green Drives Computer Vision Based 3D Augmented Reality Robot Assisted Partial Nephrectomy: The Beginning of Automatic Overlapping Era. Urology. 2022 Jun;164:e312–e316. doi: https://doi.org/10.1016/j.urology.2021.10.053. Epub 2022 Jan 19. PMID: 35063460.
4. Antonelli A, et al. Holographic reconstructions for preoperative planning before partial nephrectomy: a head-to-head comparison with standard CT scan. Urologia Internationalis S Karger AG. 2019;102(2):212–7. https://doi.org/10.1159/000495618.
5. Aoun F, et al. Indocyanine greenfluorescence-guidedsentinel lymph node identification in urologic cancers: a systematic review and meta-analysis. Minerva Urologica e Nefrologica. Edizioni Minerva Medica 2018;361–9. https://doi.org/10.23736/S0393-2249.17.02932-0.
6. Atalay HA, et al. Impact of personalized three-dimensional (3D) printed pelvicalyceal system models on patient information in percutaneous nephrolithotripsy surgery: a pilot study. Braz Soc Urol. 2017;43(3):470–5. https://doi.org/10.1590/S1677-5538.IBJU.2016.0441.
7. Autorino R, et al. Precision surgery and genitourinary cancers. Eur J Surg Oncol (W.B. Saunders Ltd.). 2017;43(5):893–908. https://doi.org/10.1016/j.ejso.2017.02.005.
8. Basile G, et al. Comparison between near-infrared fluorescence imaging with indocyanine green and infrared imaging: on-bench trial for kidney perfusion analysis. A project

of the ESUT-YAUWP group. Minerva Urologica e Nefrologica. Edizioni Minerva Medica 2019;71(3):280–5. https://doi.org/10.23736/S0393-2249.19.03353-8.
9. Bertolo R, Fiori C, et al. Assessment of the relationship between renal volume and renal function after minimally-invasive partial nephrectomy: the role of computed tomography and nuclear renal scan. Minerva Urologica e Nefrologica Edizioni Minerva Medica. 2018;70(5):509–17. https://doi.org/10.23736/S0393-2249.18.03140-5.
10. Bertolo RG, et al. Estimated glomerular filtration rate, renal scan and volumetric assessment of the kidney before and after partial nephrectomy: a review of the current literature. Minerva Urologica e Nefrologica. Edizioni Minerva Medica 2017;539–47. https://doi.org/10.23736/S0393-2249.17.02865-X.
11. Bertolo R, Autorino R, et al. Outcomes of robot-assisted partial nephrectomy for clinical T2 renal tumors: a multicenter analysis (ROSULA Collaborative Group). Eur Urol (Elsevier B.V.). 2018;74(2):226–32. https://doi.org/10.1016/j.eururo.2018.05.004.
12. Bric JD, et al. Current state of virtual reality simulation in robotic surgery training: a review. Surg Endosc. Springer, New York LLC, 2016. p. 2169–78. https://doi.org/10.1007/s00464-015-4517-y.
13. Carrion DM, et al. Current status of urological training in Europe. Archivos espanoles de urologia, 2018;71(1):11–7. http://www.ncbi.nlm.nih.gov/pubmed/29336327.
14. Carrion DM, et al. Current status of urology surgical training in Europe: an ESRU–ESU–ESUT collaborative study. World J Urol (Springer). 2020;38(1):239–46. https://doi.org/10.1007/s00345-019-02763-1.
15. Checcucci E, Amparore D, et al. 3D imaging applications for robotic urologic surgery: an ESUT YAUWP review. World J Urol (Springer). 2020;38(4):869–81. https://doi.org/10.1007/s00345-019-02922-4.
16. Checcucci E, et al. 3D mixed reality holograms for preoperative surgical planning of nephron-sparing surgery: evaluation of surgeons' perception. Minerva urologica e nefrologica = The Italian Journal of Urology and Nephrology. Minerva Urol Nefrol. 2019. https://doi.org/10.23736/S0393-2249.19.03610-5.
17. Checcucci E, De Cillis S, et al. Applications of neural networks in urology: a systematic review. Curr Opinion Urol (NLM (Medline)). 2020;30(6):788–807. https://doi.org/10.1097/MOU.0000000000000814.
18. Checcucci E, Autorino R, et al. Artificial intelligence and neural networks in urology: current clinical applications. Minerva Urologica e Nefrologica. Edizioni Minerva Medica. 2020;49–57. https://doi.org/10.23736/S0393-2249.19.03613-0.
19. Checcucci E, De Cillis S, Porpiglia F. 3D-printed models and virtual reality as new tools for image-guided robot-assisted nephron-sparing surgery: a systematic review of the newest evidences. Curr. Opinion Urol (Lippincott Williams and Wilkins). 2020;55–64. https://doi.org/10.1097/MOU.0000000000000686.
20. Feußner H, Park A. Surgery 4.0: the natural culmination of the industrial revolution? Innov. Surg Sci (Walter de Gruyter GmbH). 2017;2(3):105–8. https://doi.org/10.1515/iss-2017-0036.
21. Goh AC, et al. Global evaluative assessment of robotic skills: validation of a clinical assessment tool to measure robotic surgical skills. J Urol. 2012;187(1):247–52. https://doi.org/10.1016/j.juro.2011.09.032.
22. Grivas N, et al. Robot-assisted versus open partial nephrectomy: comparison of outcomes. A systematic review. Minerva Urologica e Nefrologica. Edizioni Minerva Medica, 2019; p. 113–20. https://doi.org/10.23736/S0393-2249.19.03391-5.
23. Lin C, et al. When to introduce three-dimensional visualization technology into surgical residency: a randomized controlled trial. J Med Syst (Springer New York LLC). 2019;43(3). https://doi.org/10.1007/s10916-019-1157-0.
24. Nosrati MS, et al. Simultaneous multi-structure segmentation and 3D nonrigid pose estimation in image-guided robotic surgery. IEEE Trans Med Imaging (Institute of Electrical and Electronics Engineers Inc.). 2016;35(1):1–12. https://doi.org/10.1109/TMI.2015.2452907.

25. Porpiglia F, Amparore D, et al. Current use of three-dimensional model technology in urology: a road map for personalised surgical planning. Eur Urol Focus (Elsevier B.V.). 2018; pp. 652–6. https://doi.org/10.1016/j.euf.2018.09.012.
26. Porpiglia F, Bertolo R, et al. Development and validation of 3D printed virtual models for robot-assisted radical prostatectomy and partial nephrectomy: urologists' and patients' perception. World J Urol (Springer). 2018;36(2):201–7. https://doi.org/10.1007/s00345-017-2126-1.
27. Porpiglia F, Fiori C, et al. Hyperaccuracy three-dimensional reconstruction is able to maximize the efficacy of selective clamping during robot-assisted partial nephrectomy for complex renal masses. Eur Urol (Elsevier B.V.). 2018;74(5):651–60. https://doi.org/10.1016/j.eururo.2017.12.027.
28. Porpiglia F, et al. Three-dimensional augmented reality robot-assisted partial nephrectomy in case of complex tumours (PADUA ≥ 10): a new intraoperative tool overcoming the ultrasound guidance. Eur Urol (Elsevier B.V.). 2020;78(2):229–38. https://doi.org/10.1016/j.eururo.2019.11.024.
29. Portelli M, et al Virtual reality training compared with apprenticeship training in laparoscopic surgery: a meta-analysis. Ann Royal Coll Surg Engl (Royal College of Surgeons of England). 2020; p. 672–84. https://doi.org/10.1308/RCSANN.2020.0178.
30. Shirk JD, et al. Effect of 3-dimensional virtual reality models for surgical planning of robotic-assisted partial nephrectomy on surgical outcomes: a randomized clinical trial. JAMA Netw Open (American Medical Association). 2019;2(9). https://doi.org/10.1001/jamanetworkopen.2019.11598.
31. Singla, R., et al. Intra-operative ultrasound-based augmented reality guidance for laparoscopic surgery. In: Healthcare technology letters. Institution of Engineering and Technology;2017. p. 204–9. https://doi.org/10.1049/htl.2017.0063.
32. Su LM, et al. Augmented reality during robot-assisted laparoscopic partial nephrectomy: toward real-time 3D-CT to stereoscopic video registration. Urology. 2009;73(4):896–900. https://doi.org/10.1016/j.urology.2008.11.040.

Open Partial Nephrectomy: Current Status in the Minimally-Invasive Surgery Era

13

Riccardo Campi, Selcuk Erdem, Onder Kara, Umberto Carbonara, Michele Marchioni, Alessio Pecoraro, Riccardo Bertolo, Alexandre Ingels, Maximilian Kriegmair, Nicola Pavan, Eduard Roussel, Angela Pecoraro, and Daniele Amparore

Partial nephrectomy (PN) is recommended as standard treatment for technically feasible all clinical T1 renal tumors, by the guidelines [1, 2]. Since its first description at the beginning of 1950s, open partial nephrectomy (OPN) has been widely used in the treatment of localized renal cancer for more than seven decades [3]. In parallel with technological improvements, almost all steps of OPN were successfully adapted in

---

R. Campi (✉) · A. Pecoraro
Unit of Urological Robotic Surgery and Renal Transplantation, University of Florence, Careggi Hospital, Florence, Italy
e-mail: riccardo.campi@unifi.it

R. Campi
Department of Experimental and Clinical Medicine, University of Florence, Florence, Italy

S. Erdem
Division of Urologic Oncology, Department of Urology, Istanbul University Istanbul Faculty of Medicine, Istanbul, Turkey

O. Kara
Department of Urology, Kocaeli University School of Medicine, Kocaeli, Turkey

U. Carbonara
Department of Emergency and Organ Transplantation-Urology, Andrology and Kidney Transplantation Unit, University of Bari, Bari, Italy

M. Marchioni
Department of Medical, Oral and Biotechnological Sciences, Laboratory of Biostatistics, University "G. D'Annunzio" Chieti-Pescara, Chieti, Italy

Department of Urology, SS Annunziata Hospital, "G. D'Annunzio" University of Chieti, Chieti, Italy

R. Bertolo
Department of Urology, San Carlo Di Nancy Hospital, Rome, Italy

© The Author(s), under exclusive license to Springer Nature Switzerland AG 2022
S. S. Goonewardene et al. (eds.), *Robotic Surgery for Renal Cancer*, Management of Urology, https://doi.org/10.1007/978-3-031-11000-9_13

laparoscopic PN (LPN) and robotic-assisted PN after their first description at 1993 and 2004, respectively [4, 5].

Despite a rising trend on minimal invasive PN (MIPN) preference which is primarily attributed the increased use of RAPN, especially in developed countries with available technologies and surgical experience, there still exists windows for performing OPN which is still considered as standard of care [6–8]. In parallel, the statement of European Association of Urology (EAU) Guideline with strong recommendation (*'Do not perform minimally invasive radical nephrectomy in patients with T1 tumours for whom a PN is feasible by any approach, including open'*), specifically highlighted the role and importance of OPN in minimal invasive era [1].

Accordingly, this chapter will particularly focus on indications, critical technical details, and oncological and functional outcomes of OPN, on the basis of the comparison with MIPNs.

13.1 Indications

Patients with solitary kidney, high complexity tumors, preexisting chronic kidney disease (CKD), and multiple renal tumors in hereditary genetic kidney cancer syndromes should be considered as optimal candidates for open partial nephrectomy.

A. Ingels
Department of Urology, University Hospital Henri Mondor, APHP, 51 Avenue du Maréchal de Lattre de Tassigny, 94010 Créteil, France

Biomaps, UMR1281, INSERM, CNRS, CEA, Université Paris Saclay, Villejuif, France

M. Kriegmair
Department of Urology, University Medical Centre Mannheim, Mannheim, Germany

N. Pavan
Department of Medical, Surgical and Health Science, Urology Clinic, University of Trieste, Trieste, Italy

E. Roussel
Department of Urology, University Hospitals Leuven, Leuven, Belgium

A. Pecoraro
Division of Urology, Department of Oncology, School of Medicine, University of Turin, San Luigi Hospital, Orbassano, Turin, Italy

D. Amparore
Division of Urology, Department of Oncology, School of Medicine, San Luigi Hospital, University of Turin, Orbassano, Turin, Italy

Renal tumor in anatomically or functionally solitary kidney is one of the imperative indication for performing PN. Recently, EAU Guideline on Renal Cell Carcinoma recommended PN for solitary kidney even in patients with T2 renal tumor [1]. Although it is not determined with only clinical staging, tumor complexity is often associated with increased T stage [9, 10]. From this point of view, managing more complex tumor in partial nephrectomy might be more feasible in open technique with compared to minimal invasive ones. A multi-institutional retrospective study found that the proportions of OPN were higher than RAPN (61.2% vs. 25%, p = 0.001) in more complex tumor (R.E.N.A.L. Nephrometry Scores of 9–12) in patients with solitary kidney [11]. Furthermore, there were no difference between two techniques with regard to trifecta outcomes including overall intraoperative/postoperative complications, positive surgical margin rates and renal function at postoperative 1 month. Similar results favoring OPN for more complex tumor in solitary kidney were reported when compared to LPN [12]. It might be interpreted that OPN provides feasibility in high complex tumor for achieving similar trifecta outcomes obtained via MIPN in relatively low complex tumors.

Patients with preexisting CKD are the special population those more benefit from PN. Despite nephron sparing advantage of PN, prolonged intraoperative ischemia may threaten kidney for irreversible functional damage [13]. In a recent analysis, OPN is reported to be the preferred treatment approach in patients with CKD, despite an overall increase on use of RAPN which was shown to significantly decrease ischemia time with compared to LPN [14]. Interestingly, surgeons with high volume of RAPN experience also showed similar tendency toward OPN preference in CKD patients. The application of intraoperative cooling and parenchymal compression, those will be discussed in technical points, might encourage surgeons to prefer OPN more, with the intent of minimizing ischemia time and maximizing renal perfusion.

Hereditary genetic kidney cancer syndromes might be another main area of subject for OPN [15]. Von Hippel-Lindau (VHL) Syndrome, Tuberosclerosis, Birt-Hugg-Dube Syndrome are well known familial genetic kidney cancer syndromes [16, 17]. Bilateral, synchronous and multiple renal tumors are typical manifestation of these syndromes. The decision of surgical treatment in hereditary genetic kidney cancers is generally based on the size of index tumor. If the size of index tumor is 3 cm or greater, performing PN is recommended not only for index tumor but also for all tumors smaller than 3 cm in ipsilateral kidney [18]. In addition to renal tumors, renal cysts those have malign potential for developing renal cancer in the future is suggested to be removed and/or decorticated at the same surgery. In the vast majority of cases, there are a lot of renal tumors and cysts those need to be treated, especially in index cases of syndromic family or in syndromic individuals those are not under regular follow-up. Open technique make more easier the control of affected kidney in cases with such higher number of renal tumors and cysts, with compared to MIPNs. It was reported that a median of 27 (up to 70) tumors and cysts were removed via open technique in patients with hereditary genetic kidney cancer syndromes [19].

Even the vast majority of cases are successfully completed via minimal invasive approach in experienced centers, conversion to open surgery and/or necessity on finalizing the operation via open approach should always be kept in mind, regardless from surgical experience on MIPN. The open conversion rate at MIPN was reported to vary from 3 to 13%, despite a decreasing trend exists with the contemporary use of robotics [20–25]. Intraoperative complications, technical problems on the devices and equipments used in MIPNs, patient intolerance against continuous pneumoperitoneum in elongated operative times, or any other unexpected circumstances during MIPNs might cause inevitable necessity of conversion to open surgery [23]. Therefore, the basic principles of OPN should be recommended to be learned and utilized by all urologists performing MIPN.

13.2 Technical Points

Open partial nephrectomy has several technical points in each steps (Fig. 13.1). Herein, some of these technical details differing OPN from MIPN will be highlighted.

Flank incision has been traditionally accepted approach in OPN. Direct access to kidney and being feasible for obese patients and patients with prior abdominal surgeries are advantages attributed to flank incision [26]. Furthermore, it is more preferable as because surgical complications such as urine leakage, abscesses, bleeding and hematoma are confined into the extraperitoneal space [27]. A miniflank incision might be utilized to decrease postoperative analgesic requirements and flank bulging after surgery [28, 29]. Non-flank incisions (subcostal, midline and thoracoabdominal) might be considered as alternatives of flank incision, in some extraordinary circumstances such as larger tumor size, prior flank incision, renal anomalies such as horseshoe kidney, vascular variations and abnormalities, physical disability for flank position (such as scoliosis), and require of simultaneous surgery [30, 31]. In a large retrospective analysis of Cleveland Clinic, 2671 (97.2%) OPN were reported to be done via flank incision while only 76 ones (2.8%) were performed via non-flank incision at same period due to above-mentioned extraordinary circumstances [31].

Renal hypothermia with intraoperative cooling reduces the risk of irreversible ischemic damage in kidney [32]. Open technique allows routine application of intraoperative cooling by using ice slush easily, which might be considered as another advantage of OPN with compared to MIPN. Despite the feasibility of several methods were suggested for intraoperative cooling in both LPN and RAPN, their use could not be generalized as routinely performed in OPN [33–35].

Parenchymal compression in OPN is the other technical point needs to be mentioned. Although several compression modifications and tourniquet methods were defined in MIPN, it is more feasible with a full parenchymal control of whole kidney in OPN [36–38]. Renal parenchymal compression may be considered in OPN as it allows to minimize ischemia related renal dysfunction in remaining renal remnant tissue. A few studies with limited cohort showed a marginal benefit on preserving postoperative renal function in cases with parenchymal compression, with compared to renal hilar clamping [39, 40].

Open surgery has been accepted as standard of care and the optimization of MIPN techniques is primarily measured by how the basic principles defined via open technique were successfully duplicated and standardized. However, open surgery and minimal invasive surgeries are in relation with an ongoing interactions. For example, several surgical technologies those were developed as response to needs of MIPN, such as self-retaining sutures, clips, hemostatic agents have been successfully adapted into OPN [41–43].

13.3 Open Versus Minimally-Invasive Partial Nephrectomy: Comparison of Oncological, Functional and Perioperative Outcomes

Briefly, no obvious superiority might be attributed to OPN or MIPNs, in terms of positive surgical margins, oncological and survival outcomes [44, 45].

Similarly, renal functional preservation on long term do not differ between OPN and MIPN, although there exists controversial outcomes particularly in early renal functions, those probably vary due to heterogeneity of the studies [46].

The outcomes on perioperative either overall- or major- complications are comparable between OPN and MIPNs, even if slight increased tendency was reported in LPNs series [47–50].

On the other hand, there is a large consensus supported by great amount of evidences on the association between OPN and increased postoperative analgesic requirements and longer hospital stay [47–49, 51]. However, a significant lower costs is generally associated with OPN, with compared to LPN and RAPN [52].

In minimal invasive technology era, OPN still remains as standard of care especially in centers where MIPN can not routinely been performed. Despite its disadvantages on postoperative convalescence, OPN should strongly be kept in mind in anywhere it serves with its nephron sparing advantages. Patients with solitary kidney, high complex tumor, preexisting CKD and hereditary genetic kidney cancer syndromes are more proned to be managed via OPN. Confining perioperative complications into extraperitoneal space, optimal intraoperative renal hypothermia and feasible renal parenchymal compression might be shown as technical advantages (Fig. 13.1).

Case 1: 40 years old male with a horseshoe kidney anomaly, 5.8 cm kidney tumor at left sided parenchyma, open partial nephrectomy via mid-line incision, tumor excision and renorraphy under cold ischemia (32 min) and renal parenchymal compression on isthmus of horsehoe kidney, histopathology: pT1b, chromophobe renal cell carcinoma, negative surgical margin; **Case 2**: 48 years old male, a member of family with Von Hippel-Lindau Syndrome, previous left partial nephrectomy (clear cell RCC, WHO/ISUP Grade 2), a numerous number of renal tumors and cysts at right kidney, open partial nephrectomy via right flank incision, a total of 8 tumor excision and 18 cysts decortication and fulgaration under cold ischemia (42 min), histopathology: pT1a, clear cell RCC, WHO/ISUP

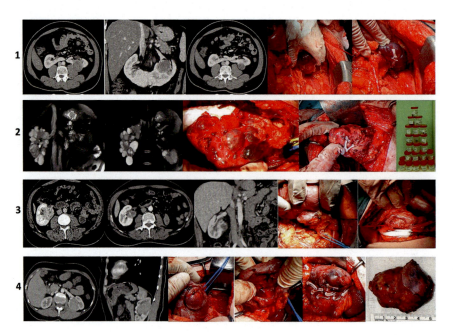

Fig. 13.1 Graphical overview of the main steps of open partial nephrectomy

Grade 2, negative surgical margin; **Case 3**: 46 years old male, previous left radical nephrectomy 13 years ago (11 cm, pT3a, clear cell RCC, Fuhrmann Grade 3), 5.1 cm perihilar high complex tumor at right kidney (PADUA: 12, R.E.N.A.L.: 10), Tru-Cut biopsy: clear cell RCC, pazopanib treatment for 6 months before surgery, 4.1 cm (PADUA: 12, RENAL: 10, 2nd CT image) tumor at 3rd months of pazopanib treatment, 3.6 cm (PADUA: 10, RENAL: 9, 3rd CT image) tumor at 6th months of pazopanib treatment, open partial nephrectomy via right flank incision, tumor excision and renorraphy under cold ischemia (30 min) histopathology: 3.8 cm, pT3a (pericapsular invasion), clear cell carcinoma, WHO/ISUP Grade 2, negative surgical margin; **Case 4**: 53 years old female, insidentally detected sporadic left renal mass, 5.2 cm high complex tumor (PADUA: 12, R.E.N.A.L.: 10), open partial nephrectomy via left flank incision, tumor excision and renorraphy under cold ischemia (29 min), histopathology: pT1b, chromophobe renal cell carcinoma, negative surgical margin.

References

1. Ljungberg B, Albiges L, Bedke J, et al. EAU Guidelines on RCC. Version 2021. http://uroweb.org/guidelines/compilations-of-all-guidelines/.
2. Campbell S, Uzzo RG, Allaf ME, et al. Renal mass and localized renal cancer: AUA guideline. J Urol. 2017;198(3):520–9. https://doi.org/10.1016/j.juro.2017.04.100 Epub 2017 May 4.

3. Vermooten V. Indications for conservative surgery in certain renal tumors: a study based on the growth pattern of the cell carcinoma. J Urol. 1950;64(2):200–8. https://doi.org/10.1016/s0022-5347(17)68620-8.
4. Winfield HN, Donovan JF, Godet AS, et al. Laparoscopic partial nephrectomy: initial case report for benign disease. J Endourol. 1993;7(6):521–6. https://doi.org/10.1089/end.1993.7.521.
5. Gettman MT, Blute ML, Chow GK, et al. Robotic-assisted laparoscopic partial nephrectomy: technique and initial clinical experience with DaVinci robotic system. Urology. 2004;64(5):914–8. https://doi.org/10.1016/j.urology.2004.06.049.
6. Xia L, Talwar R, Taylor BL, et al. National trends and disparities of minimally invasive surgery for localized renal cancer, 2010 to 2015. Urol Oncol. 2019;37(3):182.e17–182.e27. https://doi.org/10.1016/j.urolonc.2018.10.028.
7. Shah PH, Alom MA, Leibovich BC, et al. The temporal association of robotic surgical diffusion with overtreatment of the small renal mass. J Urol. 2018;200(5):981–8. https://doi.org/10.1016/j.juro.2018.05.081.
8. Mohapatra A, Potretzke AM, Weaver J, et al. Trends in the management of small renal masses: a survey of members of the endourological society. J Kidney Cancer VHL. 2017;4(3):10–9. https://doi.org/10.15586/jkcvhl.2017.82.
9. Ficarra V, Novara G, Secco S, et al. Preoperative aspects and dimensions used for an anatomical (PADUA) classification of renal tumours in patients who are candidates for nephron-sparing surgery. Eur Urol. 2009;56(5):786–93. https://doi.org/10.1016/j.eururo.2009.07.040.
10. Kutikov A, Uzzo RG. The R.E.N.A.L. Nephrometry score: a comprehensive standardized system for quantitating renal tumor size, location and depth. J Urol. 2009:182(3):844–53. https://doi.org/10.1016/j.juro.2009.05.035.
11. Zargar H, Bhayani S, Allaf ME, et al. Comparison of perioperative outcomes of robot-assisted partial nephrectomy and open partial nephrectomy in patients with a solitary kidney. J Endourol. 2014;28(10):1224–30. https://doi.org/10.1089/end.2014.0297.
12. Lane BR, Novick AC, Babineau D, et al. Comparison of laparoscopic and open partial nephrectomy for tumor in a solitary kidney. J Urol. 2008;179(3):847–51; discussion 852. https://doi.org/10.1016/j.juro.2007.10.050.
13. Mir MC, Ercole C, Takagi T, et al. Decline in renal function after partial nephrectomy: etiology and prevention. J Urol. 2015;193(6):1889–98. https://doi.org/10.1016/j.juro.2015.01.093.
14. Khandwala YS, Jeong IG, Han DH, et al. Surgeon preference of surgical approach for partial nephrectomy in patients with baseline chronic kidney disease: a nationwide population-based analysis in the USA. Int Urol Nephrol. 2017;49(11):1921–7. https://doi.org/10.1007/s11255-017-1688-6.
15. Linehan WM, Srinivasan R, Schmidt LS. The genetic basis of kidney cancer: a metabolic disease. Nat Rev Urol. 2010;7(5):277–85. https://doi.org/10.1038/nrurol.2010.47.
16. Sidana A, Srinivasan R. Therapeutic strategies for hereditary kidney cancer. Curr Oncol Rep. 2016;18(8):50. https://doi.org/10.1007/s11912-016-0537-6.
17. Capitanio U, Rosiello G, Erdem S, et al. Clinical, surgical, pathological and follow-up features of kidney cancer patients with Von Hippel-Lindau syndrome: novel insights from a large consortium World J Urol. 2021. https://doi.org/10.1007/s00345-020-03574-5.
18. Duffey BG, Choyke PL, Glenn G, et al. The relationship between renal tumor size and metastases in patients with von Hippel-Lindau disease. J Urol. 2004;172(1):63–5. https://doi.org/10.1097/01.ju.0000132127.79974.3f.
19. Fadahunsi AT, Sanford T, Linehan WM, et al. Feasibility and outcomes of partial nephrectomy for resection of at least 20 tumors in a single renal unit. J Urol. 2011;185(1):49–53. https://doi.org/10.1016/j.juro.2010.09.032.
20. Bahrami SR, Lima GC, Varkarakis IM, et al. Intraoperative conversion of laparoscopic partial nephrectomy. J Endourol. 2006;20(3):205–8. https://doi.org/10.1089/end.2006.20.205.
21. Rowley MW, Wolf JS Jr. Risk factors for conversion to hand assisted laparoscopy or open surgery during laparoscopic renal surgery. J Urol. 2011;185(3):940–4. https://doi.org/10.1016/j.juro.2010.10.063.

22. Richstone L, Seideman C, Baldinger L, et al. Conversion during laparoscopic surgery: frequency, indications and risk factors. 2008;180(3):855–9. https://doi.org/10.1016/j.juro.2008.05.026.
23. Luzzago S, Rosiello G, Pecoraro A, et al. Contemporary rates and predictors of open conversion during minimally invasive partial nephrectomy for kidney cancer. Surg Oncol. 2021;36:131–7. https://doi.org/10.1016/j.suronc.2020.12.004.
24. Khanna A, Campbell SC, Murthy PB, et al. Unplanned conversion from minimally invasive to open kidney surgery: the impact of robotics. J Endourol. 2020;34(9):955–63. https://doi.org/10.1089/end.2020.0357.
25. Klein G, Wang H, Elshabrawy A, et al. Analyzing national incidences and predictors of open conversion during minimally invasive partial nephrectomy for cT1 Renal Masses. 2021;35(1):30–8. https://doi.org/10.1089/end.2020.0161.
26. Russo P. Open partial nephrectomy. Personal technique and current outcomes. Arch Esp Urol. 2011;64(7):571–93.
27. Campbell SC, Novick AC, Streem SB, et al. Complications of nephron sparing surgery for renal tumors. J Urol. 1994;151(5):1177–80. https://doi.org/10.1016/s0022-5347(17)35207-2.
28. Wang H, Zhou L, Guo J, et al. Mini-flank supra-12th rib incision for open partial nephrectomy compared with laparoscopic partial nephrectomy and traditional open partial nephrectomy. PLoS ONE. 2014;9(2):e89155. https://doi.org/10.1371/journal.pone.0089155.
29. Diblasio CJ, Snyder ME, Russo P. Mini-flank supra-11th rib incision for open partial or radical nephrectomy. BJU Int. 2006;97(1):149–56. https://doi.org/10.1111/j.1464-410X.2006.05882.x.
30. Roussel E, Tasso G, Campi R, et al. Surgical management and outcomes of renal tumors arising from horseshoe kidneys: results from an international multicenter collaboration. Eur Urol. 2021;79(1):133–40. https://doi.org/10.1016/j.eururo.2020.09.012.
31. Caraballo ER, Palacios DA, Ouichai CS, et al. Open partial nephrectomy when a non-flank approach is required: indications and outcomes. World J Urol. 2019;37(3):515–22. https://doi.org/10.1007/s00345-018-2414-4.
32. Lane BR, Russo P, Uzzo RG, et al. Comparison of cold and warm ischemia during partial nephrectomy in 660 solitary kidneys reveals predominant role of nonmodifiable factors in determining ultimate renal function. J Urol. 2011;185(2):421–7. https://doi.org/10.1016/j.juro.2010.09.131.
33. Gill IS, Abreu SC, Desai MM, et al. Laparoscopic ice slush renal hypothermia for partial nephrectomy: the initial experience. J Urol. 2003;170(1):52–6. https://doi.org/10.1097/01.ju.0000072332.02529.10.
34. Abe T, Sazawa A, Harabayashi T, et al. Renal hypothermia with ice slush in laparoscopic partial nephrectomy: the outcome of renal function. J Endourol. 2012;26(11):1483–8. https://doi.org/10.1089/end.2012.0122.
35. Kaouk JH, Samarasekera D, Krishnan J, et al. Robotic partial nephrectomy with intracorporeal renal hypothermia using ice slush. Urology. 2014;84(3):712–8. https://doi.org/10.1016/j.urology.2014.05.008.
36. Castillo OA, Carlin AR, Fontana GL, et al. Robotic partial nephrectomy with selective parenchymal compression (Simon clamp). Actas Urol Esp. 2013;37(7):425–8. https://doi.org/10.1016/j.acuro.2012.11.009 Epub 2013 Feb 22.
37. Viprakasit DP, Altamar HO, Miller NL, et al. Selective renal parenchymal clamping in robotic partial nephrectomy: initial experience. Urology. 2010;76(3):750–3. https://doi.org/10.1016/j.urology.2010.03.051.
38. Cadeddu JA, Corwin TS, Traxer O, et al. Hemostatic laparoscopic partial nephrectomy: cable-tie compression. Urology. 2001;57(3):562–6. https://doi.org/10.1016/s0090-4295(00)01009-8.
39. Covarrubias FR, Gabilondo B, Borgen JL, et al. Partial nephrectomy for renal tumors using selective parenchymal clamping. Int Nephrol Urol. 2007;39(1):43–6. https://doi.org/10.1007/s11255-006-9069-6.

40. Ko YH, Choi H, Kang SG, et al. Efficacy of parenchymal compression in open partial nephrectomies: a comparison with conventional vascular clamping. Korean J Urol. 2010;51(1):8–14. https://doi.org/10.4111/kju.2010.51.1.8.
41. Erdem S, Tefik T, Mammadov A, et al. The use of self-retaining barbed suture for inner layer renorrhaphy significantly reduces warm ischemia time in laparoscopic partial nephrectomy: outcomes of a matched-pair analysis. J Endourol. 2013;27(4):452–8. https://doi.org/10.1089/end.2012.0574.
42. Bertolo R, Campi R, Klatte T, et al. Suture techniques during laparoscopic and robot-assisted partial nephrectomy: a systematic review and quantitative synthesis of peri-operative outcomes. BJU Int. 2019;123(6):923–46. https://doi.org/10.1111/bju.14537.
43. Pacheco M, Barros AA, Aroso IM, et al. Use of hemostatic agents for surgical bleeding in laparoscopic partial nephrectomy: biomaterials perspective. J Biomed Mater Res B Appl Biomater. 2020;108(8):3099–123. https://doi.org/10.1002/jbm.b.34637.
44. Lane BR, Gill IS. 7-year oncological outcomes after laparoscopic and open partial nephrectomy. J Urol. 2010;183(2):473–9. https://doi.org/10.1016/j.juro.2009.10.023.
45. Chang DK, Raheem AA, Kim KH, et al. Functional and oncological outcomes of open, laparoscopic and robot-assisted partial nephrectomy: a multicentre comparative matched-pair analyses with a median of 5 years' follow-up. BJU Int. 2018;122(4):618–26. https://doi.org/10.1111/bju.14250.
46. Xia L, Wang X, Xu T, et al. Systematic review and meta-analysis of comparative studies reporting perioperative outcomes of robot assisted partial nephrectomy versus open partial nephrectomy. J Endourol. 2017;31(9):893–909. https://doi.org/10.1089/end.2016.0351.
47. Seveso M, Grizzi F, Bozzini G, et al. Open partial nephrectomy: ancient art or currently available technique? Int Urol Nephrol. 2015;47(12):1923–32.
48. Gill IS, Kavoussi LR, Lane BR, et al. Comparison of 1,800 laparoscopic and open partial nephrectomies for single renal tumors. J Urol. 2007;178(1):41–6. https://doi.org/10.1016/j.juro.2007.03.038.
49. Lane BR, Novick AC, Babineau D, et al. Comparison of laparoscopic and open partial nephrectomy for tumor in a solitary kidney. J Urol. 2008;179(3):847–51; discussion 852.https://doi.org/10.1016/j.juro.2007.10.050.
50. Liu Z, Wang P, Xia D, et al. Comparison between laparoscopic and open partial nephrectomy: surgical, oncologic, and functional outcomes. Kaohsiung J Med Sci. 2013;29(11):624–8. https://doi.org/10.1016/j.kjms.2013.01.021.
51. Minervini A, Vittori G, Antonelli A, et al. Open versus robotic-assisted partial nephrectomy: a multicenter comparison study of perioperative results and complications. World J Urol. 2014;32(1):287–93. https://doi.org/10.1007/s00345-013-1136-x.
52. Alemozaffar M, Chang SL, Kacker R, et al. Comparing costs of robotic, laparoscopic, and open partial nephrectomy. J Endourol. 2013;27(5):560–5. https://doi.org/10.1089/end.2012.0462.

Decision-Making for Patients with Localized Renal Masses

14

Riccardo Campi, Selcuk Erdem, Onder Kara, Umberto Carbonara, Michele Marchioni, Alessio Pecoraro, Riccardo Bertolo, Alexandre Ingels, Maximilian Kriegmair, Nicola Pavan, Eduard Roussel, Angela Pecoraro, and Daniele Amparore

Renal cell carcinoma (RCC) represents approximately 2% of all diagnosed cancers and is the third most common genitourinary malignancy following prostate and bladder cancer [1].

The increased use of cross-sectional imaging has led to an increased incidence of incidentally detected localized renal masses, making personalized decision-making a compelling priority for clinicians, multidisciplinary teams and researchers [2].

R. Campi (✉) · A. Pecoraro
Unit of Urological Robotic Surgery and Renal Transplantation, University of Florence, Careggi Hospital, Florence, Italy
e-mail: riccardo.campi@unifi.it

R. Campi
Department of Experimental and Clinical Medicine, University of Florence, Florence, Italy

S. Erdem
Division of Urologic Oncology, Department of Urology, Istanbul University Istanbul Faculty of Medicine, Istanbul, Turkey

O. Kara
Department of Urology, Kocaeli University School of Medicine, Kocaeli, Turkey

U. Carbonara
Department of Emergency and Organ Transplantation-Urology, Andrology and Kidney Transplantation Unit, University of Bari, Bari, Italy

M. Marchioni
Department of Medical, Oral and Biotechnological Sciences, Laboratory of Biostatistics, University "G. D'Annunzio" Chieti-Pescara, Chieti, Italy

Department of Urology, SS Annunziata Hospital, "G. D'Annunzio" University of Chieti, Chieti, Italy

R. Bertolo
Department of Urology, San Carlo Di Nancy Hospital, Rome, Italy

© The Author(s), under exclusive license to Springer Nature Switzerland AG 2022
S. S. Goonewardene et al. (eds.), *Robotic Surgery for Renal Cancer*, Management of Urology, https://doi.org/10.1007/978-3-031-11000-9_14

Importantly, the epidemiological signature of RCC shows a sustained increase in incidence coupled with stable mortality [3], suggesting overdetection of renal cancers not destined to cause death superimposed on stable occurrence. In addition, while new imaging and other diagnostic methods allow earlier diagnosis with subsequent stage migration [4], they may also reveal benign renal masses and cancers that would otherwise not become clinically evident. Lastly, up to one-third of small tumours after nephrectomy are benign [5] and the vast majority of patients with localised renal masses pursue management without knowledge of histology [6].

While the gold standard for RCC diagnosis remains histopathological analysis of surgical or biopsy specimens, to date, a recent systematic review found that no serum or urinary biomarkers or innovative imaging modalities (including radiomics and deep-learning algorithms) have been validated or have shown clinical utility to better diagnose renal cancer (discriminating it from benign renal masses at the time of the decision-making process regarding the right treatment for the right patient).

In this scenario, pursuing an individualized decision-making algorithm in patients with localized renal masses is becoming increasingly important for urologists, given its potential consequences on the ultimate goals of care, namely oncologic efficacy, nephron preservation, and minimization of treatment-related morbidity. Localized RCC, often defined as clinical T1–2N0M0 RCC, is a disease that has indeed historically been managed with surgery. Of note, Chandrasekar et al. [1] recently provided a comprehensive overview of the influence of patient, kidney, tumour, and provider factors on three key decision points in the contemporary management of localized renal masses (LRM): (1) the decision on AS versus treatment; (2) the decision on treatment modality (tumour ablation [TA], partial nephrectomy [PN], or radical nephrectomy [RN]); and (3) the decision on surgical

---

A. Ingels
Department of Urology, University Hospital Henri Mondor, APHP, 51 Avenue du Maréchal de Lattre de Tassigny, 94010 Créteil, France

Biomaps, UMR1281, INSERM, CNRS, CEA, Université Paris Saclay, Villejuif, France

M. Kriegmair
Department of Urology, University Medical Centre Mannheim, Mannheim, Germany

N. Pavan
Department of Medical, Surgical and Health Science, Urology Clinic, University of Trieste, Trieste, Italy

E. Roussel
Department of Urology, University Hospitals Leuven, Leuven, Belgium

A. Pecoraro
Division of Urology, Department of Oncology, School of Medicine, University of Turin, San Luigi Hospital, Orbassano, Turin, Italy

D. Amparore
Division of Urology, Department of Oncology, School of Medicine, San Luigi Hospital, University of Turin, Orbassano, Turin, Italy

approach. Overall, this review unveils the inherent complexity of the decision-making schemes, grounded in the uncertainty regarding the biology of renal masses and patients, and traces the path to highlight the steps required to improve on value towards a patient-centered model of care for LRMs [7]. In reality, treatment decisions for patients with LRMs must balance several, often competing, priorities, and are grounded into a careful assessment of several patient-, tumor- and provider-related factors (Fig. 14.1).

Among patient-related factors, age remains an important consideration in the decision for treatment of patients with LRMs. Active surveillance (AS) with delayed intervention (DI) is a safe treatment option, especially for older patients, given the relatively low risk of metastatic progression in appropriately selected patients [8]. Yet, multiple studies confirmed the feasibility and safety of surgery (partial or radical nephrectomy) or ablation in older patients, if performed by experienced teams [1]. In recent years, patient comorbidity burden (assessed using established comorbidity indices, such as the Charlson Comorbidity Index and American Society of Anesthesiologists physical status) and patient frailty (defined as "a state of vulnerability to stressors") have also been increasingly recognized as important predictors of cancer treatment outcomes, with highly comorbid/frail patients considered candidates for AS or less aggressive treatment options such as ablation [1]. Additional relevant patient-related factors impacting on the key decision-points in patients with LRMs include: presence of familial/genetic syndromes (that may warrant modification to treatment and surveillance approaches

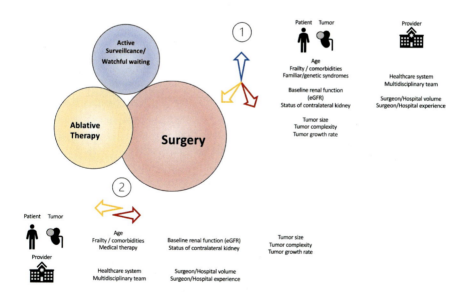

Fig. 14.1 Overview of the patient-, tumor- and provider-related factors influencing treatment decisions (active surveillance vs. treatment; ablation vs. surgery; partial vs. radical nephrectomy) for patients with localized renal masses

given the lower patient age and higher risk of tumor multifocality); anticoagulation/antiplatelet agent dependence and coagulopathy (e.g. patient utilization of anticoagulants and antiplatelet agents); history of previous surgery, and risk of COVID-19 morbidity. Notably, patient preferences and values regarding the goals of treatment also play a key role in shared decision-making.

Among kidney-related factors, the status of the contralateral kidney and the patient's baseline estimated (or measured) glomerular filtration rate may significantly influence on several decision-points in patients with LRMs. In fact, long-term preservation of kidney function is a critical consideration in the management of patients with localized RCC [1], and even patients on AS can experience a decline in the estimated glomerular filtration rate (eGFR). Importantly, the concept of surgical chronic kidney disease (CKD) has been introduced, suggesting that surgically induced renal dysfunction may have a different long-term prognosis than medically induced CKD. Overall, the risks of long-term harm related to CKD from surgical resection are controversial and must be balanced against immediate risks of more complex surgery (i.e. partial versus radical nephrectomy), especially among older/frailer patients or in patients with anatomically complex renal masses [1]. Lastly, even in patients with normal baseline eGFR, consideration should be given to future eGFR decline in those with concomitant medical comorbidities (i.e. favoring partial nephrectomy, AS or tumor ablation over radical nephrectomy).

Among tumor-related factors, tumor size, characterized by clinical T stage, tumor location and anatomic complexity (as objectified by the various proposed nephrometry scoring systems) and tumor growth pattern and kinetics remain critical factors contributing to treatment choice. This concept is well reported in the most recent Guidelines by the European Association of Urology (EAU) and American Urological Association (AUA) [9, 10].

Notably, tumor growth is not associated with the risk of malignancy, as (benign) oncocytomas may also demonstrate lesion growth. Tumor growth kinetics should be incorporated into the decision for a patient to remain on AS or proceed to DI, as it may be a predictor for metastatic progression [6]. Moreover, an infiltrative tumor growth pattern may point to more aggressive histology, and therefore favor more aggressive therapy [1]. Finally, tumor multifocality and bilateral renal lesions may significantly influence the decision-making strategy toward a careful balance between oncologic efficacy and renal function preservation.

It is important to stress that renal tumor biopsy may significantly influence on treatment decisions, despite its role in routine clinical practice is still controversial [11]. Percutaneous renal tumor biopsy can indeed help to reduce overtreatment and has been shown to be a safe and effective technique to sample indeterminate renal masses for which histology may impact treatment choice [1]. Nevertheless, in patients for whom AS is the only treatment choice, its impact on treatment decisions is still object of debate.

Aiming to solve the "biopsy always" versus "biopsy never" debate, liquid biomarkers and artificial intelligence (AI)-based imaging have been proposed to implement noninvasive diagnosis of RCC [11].

Beyond patient-, kidney- and tumor-related factors, the contemporary decision-making schemes for patients with LRMs are also highly influenced by healthcare system models, surgeons' and medical Centers' characteristics (such as experience, skills, and volume), as well as the availability and expertise of multidisciplinary tumour boards [1]. In particular, it has been shown that there is significant between-surgeon variability in outcomes after partial nephrectomy, even after adjusting for patient characteristics [12], and that the decisions regarding radical vs partial nephrectomy or open vs minimally-invasive surgical approach for highly complex or larger (cT1b-cT2) renal masses are often dependent on the surgeon's training and skills set.

Of note, medical care is increasingly being centralized to centers of excellence, based on robust evidence showing a volume-outcome relationship [13]. The data in RCC similarly support centralization [1].

In conclusion, treatment decision-making for patients with localized solid renal tumors has become complex and nuanced. To optimize treatment decisions and to realize the paradigm of precision oncology in patients with LRMs, integration of several patient-, kidney, tumor- and provider-related variables is mandatory and should be the goal of multidisciplinary tumour boards. Development of stronger predictive models, increased adoption of patient decision-aids and incorporation of patient preferences and values into routine decision-making schemes may improve care delivery in the future, toward the mission of patient-centered care for renal cancer [1, 11].

References

1. Chandrasekar T, Boorjian SA, Capitanio U, et al. Collaborative review: factors influencing treatment decisions for patients with a localized solid renal mass. Eur Urol. 2021;S0302-2838(21):00060-9. https://doi.org/10.1016/j.eururo.2021.01.021.
2. Rossi SH, Blick C, Handforth C, et al. Renal cancer gap analysis collaborative. essential research priorities in renal cancer: a modified delphi consensus statement. Eur Urol Focus. 2020;6(5):991-8. https://doi.org/10.1016/j.euf.2019.01.014.
3. Welch HG, Kramer BS, Black WC. Epidemiologic signatures in cancer. N Engl J Med. 2019;381(14):1378-86. https://doi.org/10.1056/NEJMsr1905447.
4. Patel HD, Gupta M, Joice GA, et al. Clinical stage migration and survival for renal cell carcinoma in the United States. Eur Urol Oncol. 2019;2(4):343-8. https://doi.org/10.1016/j.euo.2018.08.023.
5. Kim JH, Li S, Khandwala Y, et al. Association of prevalence of benign pathologic findings after partial nephrectomy with preoperative imaging patterns in the United States from 2007 to 2014. JAMA Surg. 2019;154(3):225-31. https://doi.org/10.1001/jamasurg.2018.4602.
6. Campi R, Sessa F, Corti F, et al. European Society of Residents in Urology (ESRU) and the EAU Young Academic Urologists (YAU) renal cancer group. Triggers for delayed intervention in patients with small renal masses undergoing active surveillance: a systematic review. Minerva Urol Nefrol. 2020;72(4):389-407. https://doi.org/10.23736/S0393-2249.20.03870-9.
7. Campi R, Mari A, Minervini A, et al. L'Essentiel est invisible pour les yeux: the art of decision-making and the mission of patient-centred care for patients with localised renal masses. Eur Urol. 2021;S0302-2838(21):00147. https://doi.org/10.1016/j.eururo.2021.02.027.

8. Klatte T, Berni A, Serni S, et al. Intermediate- and long-term oncological outcomes of active surveillance for localized renal masses: a systematic review and quantitative analysis. BJU Int. 2021. https://doi.org/10.1111/bju.15435.
9. Ljungberg B, Albiges L, Bedke J, et al. European Association of Urology (EAU) guidelines on Renal Cell Carcinoma (RCC). Version 2021. https://uroweb.org/guideline/renal-cell-carcinoma/.
10. Campbell S, Uzzo RG, Allaf ME, et al. Renal mass and localized renal cancer: AUA guideline. J Urol. 2017;198(3):520–9. https://doi.org/10.1016/j.juro.2017.04.100. Epub 2017 May 4.
11. Campi R, Stewart GD, Staehler M, et al. Novel liquid biomarkers and innovative imaging for kidney cancer diagnosis: what can be implemented in our practice today? A systematic review of the literature. Eur Urol Oncol. 2021;4(1):22–41. https://doi.org/10.1016/j.euo.2020.12.011.
12. Dagenais J, Bertolo R, Garisto J, et al. Variability in partial nephrectomy outcomes: does your surgeon matter? Eur Urol. 2019;75(4):628–34. https://doi.org/10.1016/j.eururo.2018.10.046.
13. Grande P, Campi R, Rouprêt M. Relationship of surgeon/hospital volume with outcomes in uro-oncology surgery. Curr Opin Urol. 2018;28(3):251–9. https://doi.org/10.1097/MOU.0000000000000490.

15

Management of Localized Renal Masses: The European Association of Urology (EAU), American Urological Association (AUA) and American Society of Clinical Oncology (ASCO) Guidelines' Perspective

Riccardo Campi, Selcuk Erdem, Onder Kara, Umberto Carbonara, Michele Marchioni, Alessio Pecoraro, Riccardo Bertolo, Alexandre Ingels, Maximilian Kriegmair, Nicola Pavan, Eduard Roussel, Angela Pecoraro, and Daniele Amparore

According to the European Association of Urology (EAU), American Urology Association (AUA) and American Society of Clinical Oncology (ASCO) Guidelines, the contemporary management options for patients with localized renal masses include: active surveillance, partial nephrectomy, radical nephrectomy, and thermal ablation.

R. Campi (✉) · A. Pecoraro
Unit of Urological Robotic Surgery and Renal Transplantation, University of Florence, Careggi Hospital, Florence, Italy
e-mail: riccardo.campi@unifi.it

R. Campi
Department of Experimental and Clinical Medicine, University of Florence, Florence, Italy

S. Erdem
Division of Urologic Oncology, Department of Urology, Istanbul University Istanbul Faculty of Medicine, Istanbul, Turkey

O. Kara
Department of Urology, Kocaeli University School of Medicine, Kocaeli, Turkey

U. Carbonara
Department of Emergency and Organ Transplantation-Urology, Andrology and Kidney Transplantation Unit, University of Bari, Bari, Italy

© The Author(s), under exclusive license to Springer Nature Switzerland AG 2022
S. S. Goonewardene et al. (eds.), *Robotic Surgery for Renal Cancer*, Management of Urology, https://doi.org/10.1007/978-3-031-11000-9_15

A detailed overview of the most recent Guidelines recommendations on the management of localized renal masses (LMR) is shown in Fig. 15.1.

Active surveillance is reported as a safety and effective option for small renal masses in well-selected patients [1, 2]. Particularly, in frail or comorbid patients with a limited life expectancy, physicians should prefer active surveillance when the potential risks of intervention outweigh the oncological benefits of intervention. Clearly, in case of clinical progression during follow-up, patients should be reassessed for potential delayed active treatment.

As such, all Guidelines underline that active surveillance should be considered for specific patient and/or tumour populations (Fig. 15.1).

Regarding surgical treatment of LRMs, all Guidelines recognize the pivotal role of partial nephrectomy as the gold standard treatment of all cT1 renal masses, if technically feasible and oncologically safe, given its advantages over radical nephrectomy in terms of renal function preservation [3, 4].

Furthermore, the latest EAU Guidelines also recommended to consider partial nephrectomy for selected patients with cT2 renal masses if affected by chronic kidney disease or with a solitary kidney [5]. Of note, the latest AUA Guidelines stress that clinicians should prioritize nephron-sparing approaches for patients with solid or Bosniak 3/4 complex cystic renal masses and an anatomic or functionally solitary kidney, bilateral tumors, known familial RCC, preexisting CKD,

---

M. Marchioni
Department of Medical, Oral and Biotechnological Sciences, Laboratory of Biostatistics, University "G. D'Annunzio" Chieti-Pescara, Chieti, Italy

Department of Urology, SS Annunziata Hospital, "G. D'Annunzio" University of Chieti, Chieti, Italy

R. Bertolo
Department of Urology, San Carlo Di Nancy Hospital, Rome, Italy

A. Ingels
Department of Urology, University Hospital Henri Mondor, APHP, 51 Avenue du Maréchal de Lattre de Tassigny, 94010 Créteil, France

Biomaps, UMR1281, INSERM, CNRS, CEA, Université Paris Saclay, Villejuif, France

M. Kriegmair
Department of Urology, University Medical Centre Mannheim, Mannheim, Germany

N. Pavan
Department of Medical, Surgical and Health Science, Urology Clinic, University of Trieste, Trieste, Italy

E. Roussel
Department of Urology, University Hospitals Leuven, Leuven, Belgium

A. Pecoraro · D. Amparore
Division of Urology, Department of Oncology, School of Medicine, University of Turin, San Luigi Hospital, Orbassano, Turin, Italy

Treatment	European Association of Urology (EAU)	American Urological Association (AUA)	ASCO American Society of Clinical Oncology
Active Surveillance (AS)	• Offer AS or TA to frail and/or comorbid patients with small renal masses. **(weak)** • When TA or AS are offered, discuss with patients about the harms/benefits with regards to oncological outcomes and complications. **(strong)**	• For patients with a solid renal mass < 2cm, or those that are complex but predominantly cystic, clinicians may elect AS with potential for delayed intervention for initial management. **(Conditional Recommendation; Evidence Level: Grade C)** • [...] AS with potential for delayed intervention may be pursued only if the patient understands and is willing to accept the associated oncologic risks. [...]. **(Moderate Recommendation; Evidence Level: Grade C)**	• AS should be an initial management option for patients who have significant comorbidities and limited life expectancy. **(type: evidence based; evidence quality: intermediate; strength of recommendation: moderate)**
Partial Nephrectomy (PN)	• Offer PN to patients with T1 tumours. **(strong)** • Offer PN to patients with T2 tumours and a solitary kidney or chronic kidney disease, if technically feasible. **(weak)**	• Clinicians should prioritize PN for the management of the cT1a renal mass when intervention is indicated. [...]. **(Moderate Recommendation; Evidence Level: Grade B)** • Clinicians should prioritize nephron-sparing approaches for patients with solid or Bosniak 3/4 complex cystic renal masses and an anatomic or functionally solitary kidney, bilateral tumors, known familial RCC, preexisting CKD, or proteinuria. **(Moderate Recommendation; Evidence Level: Grade C)** • Nephron-sparing approaches should be considered for patients with solid or Bosniak 3/4 complex cystic renal masses who are young, have multifocal masses, or comorbidities that are likely to impact renal function in the future [...]. **(Moderate Recommendation; Evidence Level: Grade C)**	• PN for small renal masses is the standard treatment that should be offered to all patients for whom an intervention is indicated and who possess a tumour that is amenable to this approach. **(type: evidence based; evidence quality: intermediate; strength of recommendation: strong)**
Radical Nephrectomy (RN)	• Offer laparoscopic RN to patients with T2 tumours and localised masses not treatable by PN. **(strong)**	• Clinicians should consider RN for patients with a solid or Bosniak 3/4 complex cystic renal mass whenever increased oncologic potential is suggested by tumor size, renal mass biopsy (if obtained), and/or imaging. **(Moderate Recommendation; Evidence Level: Grade B)**	• RN for small renal masses should be reserved only for patients who possess a tumor of significant complexity that is not amenable to PN [...] **(type: evidence based; evidence quality: intermediate; strength of recommendation: strong)**
Minimally Invasive Surgical Approach	• Do not perform minimally invasive surgery if this approach may compromise oncological-, functional- and peri-operative outcomes. **(strong)**	• In patients undergoing surgical excision of a renal mass, a minimally invasive approach should be considered when it would not compromise oncologic, functional, and perioperative outcomes. **(Expert Opinion)**	Not reported.
Thermal Ablation (TA)	• Do not routinely offer TA for tumours > 3 cm and cryoablation for tumours > 4 cm. **(weak)** • Offer AS or TA to frail and/or comorbid patients with small renal masses. **(weak)** • Perform a percutaneous renal mass biopsy prior to, and not concomitantly with, TA. **(strong)** • When TA or AS are offered, discuss with patients about the harms/benefits with regards to oncological outcomes and complications. **(strong)**	• Clinicians should consider TA as an alternate approach for the management of cT1a solid renal masses <3 cm in size [...]. **(Moderate Recommendation; Evidence Level: Grade C)** • Both radiofrequency ablation (RFA) and cryoablation may be offered as options for patients who elect TA. **(Conditional Recommendation; Evidence Level: Grade C)** • A renal mass biopsy should be performed prior to (preferred) or at the time of ablation to provide pathologic diagnosis and guide subsequent surveillance. **(Expert Opinion)** • Counseling about TA should include information regarding an increased likelihood of tumor persistence or local recurrence after primary TA relative to surgical excision [...]. **(Strong Recommendation; Evidence Level: Grade B)**	• Percutaneous TA should be considered an option for patients who possess tumours such that complete ablation will be achieved. A biopsy should be obtained before or at the time of ablation. **(type: evidence based; evidence quality: intermediate; strength of recommendation: moderate)**

Fig. 15.1 Overview of the most recent European Association of Urology (EAU), American Urological Association (AUA) and American Society of Clinical Oncology (ASCO) Guidelines' recommendations on the management of localized renal masses

or proteinuria, as well as for those who are young, have multifocal masses, or comorbidities that are likely to impact renal function in the future.

While radical nephrectomy has still a valuable role for specific patient characteristics, especially when partial nephrectomy is not technically feasible, it is however associated with a detrimental impact on postoperative renal function and a potential risk of overtreatment [6]. A detailed overview of the contemporary decision-making schemes regarding partial versus radical nephrectomy in patients is discussed in the previous sub-chapter. Regardless from the indication to perform radical nephrectomy, all Guidelines coherently recommend to perform a minimally invasive (laparoscopic or robotic) procedure, provided that this approach does not jeopardize perioperative, functional or oncological outcomes [7]. Yet, the well-known possible advantages of robotic-assisted and laparoscopic approaches for partial and radical nephrectomy in terms of hospital stay and blood loss (as compared to the open counterpart) are recognized by all Guideline panels. If preoperative imaging and intraoperative findings suggest an organ-confined disease, ipsilateral adrenalectomy and extended lymph node dissection should be avoided at the time of nephrectomy.

Notably, all international Guidelines recognize a role for percutaneous tumor ablation in select patients with LRMs (Fig. 15.1). In detail, while clinicians may offered thermal ablation to frail/comorbid patients with small renal masses, the EAU Guidelines strongly recommend to perform renal tumor biopsy *before* the procedure to optimize decision-making, and to avoid tumor ablation for tumours >3 cm and cryoablation for tumours >4 cm. Both radiofrequency ablation (RFA) and cryoablation may be offered as options for patients who elect TA. Of note, counseling about tumor ablation should include information regarding an increased likelihood of tumor persistence or local recurrence after relative to surgical excision [8]. According to EAU and AUA guidelines, when thermal ablation is planned, physicians should discuss with patients all potential benefits and harms of the procedure, considering the results of renal mass biopsy previously performed. Patients must be informed about oncological outcomes, especially about the higher risk of recurrence and persistence of tumor compared to partial nephrectomy [9].

In conclusion, the management of LRMs is an evolving field and is object of increasing interest among clinicians, surgeons, and researchers. Although different therapeutic strategies are available, the ultimate goal of treatment is to achieve the *Trifecta* (oncologic efficacy, renal function preservation, and minimization of treatment-related morbidity) while improving patient's quality of life. The current Guidelines from the major international Urological Associations reflect this concept and provide a framework to pursue a patient-centered, value-based model of care in routine clinical practice.

References

1. Jewett MA, Mattar K, Basiuk J, et al. Active surveillance of small renal masses: progression patterns of early stage kidney cancer. Eur Urol. 2011;60(1):39–44. https://doi.org/10.1016/j.eururo.2011.03.030.
2. Pierorazio PM, Johnson MH, Ball MW, et al. Five-year analysis of a multi-institutional prospective clinical trial of delayed intervention and surveillance for small renal masses: the DISSRM registry. Eur Urol. 2015;68(3):408–15. https://doi.org/10.1016/j.eururo.2015.02.001.
3. MacLennan S, Imamura M, Lapitan MC, et al. UCAN systematic review reference group; EAU renal cancer guideline panel. Systematic review of perioperative and quality-of-life outcomes following surgical management of localised renal cancer. Eur Urol. 2012;62(6):1097–117. https://doi.org/10.1016/j.eururo.2012.07.028.
4. Van Poppel H, Da Pozzo L, Albrecht W, et al. A prospective, randomised EORTC intergroup phase 3 study comparing the oncologic outcome of elective nephron-sparing surgery and radical nephrectomy for low-stage renal cell carcinoma. Eur Urol. 2011;59(4):543–52. https://doi.org/10.1016/j.eururo.2010.12.013.
5. Mir MC, Derweesh I, Porpiglia F, et al. Partial nephrectomy versus radical nephrectomy for clinical T1b and T2 renal tumors: a systematic review and meta-analysis of comparative studies. Eur Urol. 2017;71(4):606–17. https://doi.org/10.1016/j.eururo.2016.08.060.
6. Lane BR, Campbell SC, Demirjian S, et al. Surgically induced chronic kidney disease may be associated with a lower risk of progression and mortality than medical chronic kidney disease. J Urol. 2013;189(5):1649–55. https://doi.org/10.1016/j.juro.2012.11.121.
7. Wang L, Wang L, Yang Q, et al. Retroperitoneal laparoscopic and open radical nephrectomy for T1 renal cell carcinoma. J Endourol. 2009;23(9):1509–12. https://doi.org/10.1089/end.2009.0381.
8. Campbell S, Uzzo RG, Allaf ME, et al. Renal mass and localized renal cancer: AUA guideline. J Urol. 2017;198(3):520–9. https://doi.org/10.1016/j.juro.2017.04.100 Epub 2017 May 4.
9. Pierorazio PM, Johnson MH, Patel HD, et al. Management of renal masses and localized renal cancer: systematic review and meta-analysis. J Urol. 2016;196(4):989–99. https://doi.org/10.1016/j.juro.2016.04.081.

Active Surveillance and Watchful Waiting in Renal Cancer

16

Riccardo Campi, Selcuk Erdem, Onder Kara, Umberto Carbonara, Michele Marchioni, Alessio Pecoraro, Riccardo Bertolo, Alexandre Ingels, Maximilian Kriegmair, Nicola Pavan, Eduard Roussel, Angela Pecoraro, and Daniele Amparore

Due to the diffusion and large use of abdominal imaging small renal masses are more frequently diagnosed in the last few years [1]. However, a not negligible proportion of these lesions represent pathologically benign tumors (up to 30%) or tumors with low malignant potential [1, 2]. Indeed, even in presence of malignant histology large population-based studies showed that in presence of localized renal cell carcinoma the 5-year overall survival rates exceed 90% [3].

R. Campi (✉) · A. Pecoraro
Unit of Urological Robotic Surgery and Renal Transplantation, University of Florence, Careggi Hospital, Florence, Italy
e-mail: riccardo.campi@unifi.it

R. Campi
Department of Experimental and Clinical Medicine, University of Florence, Florence, Italy

S. Erdem
Division of Urologic Oncology, Department of Urology, Istanbul University Istanbul Faculty of Medicine, Istanbul, Turkey

O. Kara
Department of Urology, Kocaeli University School of Medicine, Kocaeli, Turkey

U. Carbonara
Department of Emergency and Organ Transplantation-Urology, Andrology and Kidney Transplantation Unit, University of Bari, Bari, Italy

M. Marchioni
Department of Medical, Oral and Biotechnological Sciences, Laboratory of Biostatistics, University "G. D'Annunzio" Chieti-Pescara, Chieti, Italy

Department of Urology, SS Annunziata Hospital, "G. D'Annunzio" University of Chieti, Chieti, Italy

R. Bertolo
Department of Urology, San Carlo Di Nancy Hospital, Rome, Italy

© The Author(s), under exclusive license to Springer Nature Switzerland AG 2022
S. S. Goonewardene et al. (eds.), *Robotic Surgery for Renal Cancer*, Management of Urology, https://doi.org/10.1007/978-3-031-11000-9_16

In these specific group of patients overdiagnosis and overtreatment should be considered as dangerous as wrong treatment choice. Indeed, even when nephron sparing surgery is used, these patients might undergo unnecessary care, psychological stress, surgical complications, superfluous financial expenses and loss of kidney function with no reasonable survival benefit [1]. This scenario is even worse when considering that more than half of patients with pT1a tumors are treated with radical nephrectomy [4].

Considering that, new strategies have been proposed and tested to reduce the overdiagnosis and overtreatment of small renal masses. Such strategies include a limitation of superfluous imaging in order to reduce the overdiagnosis and a combination of treatments to reduce the overtreatment. Alternative strategies to surgery (radical or partial nephrectomy as well as tumor ablation) are represented by active surveillance and delayed treatment or watchful waiting. These approaches could be used in combination with renal biopsy in order to improve patient's selection [1].

Active surveillance and delayed treatment have been prospectively explored by the Johns Hopkins's group within the Delayed Intervention and Surveillance for Small Renal Masses (DISSRM) registry. Authors developed a diagnostic and therapeutic algorithm where all adult patients with asymptomatic small renal cortical tumors (≤4 cm) at axial imaging were proposed to be enrolled in the DISSRM. Patients could either be treated with intervention (partial nephrectomy or tumor ablation) or undergo surveillance. The observational protocol included ultrasound every 6 months for the first two years and every 12 months for the subsequent 3 years. Patients who experienced a mass growth rate >0.5 cm/year or with a mass >4 cm or developed hematuria were differed to delayed intervention [5]. At 5 years 223 patients were followed in the active surveillance arm and only the 9% crossed over to delayed treatment. Cancer specific survival was approximately 100% in both groups and overall survival rates at

---

A. Ingels
Department of Urology, University Hospital Henri Mondor, APHP, 51 Avenue du Maréchal de Lattre de Tassigny, 94010 Créteil, France

Biomaps, UMR1281, INSERM, CNRS, CEA, Université Paris Saclay, Villejuif, France

M. Kriegmair
Department of Urology, University Medical Centre Mannheim, Mannheim, Germany

N. Pavan
Department of Medical, Surgical and Health Science, Urology Clinic, University of Trieste, Trieste, Italy

E. Roussel
Department of Urology, University Hospitals Leuven, Leuven, Belgium

A. Pecoraro · D. Amparore
Division of Urology, Department of Oncology, School of Medicine, University of Turin, San Luigi Hospital, Orbassano, Turin, Italy

5 year were similar too (92% vs. 75% in the primary intervention vs. active surveillance arm, respectively; p = 0.06) [5]. For those treated with delayed intervention the median time on active surveillance is about 12 months [2]. Main reasons for switching to intervention were growth rate >0.5 cm/year (50%) and patients' choice (47.8%). Moreover, a radical nephrectomy was necessary only in 10.9% of patients, confirming the feasibility of a nephron sparing approach also when treatment is delayed [2]. In addition, none of the included patient died for the cancer or had a metastatic progression [2]. Similar results were reported by Uzzo's group [6]. Authors also showed no association with differed treatment and overall survival when compared to active surveillance (HR: 1.34; p = 0.3) [6]. More important cancer specific mortality rates were reported to be about 1.2% in the examined cohort with no difference in terms of treatment choice [6]. Previous studies showed that active surveillance patients are generally older or with higher comorbidity burden [7]. Even DISSRM group suggested a tool based on comorbidities and age to select patients most suitable for active surveillance [8]. Such strategies are justified by the results of various studies showing no detrimental effect of active surveillance in elderly when compared to active treatments [9]. However, most recent evidence from the DISSRM support the use of active surveillance as primary strategy also in younger patients [10]. Indeed, in 60 or younger delayed intervention is necessary only in about one third of cases [10]. Overall survival also exceeds 90% with no meaningful or statistically significant differences between the groups (Metcalf MR). In addition, cancer specific survival remains 100% independently from the treatment approach (Metcalf MR).

The cornerstones for active surveillance strategies remain patients' selection and follow-up strategies. For patients' selection the DISSRM tool seems to offer a handful help to clinicians, however it is our opinion that, for patients who are candidate to active surveillance renal mass biopsy should be recommended since the low complication rates (<0.4%) [11]. On the other hand, the follow-up of these patients is still matter of debate. However, ultrasound seems to be a good choice, considering its safety profile and that no radiations are employed. Even though approximately 5% of small renal masses on active surveillance might not be optimally followed by ultrasound and could "disappear" [12]. This is the case in particular with really small renal masses (<1 cm), but after considering the indolent nature of these lesions it seems reasonable to not change the therapeutic and diagnostic approach even in those with "phantom lesions" [12]. The timing for delayed treatment is also of importance. Growth rate is the suggested parameter in several cases, however linear growth rate has shown low accuracy in predicting overall survival [6]. So new studies should be designed to find the best predictor of progression and survival in order to tailor the treatment choice on patients' characteristics.

Finally, an approach that do not include any possible differed or primary treatment or surveillance protocol, such as watchful waiting, should be used only in patients that are not eligible for any curative approach, such as those with short life expectancy. Indeed, even if small a certain probability of metastases or local spreading is possible also for renal masses <4 cm.

References

1. Sohlberg EM, Metzner TJ, Leppert JT. The harms of overdiagnosis and overtreatment in patients with small renal masses: a mini-review. Eur Urol Focus. 2019;5(6):943–5. https://doi.org/10.1016/j.euf.2019.03.006.
2. Gupta M, Alam R, Patel HD, et al. Use of delayed intervention for small renal masses initially managed with active surveillance. Urol Oncol. 2019;37(1):18–25. https://doi.org/10.1016/j.urolonc.2018.10.001.
3. Siegel RL, Miller KD, Fuchs HE, et al. Cancer Statistics, 2021. CA Cancer J Clin. 2021;71(1):7–33. https://doi.org/10.3322/caac.21654.
4. Marchioni M, Preisser F, Bandini M, et al. Comparison of partial versus radical nephrectomy effect on other-cause mortality, cancer-specific mortality, and 30-day mortality in patients older than 75 years. Eur Urol Focus. 2019;5(3):467–73. https://doi.org/10.1016/j.euf.2018.01.007.
5. Pierorazio PM, Johnson MH, Ball MW, et al. Five-year analysis of a multi-institutional prospective clinical trial of delayed intervention and surveillance for small renal masses: the DISSRM registry. Eur Urol. 2015;68(3):408–15. https://doi.org/10.1016/j.eururo.2015.02.001.
6. McIntosh AG, Ristau BT, Ruth K, et al. Active surveillance for localized renal masses: tumor growth, delayed intervention rates, and >5-yr clinical outcomes. Eur Urol. 2018;74(2):157–64. https://doi.org/10.1016/j.eururo.2018.03.011.
7. Trudeau V, Larcher A, Sun M, et al. Sociodemographic disparities in the nonoperative management of small renal masses. Clin Genitourin Cancer. 2016;14(2):e177–82. https://doi.org/10.1016/j.clgc.2015.10.011.
8. Sotimehin AE, Patel HD, Alam R, et al. Selecting patients with small renal masses for active surveillance: a domain based score from a prospective cohort study. J Urol. 2019;201(5):886–92. https://doi.org/10.1097/JU.0000000000000033.
9. Marchioni M, Cheaib JG, Takagi T, et al. Active surveillance for small renal masses in elderly patients does not increase overall mortality rates compared to primary intervention: a propensity score weighted analysis. Minerva Urol Nefrol. 2020. https://doi.org/10.23736/S0393-2249.20.03785-6.
10. Metcalf MR, Cheaib JG, Biles MJ, et al. Outcomes of active surveillance for young patients with small renal masses: prospective data from the DISSRM registry. J Urol. 2021;205(5):1286–93. https://doi.org/10.1097/JU.0000000000001575.
11. Ozambela M Jr, Wang Y, Leow JJ, et al. Contemporary trends in percutaneous renal mass biopsy utilization in the United States. Urol Oncol. 2020;38(11):835–43. https://doi.org/10.1016/j.urolonc.2020.07.022.
12. Srivastava A, Patel HD, Gupta M, et al. The incidence, predictors, and survival of disappearing small renal masses on active surveillance. Urol Oncol. 2020;38(2):42.e1–42.e6. https://doi.org/10.1016/j.urolonc.2019.10.005.

Ablative Therapies in Renal Cancer

17

Riccardo Campi, Selcuk Erdem, Onder Kara, Umberto Carbonara, Michele Marchioni, Alessio Pecoraro, Riccardo Bertolo, Alexandre Ingels, Maximilian Kriegmair, Nicola Pavan, Eduard Roussel, Angela Pecoraro, and Daniele Amparore

Current guidelines by the American Urological Association (AUA), European Association for Urology (EAU), National Comprehensive Cancer Network (NCCN) for the small renal masses (SRMs) recommend partial nephrectomy (PN) as the standard-of-care, compared to radical nephrectomy (RN) [1–3]. Nevertheless, in the last decades, ablative techniques have been increasing as an alternative

R. Campi (✉) · A. Pecoraro
Unit of Urological Robotic Surgery and Renal Transplantation, University of Florence, Careggi Hospital, Florence, Italy
e-mail: riccardo.campi@unifi.it

R. Campi
Department of Experimental and Clinical Medicine, University of Florence, Florence, Italy

S. Erdem
Division of Urologic Oncology, Department of Urology, Istanbul University Istanbul Faculty of Medicine, Istanbul, Turkey

O. Kara
Department of Urology, Kocaeli University School of Medicine, Kocaeli, Turkey

U. Carbonara
Andrology and Kidney Transplantation Unit, Department of Emergency and Organ Transplantation-Urology, University of Bari, Bari, Italy

M. Marchioni
Laboratory of Biostatistics, Department of Medical, Oral and Biotechnological Sciences, University "G. D'Annunzio" Chieti-Pescara, Chieti, Italy

Department of Urology, SS Annunziata Hospital, "G. D'Annunzio" University of Chieti, Chieti, Italy

R. Bertolo
Department of Urology, San Carlo Di Nancy Hospital, Rome, Italy

Table 17.1 EAU versus NCCN versus AUA guidelines for ablative techniques

EAU 2021	NCCN V1.2021	AUA 2017
Offer thermal ablation or cryoablation to frail and/or comorbid patients with small renal masses	Thermal ablation is an option for cT1 renal mass <3 cm	Consider thermal ablation as an alternate approach for cT1a renal masses <3 cm
When thermal ablation and cryoablation are offered, inform patients about the higher risk of local recurrence and/or tumour progression	May also be an option for masses >3 cm, but higher risk of local recurrence or persistence and complications	Both radiofrequency ablation and cryoablation are options. A percutaneous technique is preferred
Do not routinely offer thermal ablation for tumours >3 cm and cryoablation for tumours >4 cm	Biopsy confirms a diagnosis for malignancy	A renal mass biopsy should be performed prior to ablation
Biopsy is recommended before ablative therapies	Higher local recurrence rates than conventional surgery and may require multiple treatments to achieve the same oncological outcomes	Inform on the likelihood of tumor persistence or local recurrence after thermal ablation relative to surgical extirpation, which may be addressed with repeat ablation

to surgical approaches, especially in patients who are unfit for surgery or with the low probability of aggressive malignancy (Table 17.1).

The most widely used ablation therapies consist of radiofrequency ablation (RFA), cryoablation (CRA) and microwave ablation (MVA).

A. Ingels
Department of Urology, University Hospital Henri Mondor, APHP, 51 Avenue du Maréchal de Lattre de Tassigny, 94010 Créteil, France

Biomaps, UMR1281, INSERM, CNRS, CEA, Université Paris Saclay, Villejuif, France

M. Kriegmair
Department of Urology, University Medical Centre Mannheim, Mannheim, Germany

N. Pavan
Urology Clinic, Department of Medical, Surgical and Health Science, University of Trieste, Trieste, Italy

E. Roussel
Department of Urology, University Hospitals Leuven, Leuven, Belgium

A. Pecoraro · D. Amparore
Division of Urology, Department of Oncology, School of Medicine, University of Turin, San Luigi Hospital, Orbassano (Turin), Italy

17.1 Radiofrequency

Percutaneous RFA is the direct placement of one or more radiofrequency electrodes into the tumour tissue by using ultrasound, computed tomography (CT) or magnetic resonance guidance. RFA relies on radiofrequency energy that creates tissue heating. High-frequency (375–400 kHz) alternating electric current induces oscillation of ions within the tissue with a 5–20 min process repeated until the impedance threshold is reached twice. Ions oscillation results in molecular friction and heat production up to temperatures of 60–90 °C [4].

17.2 Microwave Ablation

Like RFA, MWA uses electromagnetic waves to generate heat and also kills cells by mechanisms of direct hyperthermic injury. An electromagnetic field, which is typically between 900–2500 MHz, is created through an intratumorally placed antenna. This causes polar molecules (e.g., water) to realign, which increases kinetic energy in the tissue surrounding the probe. The resulting increase in temperature ultimately causes coagulation necrosis of the target tissue. Compared to RFA, the potential size of the ablation zone is larger due to a faster tissue necrosis (10 min), limited impact of tissue impedance on energy deposition and higher temperatures created with secondary increased passive heating [5]. However, the high heat generated by MWA can lead to significant urothelial injury.

17.3 Cryoablation

In contrast to the hyperthermic techniques, CRA uses cold injury to kill tumours. CRA uses liquefied gases that cool as they expand, such as argon and relies on low temperature (between −20 and −40 °C) to induce cell death. Argon-based cryoprobes are used to cool the tumor through the Joule–Thomson principle tissue destruction occurs through both freezing and thawing (double freeze–thaw cycle) [4]. Usually, a laparoscopic approach is preferred because it allows accurate puncture of tumor with cryoprobes under direct vision [6]. Relative to RFA, CRA is less harmful to the renal collecting system and can be monitoring during the ablation with imaging (US) and it is potentially more effective for larger tumors. However, RFA has a shorter procedure time, lower bleeding complications and lower costs. The success of ablation generally is measured radiologically (as lack of contrast enhancement). However, the definition of technical success/efficacy is variable and not standardized. Overall complication rates, metastases free survival (MFS), cancer specific survival (CSS) and overall survival (OS) are similar for the two techniques. Serial axial CT or MRI imaging most commonly used during follow-up [7].

17.4 Ablation Planning

ABLATE (Table 17.2) is a practical algorithm for ablation planning based on renal tumor characteristics identifiable on pre-ablation cross-sectional imaging. By utilizing this system, it is possible to identify potential technical challenges of ablation for a specific renal mass and thereby plan the procedure accordingly to increase the odds of a successful outcome and decrease the risk of complications. This includes identification of renal tumor characteristics and locations that may require protective ablation techniques, such as hydro-displacement, retrograde pyelo-perfusion via an externalized ureteral stent, or pre-ablation arterial tumor embolization [8].

Table 17.2 The Ablate Algorithm for ablation planning

A (Axial tumor diameter)
Local treatment failures increase with increasing tumor size
Ablation-related bleeding complications increase with increasing tumor size
If the tumor is ≥3 cm in diameter, consider cryoablation
If the tumor is ≥5 cm in diameter, consider pre-ablation tumor embolization
B (Bowel proximity)
Ablation-related bowel injury may result in long-term catheter drainage or surgery
If the tumor is ≤1 cm from the colon or small bowel, patient repositioning or bowel displacement manoeuvres will likely be necessary
L (Location within kidney)
Ablation can be performed safely and effectively in locations other than just the posterior and lateral kidney
If the tumor is in the anterior kidney, hydro displacement will likely be necessary to protect adjacent bowel
If the tumor is in the anterolateral upper pole of the right kidney, a transhepatic approach may be necessary
If the tumor is in the anteromedial upper pole of the kidney near the adrenal gland, close blood pressure monitoring and even pre-ablation α-receptor blockade may be necessary
If the tumor is in the medial lower pole of the kidney, displacement techniques may be required to protect the nerves that run along the anterior surface of the psoas muscle
A (Adjacency to ureter)
Ablation-related ureteral injuries may require long-term stenting or surgery
If the tumor is ≤1 cm from the ureter, retrograde pyelo-perfusion via an externalized ureteral stent or ureteral displacement manoeuvres will likely be necessary
T (Touching renal sinus fat)
Local treatment failures are more common with treatment of central tumors (those that touch renal sinus fat)
Ablation-related renal collecting system injuries and major bleeding complications are more frequent with treatment of tumours that touch renal sinus fat
If the tumor touches renal sinus fat, consider cryoablation

Table 17.3 Complications post ablation

	Post-ablation syndrome (9%)	Fever and flu-like symptoms (myalgia, malaise, mild pain)
	Bleeding	Hematoma formation (6%)
		Transfusion rate (<1%)
	Non-target thermal Injury	Ureter (urinary fistula, ureteral obstruction)
		Bowel (perforation, fistula)
		Genitofemoral nerve (chronic pain)
		Psoas muscle (impairment of hip flexion)
		Adrenal gland (hypertensive crisis)
	Less frequent complications	Tumor seeding
		Grounding pad burns
		Infection
		Pneumothorax
		Cryoshock (theoretical)

17.5 Complications

Overall complication rate 7.8–12.9% with most complications Clavien grade <3. Tumor size, location and medical comorbidities are important predictors of complications. The main complications are reported in Table 17.3 [9].

17.6 Ablative Techniques Versus Surgery

To date, no randomized clinical trials exist on ablative techniques and surgery. Two recorded clinical trials completed the recruitment in 2015 (NCT01608165) and in 2016 (NCT02850809), but never published their results. A recent systematic review of the literature [10] compared oncologic and functional outcomes after PN and ablation for treating clinical T1a renal masses. Perioperative complications were fewer in the ablation group than in the PN group (OR = 0.76; 95% CI:0.60–0.97; p = 0.025), but ablation group was associated with increased risk of local recurrence (OR = 1.88; 95% CI:1.29–2.72; p = 0.001) and lower OS (HR = 1.53; 95% CI:1.16–2.00; p = 0.002). CSS and DFS were comparable in two groups. Decline of renal function at 6-month follow up was lower in ablation than PN (WMD = 3.32; 95% CI:0.04–6.60; p = 0.047). Besides, ablation had a trend towards lower reduction of renal function of long-term follow up (WMD = 3.06; 95% CI:2.13–8.25; p = 0.247).

Another systematic review examined current evidence for cryoablation, radiofrequency ablation, and microwave ablation of T1b renal masses. They found that CRA and MWA likely yield the best opportunity for durable oncologic efficacy, notwithstanding current evidence is heterogeneous and limited by thermal modality utilized, number of probes/antennae used, and operator technique (laparoscopic versus percutaneous, method of intraprocedural monitoring) [5]. However, as reported in a large population-based study, cryoablation should not be recommended outside of clinical trial or institutional protocols in T1b RCC patients, because of a 2.5-fold increase in CSM relative to PN [11].

Finally, the EAU Renal Cell Carcinoma (RCC) Guideline Panel performed a protocol driven systematic review on thermal ablation (TA) compared with PN for T1N0M0 renal masses, in order to provide evidence to support its recommendations. They found that the current data are inadequate to make any strong and clear conclusions regarding the clinical effectiveness of TA for treating T1N0M0 renal masses compared with PN. Therefore, TA may be cautiously considered an alternative to PN for T1N0M0 renal masses, but patients must be counselled carefully regarding the prevailing uncertainties. We recommend specific steps to improve the evidence base based on robust primary and secondary studies [12].

References

1. Ljungberg B, Albiges L, Bedke J, et al. EAU guidelines on RCC. Version 2021. Available from: http://uroweb.org/guidelines/compilations-of-all-guidelines/.
2. Campbell S, Uzzo RG, Allaf ME, et al. Renal mass and localized renal cancer: AUA guideline. J Urol. 2017;198(3):520–9. https://doi.org/10.1016/j.juro.2017.04.100. Epub 2017 May 4.
3. Motzer RJ, Jonasch E, Boyle S, et al. NCCN guidelines insights: kidney cancer, Version 1.2021. J Natl Compr Canc Netw. 2020;18(9):1160–70. https://doi.org/10.6004/jnccn.2020.0043.
4. Chu KF, Dupuy DE. Thermal ablation of tumours: biological mechanisms and advances in therapy. Nat Rev Cancer. 2014;14(3):199–208. https://doi.org/10.1038/nrc3672.
5. Welch BT, Shah PH, Thompson RH, et al. The current status of thermal ablation in the management of T1b renal masses. Int J Hyperthermia. 2019;36(2):31–6. https://doi.org/10.1080/02656736.2019.1605097.
6. Hinshaw JL, Shadid AM, Nakada SY, et al. Comparison of percutaneous and laparoscopic cryoablation for the treatment of solid renal masses. AJR Am J Roentgenol. 2008;191(4):1159–68. https://doi.org/10.2214/AJR.07.3706.
7. Ahmed M. Technology assessment committee of the society of interventional radiology. Image-guided tumor ablation: standardization of terminology and reporting criteria–a 10-year update: supplement to the consensus document. J Vasc Interv Radiol. 2014;25(11):1706–8. https://doi.org/10.1016/j.jvir.2014.09.005.
8. Schmit GD, Kurup AN, Weisbrod AJ, et al. ABLATE: a renal ablation planning algorithm. AJR Am J Roentgenol. 2014;202(4):894–903. https://doi.org/10.2214/AJR.13.11110.
9. Zargar H, Atwell TD, Cadeddu JA, et al. Cryoablation for small renal masses: selection criteria, complications, and functional and oncological results. Eur Urol. 2016;69(1):116–28. https://doi.org/10.1016/j.eururo.2015.03.027.
10. Hu X, Shao YX, Wang Y, et al. Partial nephrectomy versus ablative therapies for cT1a renal masses: a systematic review and meta-analysis. Eur J Surg Oncol. 2019;45(9):1527–35. https://doi.org/10.1016/j.ejso.2019.05.010. Epub 2019 May 10.

11. Pecoraro A, Palumbo C, Knipper S, et al. Cryoablation predisposes to higher cancer specific mortality relative to partial nephrectomy in patients with nonmetastatic pT1b kidney cancer. J Urol. 2019;202(6):1120–6. https://doi.org/10.1097/JU.0000000000000460.
12. Abu-Ghanem Y, Fernández-Pello S, Bex A, et al. Limitations of available studies prevent reliable comparison between tumour ablation and partial nephrectomy for patients with localised renal masses: a systematic review from the european association of urology renal cell cancer guideline panel. Eur Urol Oncol. 2020;3(4):433–52. https://doi.org/10.1016/j.euo.2020.02.001.

Open Radical Nephrectomy 18

Riccardo Campi, Selcuk Erdem, Onder Kara, Umberto Carbonara, Michele Marchioni, Alessio Pecoraro, Riccardo Bertolo, Alexandre Ingels, Maximilian Kriegmair, Nicola Pavan, Eduard Roussel, Angela Pecoraro, and Daniele Amparore

Open radical nephrectomy (ORN), first described by Frederic Foley in 1952 [1], includes the early ligation of the renal artery and vein, removal of the ipsilateral adrenal gland and the Gerota's fascia surrounding the kidney, and removal of the paraaortic/paracaval lymph nodes extending from the diaphragm crus to the inferior mesenteric artery [2]. Adrenalectomy is recommended in patients with large tumors and adrenal involvement on preoperative imaging [3]. Although initially

R. Campi (✉) · A. Pecoraro
Unit of Urological Robotic Surgery and Renal Transplantation, Careggi Hospital, University of Florence, Florence, Italy
e-mail: riccardo.campi@gmail.com; riccardo.campi@unifi.it

R. Campi
Department of Experimental and Clinical Medicine, University of Florence, Florence, Italy

S. Erdem
Division of Urologic Oncology, Department of Urology, Istanbul University Istanbul Faculty of Medicine, Istanbul, Turkey

O. Kara
Department of Urology, Kocaeli University School of Medicine, Kocaeli, Turkey

U. Carbonara
Department of Emergency and Organ Transplantation-Urology, Andrology and Kidney Transplantation Unit, University of Bari, Bari, Italy

M. Marchioni
Department of Medical, Oral and Biotechnological Sciences, Laboratory of Biostatistics, University "G. D'Annunzio" Chieti-Pescara, Chieti, Italy

Department of Urology, SS Annunziata Hospital, "G. D'Annunzio" University of Chieti, Chieti, Italy

R. Bertolo
Department of Urology, San Carlo Di Nancy Hospital, Rome, Italy

identified as a component of RN, the routine application of ipsilateral adrenalectomy in local or locally advanced disease is not recommended [4]. This is because patients who undergo ipsilateral adrenalectomy have lower adrenal involvement rates [5] and do not have a survival benefit compared with those who do not [6–8]. Regional lymphadenectomy is not necessary in every radical nephrectomy case, considering the overall incidence of lymph node disease is about 5% [9, 10]. Guidelines continue to recommend lymph node dissection for patients with visible lymphadenopathy on preoperative imaging, although there is no evidence of benefit [11].

Indications for ORN include locally advanced kidney tumors with invasion of the perirenal fat and adrenal gland (T3a), tumors with invasion of the renal vein or vena cava (T3b and c), tumors that extend to adjacent organs (T4), and tumors that will likely undergo a wide lymph node dissection [12, 13].

18.1 Surgical Technique

The surgical site can be reached retroperitoneally by flank incision and transperitoneally by midline or subcostal incision (Fig. 18.1). The thoracoabdominal approach may be preferred for large upper-pole tumors. Briefly, the kidney is released from the surrounding organs and tissues along with its fascia, then the artery and vein are cut after the ligation. The lengths of the renal vein on the right (shorter) and left (longer) sides should be considered. The gonadal, adrenal,

A. Ingels
Department of Urology, APHP, University Hospital Henri Mondor, 51 Avenue du Maréchal de Lattre de Tassigny, 94010 Créteil, France

Biomaps, UMR1281, INSERM, CNRS, CEA, Université Paris Saclay, Villejuif, France

M. Kriegmair
Department of Urology, University Medical Centre Mannheim, Mannheim, Germany

N. Pavan
Urology Clinic, Department of Medical, Surgical and Health Science, University of Trieste, Trieste, Italy

E. Roussel
Department of Urology, University Hospitals Leuven, Leuven, Belgium

A. Pecoraro
Division of Urology, Department of Oncology, School of Medicine, University of Turin, San Luigi Hospital, Orbassano, Turin, Italy

D. Amparore
Division of Urology, Department of Oncology, School of Medicine, San Luigi Hospital, University of Turin, Orbassano, Turin, Italy

18 Open Radical Nephrectomy

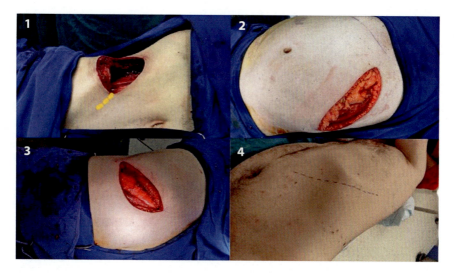

Fig. 18.1 Graphical overview of possible skin incisions for open partial nephrectomy. 1: Right flank incision; 2: Left anterior subcostal incision; 3: Right modified flank incision (Incision started from the posterior edge of 12th rib); 4: Left thoracoabdominal incision line (9th intercostal space)

and lumbar veins should also be ligated and the ureter should be ligated and cut distally to the extent possible and removed along with the Gerota's fascia of the kidney. Performing RN involving perirenal tissues as described [2] is important in preventing local recurrence because perinephric fat invasion is observed in about 25% of RN specimens [14].

18.2 Flank Approach

This approach provides easy access to the kidney and renal hilum prevents peritoneal cavity involvement, and reduces the risk of bowel injury, especially in patients with a previous history of abdominal surgery. Nevertheless, approaching the renal artery and vein is more difficult. The retroperitoneal flank approach may not provide sufficient surgical space in large tumors, upper-pole tumors, or in patients with thrombus in the inferior vena cava (IVC). It may also not be appropriate in cases where lymphadenectomy is planned. With this approach, although subcostal access may be sufficient in most cases, the subsequent division and removal of the 11th and 12th ribs may be required in tumors located in the upper pole and when the adrenal glands need to be evaluated. In this case, the rib to be removed is selected, the incision is started over that rib, and if necessary, the incision can be extended to end at the lateral edge of the rectus abdominis.

18.3 Anterior Subcostal Approach

The anterior subcostal approach provides good exposure to the renal hilum. The incision is started in front of the 12th rib and, at approximately 2 cm below the costal arch, is extended in the cranial direction along the costal arch and terminated at the level of the xiphoid bone. In tumors that are medially located and require meticulous pedicle dissection or aorta and IVC dissection, the incision can be passed to the opposite side in a "Chevron" fashion without ending at the xiphoid level. When necessary, lymphadenectomy can be performed easily, and even the opposite side can be evaluated and improved if needed by entering the retroperitoneum. In the modified approach we implement at our clinic, we perform the incision in the 45-degree lateral decubitus position, a little more forward than the classical flank approach, starting from the front of the 12th rib and extending slightly longer medially. This way, not only can we continue operating retroperitoneally but also reduce the likelihood of incisional hernia by preventing subcostal nerve injury in most patients.

18.4 Thoracoabdominal Approach

The thoracoabdominal approach reveals the upper abdomen, retroperitoneal structures, and thoracic cavity. It is used in large kidney tumors or when a mass or metastasis in the ipsilateral lung needs to be removed. The patient is placed in a semi-oblique position, and an incision is made between the 8th and 10th ribs. The incision can be made between the ribs or over the ribs, allowing them to be removed. The incision starts from the posterior axillary line, continues from the costal cartilage edge, and is advanced from the midline to the umbilicus. Performing intercostal nerve blockage while closing the surgical incision may reduce postoperative pain.

References

1. Foley FB, Mulvaney WP, Richardson EJ, et al. Radical nephrectomy for neoplasms. J Urol. 1952 Jul;68(1):39–49. https://doi.org/10.1016/s0022-5347(17):68168–0
2. Robson CJ. Radical nephrectomy for renal cell carcinoma. J Urol. 1963 Jan;89:37–42. https://doi.org/10.1016/s0022-5347(17)64494-x
3. Campbell S, Uzzo RG, Allaf ME, et al. Renal mass and localized renal cancer: AUA guideline. J Urol. 2017 Sep;198(3):520–529. https://doi.org/10.1016/j.juro.2017.04.100. Epub 2017 May 4
4. Ljungberg B, Albiges L, Bedke J, et al. European Association of Urology (EAU) Guidelines on Renal Cell Carcinoma (RCC). Version 2021. Available at: https://uroweb.org/guideline/renal-cell-carcinoma/.
5. Kletscher BA, Qian J, Bostwick DG, et al. Prospective analysis of the incidence of ipsilateral adrenal metastasis in localized renal cell carcinoma. J Urol. 1996 Jun;155(6):1844–6

6. Siemer S, Lehmann J, Kamradt J, et al. Adrenal metastases in 1635 patients with renal cell carcinoma: outcome and indication for adrenalectomy. J Urol. 2004 Jun;171(6 Pt 1):2155–9; discussion 2159. https://doi.org/10.1097/01.ju.0000125340.84492.a7
7. Leibovitch I, Raviv G, Mor Y, et al. Reconsidering the necessity of ipsilateral adrenalectomy during radical nephrectomy for renal cell carcinoma. Urology. 1995 Sep;46(3):316–20. https://doi.org/10.1016/S0090-4295(99)80213-1
8. Kozak W, Höltl W, Pummer K, et al. Adrenalectomy--still a must in radical renal surgery? Br J Urol. 1996 Jan;77(1):27–31. https://doi.org/10.1046/j.1464-410x.1996.08105.x
9. Olumi AF, Preston MA, Blute ML. Chapter 60: Open surgery of the kidney, In: Alan J. Wein, Louis R. Kavoussi, Alan W. Partin editors. Campbell-Walsh Urology. 2020;12th
10. Freedland SJ, Dekernion JB. Role of lymphadenectomy for patients undergoing radical nephrectomy for renal cell carcinoma. Rev Urol. 2003 Summer;5(3):191–5
11. Ljungberg B, Albiges L, Abu-Ghanem Y, et al. European association of urology guidelines on renal cell carcinoma: the 2019 update. Eur Urol. 2019 May;75(5):799–810. https://doi.org/10.1016/j.eururo.2019.02.011
12. Gregg JR, Scarpato KR. Chapter 8: surgical approaches for open renal surgery, including open radical nephrectomy. In: Smith JA, Howards SS, Preminger GM, et al. editors. Hinman's Atlas of Urologic Surgery. 2019;4th.
13. Van Poppel H, Becker F, Cadeddu JA, et al. Treatment of localised renal cell carcinoma. Eur Urol. 2011 Oct;60(4):662–72. https://doi.org/10.1016/j.eururo.2011.06.040. Epub 2011 Jun 29
14. Shah PH, Lyon TD, Lohse CM, et al. Prognostic evaluation of perinephric fat, renal sinus fat, and renal vein invasion for patients with pathological stage T3a clear-cell renal cell carcinoma. BJU Int. 2019 Feb;123(2):270–276. https://doi.org/10.1111/bju.14523
15. Petros FG, Angell JE, Abaza R. Outcomes of robotic nephrectomy including highest-complexity cases: largest series to date and literature review. Urology. 2015;85(6):1352–8. https://doi.org/10.1016/j.urology.2014.11.063.
16. Crocerossa F, Carbonara U, Cantiello F, et al. Robot-assisted radical nephrectomy: a systematic review and meta-analysis of comparative studies. Eur Urol. 2020; S0302–2838(20)30854-X. https://doi.org/10.1016/j.eururo.2020.10.034.
17. Abaza R, Gerhard RS, Martinez O. Robotic radical nephrectomy for massive renal tumors. J Laparoendosc Adv Surg Tech A. 2020;30(2):196–200. https://doi.org/10.1089/lap.2019.0630.

Transperitoneal and Retroperitoneal Port Placement

19

Alireza Ghoreifi, Hooman Djaladat, and Andre Luis Abreu

19.1 Introduction

Robotic partial/radical nephrectomy has become increasingly utilized for renal cancer due to the equivalent oncologic and functional outcomes and decreased morbidity when compared to open surgery [1–3]. It can be performed through different approaches, including transperitoneal and retroperitoneal, and using single or multi port techniques [4]. The choice of surgical approach should be selected based on the availability of resources, surgeon's experience, and patient/disease characteristics. Performing robotic renal surgery utilizing each of these approaches needs its own considerations including patient positioning, access obtaining, and port placement. This chapter presents an overview of access obtaining and port placement in different robotic renal surgery approaches. Furthermore, specific considerations are highlighted for the da Vinci Si® and Xi® robotic platforms. Renal sugery via single-port approach will be addressed in a different chapter.

A. Ghoreifi (✉) · H. Djaladat · A. L. Abreu
USC, Institute of Urology and Catherine and Joseph Aresty Department of Urology, Keck School of Medicine, University of Southern California, Los Angeles, California, USA
e-mail: Alireza.Ghoreifi@med.usc.edu

H. Djaladat
e-mail: djaladat@med.usc.edu

A. L. Abreu
e-mail: Andre.Abreu@med.usc.edu

19.2 General Principles of Pneumoperitoneum Obtaining

There are general considerations regarding pneumoperitoneum obtaining in robotic renal surgeries that share common principles with different robotic approaches and platforms. The main techniques include closed, open, and optical.

19.2.1 Closed Technique and Creating Pneumoperitoneum

This is the most common technique of pneumoperitoneum obtaining that is performed with the Veress needle [5]. This needle is a blunt-tipped, spring-loaded inner stylet with sharp outer needle that has 12–15 cm length and 2 mm external diameter. The most common insertion site for the Veress needle is the right/left lower quadrant, away from the epigastric vessels. Once the peritoneum is entered, the surgeon usually feels or hears the protective sheath clicking when it recoils, indicating that the cavity has been entered. Other techniques such as the aspiration test and the saline drop test are also performed to confirm the appropriate placement of the needle [6]. After the Veress needle is in place, it can be connected to an AirSeal® device, and then CO_2 gas is injected through the needle to create a pneumoperitoneum. It's imperative to ensure low pneumoperitneum pressure (1–4 mmHg) on AirSeal® at the begning of insuflation, and that the pressure is slowly increasing to a pre-set desidred pressure. In our practice we use a 15 mmHg for the pneumoperitoneum pressure.

19.2.2 Open (Hasson) Technique

In this technique, an incision is made through the abdominal wall under direct vision, passing through each of the layers until the peritoneal cavity is reached. The advantages of this technique include establishing a pneumoperitoneum and correct anatomical repair of the abdominal wall incision [5, 6]. The open technique can potentially reduce in vascular and bowel injuries related to the initial access. However, a recent Cochrane systematic review demonstrated that although open entry technique is associated with a significant reduction of failed entry compared to the closed technique, the incidence of visceral or vascular injury was similar between these two techniques [7]. Nevertheless, this techinique is recommended for patients with prior abdominal sugery in the vicinity of, or in the area/organ of interest.

19.2.3 Optical Technique

In the optical access or direct vision technique, access to the abdominal cavity is obtained with a specialized optical port that has a transparent tip, allowing each layer of the abdominal wall to be seen with a 5 mm 0-degree laparoscope. These devices are typically used for primary port placement after Veress needle abdominal insufflation or secondary port placement after establishing the pneumoperitoneum [5, 6]. This is also recommended in case of prior abdominal surgery for safety.

19.3 Robotic Nephrectomy: Transperitoneal Approach

Transperitoneal approach is the most common and widely used surgical approach for robotic partial/radical nephrectomy. It can be performed with the da Vinci Si® or Xi® robotic platforms using 3- or 4-arm techniques. Given the availability of both Si® and Xi® robotic systems in current market, we will present both plaforms in details.

19.3.1 Operative Room Setup and Patient Positioning

Under general anesthesia with endotracheal intubation, a naso- or orogastric tube is placed to decompress the stomach and avoid gastric injury during ports placement. An 18 French urethral catheter is inserted. The patient is then placed in a modified (60–70 degree) lateral decubitus position (Fig. 19.1). Care is taken to adequately pad all pressure points and place all limbs in a neutral position to minimize positioning injuries. For this purpose, an axillary roll is placed, and appropriate padding is used to support the hip and flank. Pillows are placed between the flexed lower and straight upper leg. The upper arm rests on a well-padded arm board without tension on the brachial plexus. To secure the patient, tape is used around the hips, shoulders, and thighs to ensure stability when rolling the table.

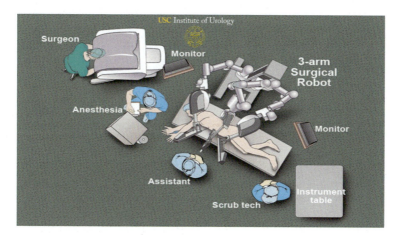

Fig. 19.1 Room setup and patient positioning for transperitoneal robotic nephrectomy using Si® robotic platform

The operative setup may vary based on surgeon preference and the type of robot used (i.e., daVinci Si® vs. Xi®). The assistant is positioned facing the patient's abdomen; the scrub technician is positioned behind the assistant. Video monitors are placed at the head and foot end of the patient on the side of the robot for easy viewing by the surgical team.

19.3.2 Port Placement for Da Vinci Xi®

Port placement is started once four-quadrant pneumoperitoneum is achieved. We prefer using the Xi® robotic platform with a 4-arm technique. There are few described techniques; however, we routinely place trocars in a "smile" fashion (Figs. 19.2 and 19.3). Trocar type and configuration may change to some extent in case of adhesions encountered and the patient's body habitus. Extra-long trocars can be used to decrease the likelihood of clashing in obese patients.

Robotic camera port: the first 8 mm trocar is inserted lateral and superior to the umbilicus, at the para-rectus line. Ideally, this trocar is placed to achieve a proper view of the kidney and tumor. The robotic camera is inserted and the peritoneal cavity inspected to ensure safe entry. Other trocars are inserted under direct visualization.

Robotic instrument trocars: an 8 mm trocar is placed at the same line but about 6 cm cephalad to the camera port. Two 8 mm trocars are placed caudal and slightly lateral to the camera port, toward the anterior superior iliac spine. All robotic trocars are palced, at least, 6 cm apart from each to avoid colisions. For the right tumors, these trocars will be hooked to the right, left, and 4th robotic arms, respectively.

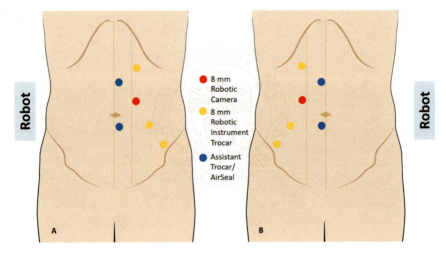

Fig. 19.2 Trocar placement for left **A** and right **B** partial/radical nephrectomy using Xi® robotic platform

19 Transperitoneal and Retroperitoneal Port Placement   177

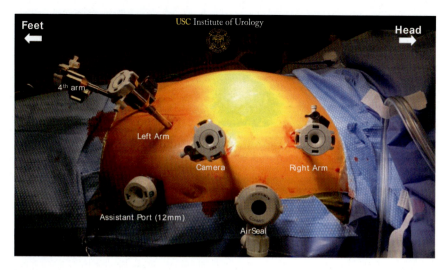

Fig. 19.3 Trocar placement and arm configuration for right nephrectomy in a patient with right renal mass using Xi® robotic platform

Assistant trocars: One or two 5–12 mm assistant ports can be placed according to the surgeon's discretion in the midline approximately 2–3 cm cranial and caudal to the umbilicus (i.e., between the camera and right/left robotic arm). We routinely use a 12 cm AirSeal® (SurgiQuest Inc, Milford, CT) as one of the assistant ports.

Liver retractor: Usually, a 5 mm trocar will need to be placed below the xiphoid sternum for right-sided procedures in order to aid with liver retraction.

19.3.3 Port Placement for Da Vinci Si®

With the Si® robotic platform, few modifications in the port placement should be considered. Firstly, a 12 mm trocar is used for the robotic camera. Secondly, the two 8 mm instrument trocars are placed more laterally (compared to the Xi® configuration) in such a configurtion that they form a broad-based triangle with the kidney/tumor, in which the tumor forms the apex of this triangle. Finally, if the surgeon decides to use the 4th arm, it will be placed through a trocar located lateral, midway from the camera and the most distal robotic trocar (Figs. 19.4 and 19.5). Also, in Si® system to expand the arms as much as possible, we recommend using long trocars for right and left arms.

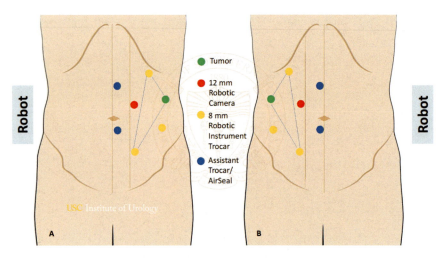

Fig. 19.4 Trocar placement for left **A** and right **B** partial/radical nephrectomy using Si® robotic platform

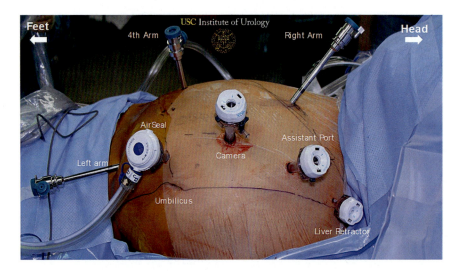

Fig. 19.5 Trocar placement and arm configuration for right nephrectomy in a patient with right renal mass using Si® robotic platform

19.3.4 Robot Docking

After completion of the port placement, the robot is docked. With the Si® platform, the robot is brought towards to the operating table at an approximately 45-degree oblique angle over the patient's shoulder. The da Vinci Xi® robot allows more flexibility than the Si® robot and can be docked from many different angles due to its unique rotating boom design. To keep the operative setup as consistent as possible, we routinely dock the Xi® robot posterior to the patient with the camera arm coming into the patient at an angle of 15-degree in line with the camera port. Robotic instruments are then inserted into the peritoneal cavity under direct vision following completion of targeting.

19.4 Robotic Nephrectomy: Retroperitoneal Approach

The retroperitoneal approach for robotic nephrectomy is suitable for two group of patients. First, patients with prior abdominal surgery in whom exposure of the kidney and retroperitoneum may be more difficult due to adhesions and/or distorted anatomy. Second, patients with posterior renal masses located in whom getting access to the tumor would require significantly more mobilization of the kidney with transperitoneal approach [8]. The retroperitoneal approach allows for direct and rapid access to the retroperitoneum and renal hilum. Nevertheless, the limitations of this approach are the smaller working space as well as limited anatomic landmarks that may cause potential disorientation and inadvertent vascular injury requiring open conversion. Contraindications of retroperitoneal approach include prior major retroperitoneal surgery, dense perirenal inflammation/fibrosis (e.g., xanthogranulomatous pyelonephritis), musculoskeletal limitations that preclude proper positioning, large tumors with extensive collaterals, and abundant perinephric fat with extensive stranding [8–10].

19.4.1 Operative Room Setup and Patient Positioning

Retroperitoneal approach in not utilized as routine as the transperitoneal approach. Increased familiarity of the operating team with the operative setup and process can potentially minimize the perioperative morbidity. Similar to the transperitoneal approach, 3- and 4-arm techniques can be used in this setting, according to the surgeon preference [11]. We prefer to use the 4-arm technique.

After induction of general endotracheal anesthesia, an 18 French urethral catheter is inserted and the patient is placed in full 90-degree flank position with the side of the renal mass up. Of note, no orogastric or nasogastric tube is required in this appraoch. After appropriate padding and securing the patient (similar to what we discussed for transperitoneal approach), the bed is fully flexed to maximize the space between the 12th rib and iliac crest.

19.4.2 Retroperitoneal Access

An open access is obtained through a transverse incision that is made in the midaxillary line, between the tip of 12th rib and iliac crest. Performing an incision too anterior or posterior can be associated with an increased risk of peritoneotomy or clashing with the posterior port, respectively. Blunt dissection is performed to penetrate the external and internal oblique as well as the transversalis fascia. The index finger is then entered the retroperitoneal space to gently sweep the peritoneum away and the surgeon should be able to feel the psoas muscle posteriorly. The balloon-dilating device is then placed into this space with the goal of achieving maximal expansion along the cranial-caudal axis posterior to the kidney. A 30-degree laparoscope is inserted into the balloon dissector, and 40 pumps are performed under direct vision. At this point, the anatomical landmarks are identified including: the transversus abdominis muscle and anterior layer of peritoneum superiorly, Gerota's fascia as it is pushed off the psoas muscle posteriorly, and the ureter inferiorly [12]. The balloon is then deflated and replaced by the 12 mm camera trocar.

19.4.3 Trocar Placement for Da Vinci Si®

Once pneumo-retroperitoneum is established and the *12 mm camera* is inserted, the remaining trocars are marked and inserted under direct vision (Fig. 19.6A).

Robotic instrument trocars: an 8 mm trocar is placed along the posterior axillary line at the apex formed by the erector spinae muscles and 12th rib. Another 8 mm trocar is placed medially along the anterior axillary line, 7–8 cm away from the camera trocar toward the umbilicus. Another 8 mm trocar is placed 7–8 cm medially. For the right tumors, these trocars will be hooked to the left, right, and 4th arms, respectively (Fig. 19.6B).

Assistant trocar: a 12 mm assistant port or AirSeal® is placed in the anterior axillary line above the anterior superior iliac spine, and 7–8 cm caudal to the medial robotic trocar.

19.4.4 Trocar Placement for Da Vinci Xi®

Trocar placement can be performed similar to the Si® template with few modifications. An 8 mm trocar is used for the robotic camera throught the balloon trocar in "port in port" fashion. The instrument trocars are placed in a line as shown in Fig. 19.7. The assistant port/AirSeal® is placed at the posterior axillary line above the iliac crest.

19 Transperitoneal and Retroperitoneal Port Placement   181

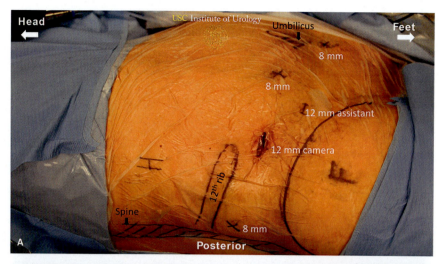

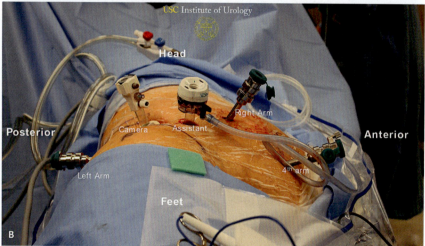

Fig. 19.6 Port planning **A** and trocar placement **B** for right nephrectomy in a patient with right renal mass using Si® robotic platform and retroperitoneal approach

19.4.5 Robot Docking

Once the port placement is completed, the robot is docked. For DaVinci Si®, the robot is docked over the patient's head, parallel to the spine. When using DaVinci Xi®, the robot is docked posteriorly to the patient, perpendicular or parallel to the bed. Robotic instruments are then inserted under direct vision.

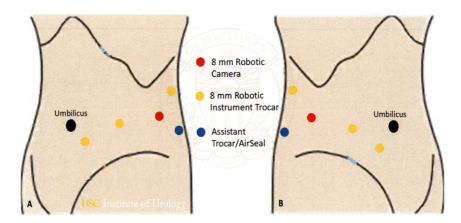

Fig. 19.7 Trocar placement for left **A** and right **B** partial/radical nephrectomy using Xi® robotic platform and retroperitoneal approach

19.5 Complications of the Port Placement

Complications related to port placement are uncommon yet can be associated with a high morbidity. Several patient- and surgeon-related risk factors can contribute to the development of these complications. Obesity and prior abdominal surgery are the main patient-related factors. The experience of the surgeon is an important factor in this context with the higher rates of complications reported in the beginners compared to experienced hands [13, 14].

In order to prevent possible injuries during port placement, different points can be considered. The use of open (Hasson) technique as well as the optic trocar can be helpful, especially in obese patient or those with a history of abdominal surgeries [5–7]. In patients with prior abdominal surgeries, initial access through the Palmer's point can also reduce the likelihood of intra-abdominal injuries. This point is located at midclavicular line, 3 cm distal to the costal rib in left upper quadrant. It has been shown that the probability of abdominal adhesions is considerably lower at this point compared to the other abdominal areas [15]. Placement of nasogastric tube and Foley catheter can decrease the risk of gastrointestinal and bladder injuries.

The most common complications during port placement include vascular and bowel injuries.

Vascular injury: These types of injuries may involve abdominal wall, retroperitoneal, or intra-abdominal vessels. Epigastric vessels are the most common site of abdominal wall vascular injuries. The abdominal wall injuries can be controlled with insertion and inflation of a Foley catheter to tamponade the site of injury. Other options include U stiches and rarely extending the incision to control the bleeding under direct vision. In case of intraabdominal major vascular injury (e.g., iliac vein, inferior vena cava) or retroperitoneal expanding hematoma, immediate open conversion is usually necessary [16, 17].

Bowel injury: These injuries should be addressed as soon as diagnosed. Depending on the extent of the injury and segment type (small vs. large bowel) they can be managed with primary repair or secondarily following ostomy creation. Unfortunately, up to 50% of the bowel injuries are not diagnosed intraoperatively. Abdominal exploration and repair of the site of injury is usually recommended in these situations [17].

Other: Liver and spleen injuries can rarely happen during port placement. Management includes direct compression and increasing the pneumoperitoneal pressure. Bladder injuries are usually managed conservatively by keeping the Foley catheter for 7–14 days after surgery. Major bladder injuries may require primary repair.

References

1. Peyronnet B, Seisen T, Oger E, et al. Comparison of 1800 robotic and open partial nephrectomies for renal tumors. Ann Surg Oncol. 2016;23(13):4277–83.
2. Leow JJ, Heah NH, Chang SL, et al. Outcomes of robotic versus laparoscopic partial nephrectomy: an updated meta-analysis of 4,919 patients. J Urol. 2016;196(5):1371–7.
3. Petros FG, Angell JE, Abaza R. Outcomes of robotic nephrectomy including highest-complexity cases: largest series to date and literature review. Urology. 2015;85(6):1352–8.
4. Kaouk J, Garisto J, Eltemamy M, et al. Pure single-site robot-assisted partial nephrectomy using the sp surgical system: initial clinical experience. Urology. 2019;124:282–5.
5. Thepsuwan J, Huang KG, Wilamarta M, et al. Principles of safe abdominal entry in laparoscopic gynecologic surgery. J Minim Invasive Gynecol. 2013;2(4):105–9.
6. Teoh B, Sen R, Abbott J. An evaluation of four tests used to ascertain Veres needle placement at closed laparoscopy. J Minim Invasive Gynecol. 2005;12(2):153–8.
7. Ahmad G, Baker J, Finnerty J, et al. Laparoscopic entry techniques. Cochrane Database Syst Rev. 2019;1(1):CD006583.
8. Hu JC, Treat E, Filson CP, et al. Technique and outcomes of robot-assisted retroperitoneoscopic partial nephrectomy: a multicenter study. Eur Urol. 2014;66(3):542–9.
9. Ghani KR, Porter J, Menon M, et al. Robotic retroperitoneal partial nephrectomy: a step-by-step guide. BJU Int. 2014;114(2):311–3.
10. Patel M, Porter J. Robotic retroperitoneal partial nephrectomy. World J Urol. 2013;31(6):1377–82.
11. Feliciano J, Stifelman M. Robotic retroperitoneal partial nephrectomy: a four-arm approach. JSLS. 2012;16(2):208–11.
12. Lee J, Porter J. Retroperitoneal robotic partial nephrectomy. In: Atlas of robotic urologic surgery. Switzerland, Springer International Publishing;2017. p. 113–4.
13. Pemberton RJ, Tolley DA, van Velthoven RF. Prevention and management of complications in urological laparoscopic port site placement. Eur Urol. 2006;50(5):958–68.
14. Parsons JK, Jarrett TJ, Chow GK, Kavoussi LR. The effect of previous abdominal surgery on urological laparoscopy. J Urol. 2002;168(6):2387–90.

15. Tüfek I, Akpınar H, Sevinç C, Kural AR. Primary left upper quadrant (Palmer's point) access for laparoscopic radical prostatectomy. Urol J. 2010;7(3):152–6.
16. Simforoosh N, Basiri A, Ziaee SA, et al. Major vascular injury in laparoscopic urology. JSLS. 2014; 18(3):e2014.00283.
17. Sánchez A, Rosciano J. Complications of port placement. In: Sotelo R, Arriaga J, Aron M, editors. Complications in robotic urologic surgery. Cham: Springer; 2018. p. 83–91.

Robot Assisted Laparoscopy for Renal Cancer: Transperitoneal Versus Retroperitoneal Approach

20

Vidyasagar Chinni, Zein Alhamdani, Damien Bolton, Nathan Lawrentschuk, and Greg Jack

20.1 Introduction

Surgical resection remains the mainstay of treatment for localized renal cell carcinoma (RCC), either via radical or partial nephrectomy. The first reported laparoscopic nephrectomy was performed by Clayman and colleagues using transperitoneal access to the kidney [1]. Subsequently Gaur and Colleagues reported successful retroperitoneoscopic nephrectomy a few years later [2]. Laparoscopic renal surgery became the mainstay of care for localised RCC with benefits of lower postoperative complications, decreased blood loss, decreased blood transfusion rate, improved time to oral intake, and shorter hospital stays and time to convalescence when compared to an open approach [3–6]. Within the past 20 years, robotic-assisted laparoscopic platforms have supplemented standard laparoscopy for renal surgery, starting with the first reported robot-assisted radical nephrectomy reported in 2001 by Guillonneau et al. [5] who performed

---

Vidyasagar Chinni and Zein Alhamdani are co-first authors

V. Chinni · Z. Alhamdani · D. Bolton · G. Jack
Department of Urology, Olivia Newton-John Cancer Research Institute, Melbourne, Australia
e-mail: Gregory.Jack@austin.org.au

Z. Alhamdani · D. Bolton · G. Jack
Department of Surgery, Austin Health, University of Melbourne, Melbourne, Australia

N. Lawrentschuk (✉)
Department of Urology, Royal Melbourne Hospital, Victoria, Australia
e-mail: nlaw@unimelb.edu.au

Department of Surgery, University of Melbourne, Melbourne, Australia

Department of Surgical Oncology, Peter MacCallum Cancer Centre, Melbourne, Australia

EJ Whitten Prostate Cancer Research Centre at Epworth, Melbourne, Australia

a retroperitoneal right radical nephrectomy whilst utilising the Zeus robotic surgical system with two arms and the Aesop robotic arm to control the camera [5]. The robotic-assisted platforms overcome the ergonomic and technical challenges that accompany standard laparoscopy and allow for completion of more technically challenging cases radical [6] and partial nephrectomy cases [4].

Cacciamani et al. [3] found that when compared to laparoscopic partial nephrectomies, robot-assisted surgery had a decrease in ischemia time, conversion rate, intraoperative outcomes, postoperative outcomes, positive margins, percentage decrease of estimated glomerular filtration rates and overall mortality. The different approaches for robotic nephrectomy are a constantly evolving area of study where additional data are needed to make any conclusions between the two techniques. The majority of robotic-assisted renal surgeries are performed transperitoneal according to multi-centre studies [4, 7, 8], but the retroperitoneoscopic approach to the kidney described in 1993 is still widely utilised and increasing in popularity. Herein we discuss the merits and considerations for the transperitoneal and retroperitoneoscopic approaches with respect to robotic-assisted surgery.

20.1.1 Indications: Transperitoneal and Retroperitoneal Robotic Surgery

Transperitoneal and retroperitoneal access are both indicated in robotic renal surgery, and the choice between them is often surgeon and patient specific.

20.2 Transperitoneal Indications

There are several factors to take into consideration when selecting a transperitoneal or retroperitoneal approach to robotic-assisted renal surgery, including location and size of tumour, training and preference of the surgeon, obliteration of surgical planes from prior procedures, and patient factors that may compromise each approach.

20.2.1 Larger Working Volume

Most cases of robotic nephrectomy are transperitoneal, owing to a shorter learning curve, larger working space, and surgeons' greater familiarity with the anatomical landmarks surrounding the kidney [4, 7, 8]. Insufflation of the peritoneal cavity offers a larger working space, typically 5–7 L of carbon dioxide insufflation volume in an adult, compared to only 1–2 L in the retroperitoneal cavity [9]. The large insufflation volume of the transperitoneal cavity allows early visualisation of surrounding organs including the colon, duodenum and liver on the right, and spleen on the left. The larger insufflation volume also allows for wider port placements to facilitate additional dexterity offered by robotic systems [10] and additional space

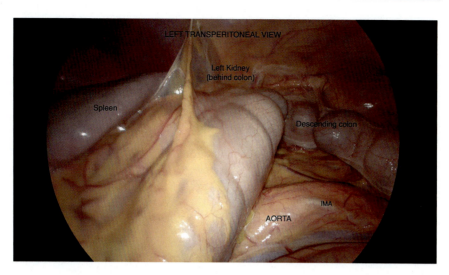

Fig. 20.1 Typical left transperitoneal view upon entry into the abdomen. Note the kidney is rarely on view on the left side

for a third robotic arm, particularly in the older generation robotic systems which utilised wider platforms. Figure 20.1 shows the large working volume, typically 5–7 L of CO^2, and familiar anatomy of the transperitoneal approach.

20.2.2 Stage 3 Tumours

The larger peritoneal working space provided by the transabdominal approach is useful in the event of very large tumours, including tumours with adhesions to the colon or surrounding organs, highly vascular tumours with parasitic vessels, and tumours with vein thrombus. Transperitoneal robot-assisted partial and radical nephrectomy has been utilised in stage 1–3 [4, 11, 12] tumours including tumours requiring renal vein or vena cava thrombectomy. The outcomes of robotic-assisted laparoscopic radical nephrectomy for stage T3 tumours are comparable with the open approach, with studies suggesting lower perioperative complication rates [13–16]. The transperitoneal robotic approach provides direct and clear visualisation of the renal vein in the event of renal vein thrombus, and multiple cases of transperitoneal robotic assisted nephrectomy with vena cava thrombectomy are described [17, 18]. The psoas muscle typically provides a safe anatomical landmark and dissection plane, and utilisation of the 4th arm or assistant port of robot allows lifting the large kidney from the psoas to provide safe passage to the hilum [19]. The larger working space of the peritoneal cavity allows for significant elevation of the large kidney and mass laterally. Robotic assistance in advanced renal cell carcinoma cases has shown benefits over traditional laparoscopy since it provides greater mobility and greater ease of intracorporeal suturing [10]. Although there

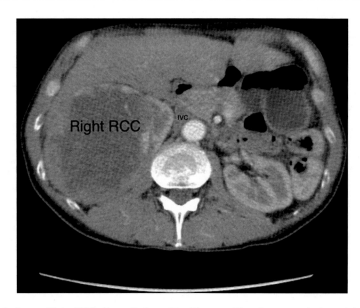

Fig. 20.2 Large Right RCC, Stage 3, in a thin 30 year old male removed via a right robotic assisted transperitoneal nephrectomy to avoid parasitic vessels and gain additional working space

is no consensus on the optimal surgical technique in the management of renal cell carcinoma with IVC thrombus [20], robotic renal surgery has enabled surgeons to remove advanced renal cell carcinomas with the benefits of minimally invasive surgery [21]. Figure 20.2 shows a large right renal tumour, removed via right transperitoneal right robotic assisted approach. Figure 20.3 demonstrates an easily visualised small renal vein thrombus.

20.2.3 Anterior and Lower Pole Tumours

Transperitoneal insufflation and port placement provides easy access to the anterior surface of the kidney, which is particularly helpful in the event of anterior tumours suitable for partial nephrectomy [9], since it allows for minimal manipulation of the kidney [22]. Lower pole tumours are also particularly suited for an transperitoneal approach, due to the natural rotation and mobility of the lower pole anteriorly. There is also lack of conflict with the anterior superior iliac spine (ASIS) which can sometimes clash with robotic instruments during a retroperitoneal approach with older and larger robotic platforms such as the DaVinci S. Figure 20.4 shows a right anterior renal tumour amenable to transperitoneal right partial nephrectomy.

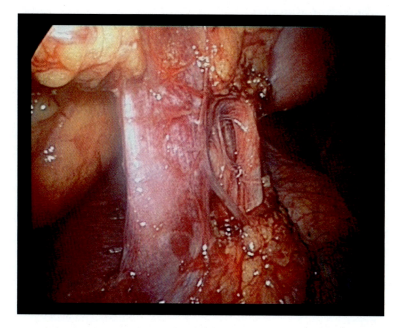

Fig. 20.3 Transperitoneal exposure of the entire renal vein in the event of vein thrombus

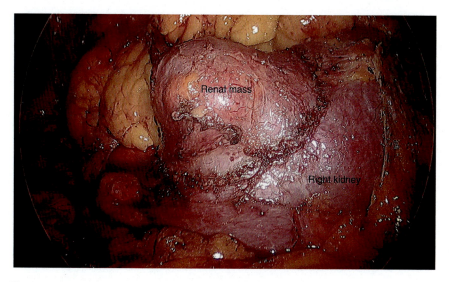

Fig. 20.4 Right anterior renal mass with transperitoneal exposure

20.2.4 Posterior Tumours

Conventionally it has been taught that posterior tumours should be resected through a retroperitoneal approach during partial nephrectomy. This is true in terms of immediate access to posterior tumours without mobilisation of the kidney [4, 7, 23], but, numerous studies have shown that posterior tumours can be safely resected via a transperitoneal robotic approach with complete mobilisation of the kidney and comparable outcomes to a retroperitoneal approach. Mclean et al. [23] suggests that the most suitable approach depends on surgeon experience and familiarity with the technique, in addition to employing a risk stratified approach depending on patient characteristics. Many surgeons will opt to perform a transperitoneal resection of posterior tumours due to familiarity and comfort with the approach [24]. Posterior tumours are subject to the surgeon's clinical judgement. Posterior tumours located in the lower and upper poles of the kidney are easy to access from an anterior approach by mobilising and rotating the desired pole anteriorly with the fourth arm of the robot or surgical assistant. Posterior tumours in the mid-zone and hilar region of the kidney (See Photo) are also accessible anteriorly, but they require complete mobilisation of the posterior surface of the kidney to flip the kidney medially to provide expose to the posterior surface of the kidney. This can be accomplished with a transperitoneal approach, but requires additional surgical time and kidney mobilisation (Fig. 20.5).

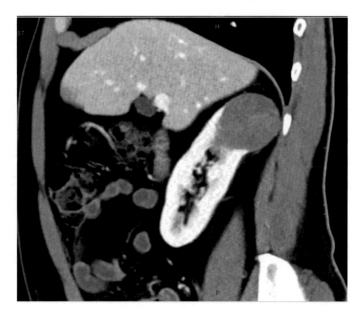

Fig. 20.5 A 6 cm papillary RCC in the posterior upper pole approached via a transperitoneal partial nephrectomy by rotating the upper pole medially on its axis, based on surgeon preference in large tumours

20.2.5 Prior Surgeries and Percutaneous Procedures

A transperitoneal approach may be beneficial in situations where the retroperitoneal plane has been obliterated or severely scarred. This includes cases of prior retroperitoneal renal surgery such as partial nephrectomy, prior percutaneous nephrolithotomy, prior nephrostomy tracts, and prior open flank incisions [19, 25, 26]. A past history of percutaneous procedures on the kidney must also be considered and may favour a transperitoneal approach. Prior percutaneous renal mass ablation [27, 28], prior nephrostomy tracts, and prior renal biopsy can cause perirenal fibrosis of the soft adipose tissue of the retroperitoneum making posterior dissection difficult during retroperitoneal surgery, and favouring a transperitoneal robotic approach, especially during a surgeons learning curve.

The transperitoneal approach can be used cautiously in patients with a history of previous abdominal surgery, however the transperitoneal robotic surgeon must be aware that prior major abdominal surgery significantly increases the chance of visceral organ injury, and prolongs operating times due to bowel adhesions, adhesiolysis, bleeding, and overall operative difficulty [29]. Many authors advocate that retroperitoneal surgery should be considered in these cases when possible, and we would agree. Figure 20.6 shows minor adhesions from peritoneal dialysis and a prior renal surgery. These can easily be taken down sharply under vision.

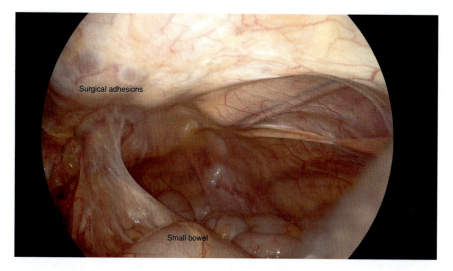

Fig. 20.6 Surgical adhesions between small bowel and the left flank wall from prior left flank incision in a patient on peritoneal dialysis. Entry into the abdomen at a site away from the incision under open Hassan technique provides safe entry into the abdomen, and the adhesions can easily be divided sharply to expose the descending colon and left kidney

20.2.6 Xanthogranulomatous Pyelonephritis

The optimal approach to xanthogranulomatous pyelonephritis is never ideal, since these kidneys can be severely inflamed and adherent to surrounding organs and vicera, with obliteration of the Gerota's planes. They are often very challenging. A transabdominal approach provides greater visibility of the local adherent organs and greater working space. Although a retrospective study by Asali and Tsivian [30] demonstrated retroperitoneal laparoscopic nephrectomy for xanthogranulomatous pyelonephritis is feasible and should be considered [30].

20.3 Retroperitoneal Indications

Retroperitoneal robotic-assisted renal surgery is easily performed for radical nephrectomy and partial nephrectomy [6, 23, 24, 31–33]. The retroperitoneal approach offers the advantage of immediate access to the renal artery (Fig. 20.7) and has been shown to decrease overall operating time and estimated blood loss with no difference in warm ischemia time, conversion to open surgery and perioperative complications [7, 8].

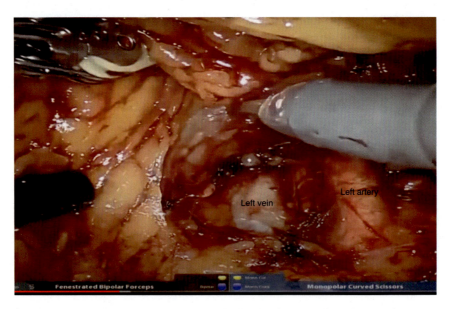

Fig. 20.7 Early exposure of the renal artery and vein with the retroperitoneal approach

20.3.1 Surgeon Experience

The retroperitoneal approach to robot-assisted laparoscopic nephrectomy is gaining popularity amongst urologists [4] coinciding with the increasing technical ability of the surgeons performing robotic surgery. Retroperitoneal access is considered more surgically challenging due to the limited working space and unconventional anatomical visability with unclear landmarks [7–9, 34–36]. In developing the retroperitoneal space with a balloon dilator, Gerota's fascia will be pushed off the psoas muscle [37]. It is key to keep the psoas muscle horizontal during the entire operation to ensure correct anatomical plane. The landmarks in the retroperitoneum is the transversus abdominus and peritoneum anteriorly, psoas tendon, ureter, vena cava posteriorly, posterior Gerota's fascia laterally and the renal artery which should be encountered before the renal vein [19]. The unconventional anatomical view has led to inadvertent injuries including breaching of the peritoneum [4], vena cava injury [34], pancreas during left partial or radical nephrectomy [38], duodenum for right sided procedures [39] since these organs are difficult to visualise and it is quite disorienting for surgeons unfamiliar to this approach particularly since they are working in a tighter environment. The awareness of these pitfalls is paramount for surgeons starting to adopt the retroperitoneal approach for robotic partial and radical nephrectomy (Fig. 20.8).

Abaza et al. assessed the feasibility of adopting a retroperitoneal approach to robotic partial nephrectomy in urologists trained in the transperitoneal approach. They found that there were no clinically significant operative outcomes when comparing estimated blood loss, warm ischemia time and operative time. As such they

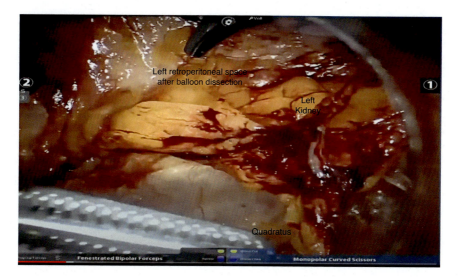

Fig. 20.8 Initial inspection of the retroperitoneal space after balloon dissection and entry can be disorientating due to the small working space and lack of visible landmarks

posit that there is no identifiable learning curve [40]. Therefore, training urologists should consider starting off with the transperitoneal approach which is more accessible due to the wider working space and more identifiable landmarks, then utilising the retroperitoneal approach in suitable situations. The use of robotics has minimised the impacts of the tight working space with the enhanced three-dimensional view of the operating field and the augmented manoeuvrability of instruments such as EndoWrist technology which simplifies complex tasks such as intracorporeal suturing while providing an ergonomic position for the surgeon [4].

20.3.2 Small Tumours (Stage T1-2)

Retroperitoneal approach is often limited to stage T2 tumours or less due to the smaller working space [6, 8], although T3 tumour resection and large radical nephrectomies have been successfully reported in the literature [6, 41, 42]. The RECORD 2 study is a large multi-centre cohort study that evaluated outcomes of T1 renal tumours across 26 Italian centres comparing a transperitoneal and retroperitoneal approach for minimally invasive partial nephrectomy found that retroperitoneal had a significantly lower rate of overall and surgical intraoperative complications, lower time of drain maintenance and postoperative stay compared to those treated with transperitoneal approach [4]. It is worth noting that there was a significant element of selection bias in the position of the tumour. The ROSULA collaborative group analysed the outcomes of stage T1-2 tumours with robot-assisted laparoscopic partial nephrectomy using both a transperitoneal approach and retroperitoneal approach over 19 sites and found that robot-assisted laparoscopic partial nephrectomy is safe with acceptable outcomes [6]. However, only 8% of the partial nephrectomies performed by this group were retroperitoneal. The outcomes of each approach will be discussed in greater depth later in the chapter.

20.3.3 Posterior Tumours

A retroperitoneal approach is the preferred approach for posterior central tumours suitable for partial nephrectomy due to the immediate access to the renal artery and the tumour above [4, 12, 22, 43–46]. The direct access to the posterior hilum has been reported to lower operation time and decrease the risk of injury during its isolation [4]. Most studies comparing transperitoneal and retroperitoneal approaches have a strong selection bias where the posterior tumours are excised through a retroperitoneal approach (Fig. 20.9).

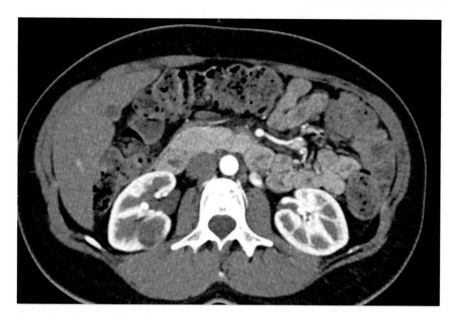

Fig. 20.9 A 30 year old female with a 3 cm RCC for partial nephrectomy. The mid pole posterior location makes this tumour suitable for retroperitoneal partial nephrectomy

20.3.4 Anterior Tumours

Numerous studies have demonstrated the feasibility of retroperitoneal robotic-assisted approaches to anterior renal tumours suitable for partial nephrectomy [12, 32]. Dell'Oglio et al. reject the hypothesis of superior outcomes when a surgical approach is chosen based on a tumour's location, and as such say that it is equally as safe and feasible to perform a retroperitoneal robot assisted partial nephrectomy for anterior tumour [32]. During retroperitoneoscopic approaches, the kidney can be completely mobilised and flipped on its hilar axis to provide exposure to the anterior surface when required. Some authors advocate this approach should be used selectively with anterior hilar tumours since the smaller working space and stripping away of the thin peritoneal membrane along the anterior surface of Gerota's fascia can lead to inadvertent peritoneal cavity entry during mobilisation, which can complicate retroperitoneoscopy due to the deterioration of the working space [4]. The retroperitoneal approach to anterior central tumours is technically challenging and is at higher risk of the inadvertent injuries to organs and peritoneum. Entry into the peritoneal cavity is common with large anterior tumours since the peritoneum is usually adherent. However, with appropriate clinical judgement by the surgeon, a retroperitoneal approach can be utilised safely and efficaciously even for large anterior tumours.

20.3.5 Prior Major Abdominal Surgery

The retroperitoneal approach has the benefit of avoiding the visceral contents of the peritoneal cavity [7]. This has significant implications for patients with prior peritoneal adhesions [47], prior peritoneal dialysis complications, and inflammatory bowel disease. In this cases avoiding entry into the peritoneum reduces the risk of iatrogenic visceral injury, particularly at initial port placement [43]. Patients with large sheets of abdominal mesh in-situ, such as ventral hernia repair, are increasing in prevalence and best served with the retroperitoneal approach. In addition, there has been some claim of an advantage of the enclosed retroperitoneal space to tamponade surgical bleeding [19] and containing urine leaks to the retroperitoneal space [48], although these claims are theoretical thus far. These complications are relatively rare in the modern era with the enhanced vision and increased suturing dexterity provided by robotic technique [49, 50].

20.4 Technical Considerations: Transperitoneal and Retroperitoneal Robotic Surgery

20.4.1 Positioning and Docking

Positioning of the patient in transperitoneal compared to a retroperitoneal approach is mostly similar [51]. While various techniques are described, in transperitoneal robotic surgery the patient is often in the flank position at 60–90 ° [52] with the table moderately flexed. In the retroperitoneal approach, the patient is typically in the full flank position with the table fully flexed to open up the small working space between the ASIS and ribs as much as possible [19]. During retroperitoneoscopic renal surgery, the robot docks over the head or shoulder with the larger DaVinci models [53], however with the da Vinci Xi it can dock from the back and pivot if the surgeon prefers [37]. Transperitoneal robotic procedures are usually docked laterally along the patients back without difficulty, regardless of the surgical platform.

20.4.2 Robotic Platform and Ports

Transperitoneal and retroperitoneal robotic renal surgery can be performed with three or four robotic ports, and typically 1–2 assistant ports. Transperitoneal robotic renal surgery can easily accommodate 4 robotic arms due to the large 5–7 L working space of the peritoneum previously discussed. Triangulation, freedom of movement, and instrument clashing may be more difficult in retroperitoneoscopic approaches, particularly when a fourth robotic arm is utilised [19]. The small working volume of 1–2 L of the retroperitoneum and proximity to the ASIS bone reduces the surface area available for retroperitoneal port placement, particularly during utilisation of the wider robotic platforms such as the da Vinci S and

Si (Intuitive surgical, Sunnyvale, California). The da Vinci S and Si and X benefit from 8 to 11 cm of port separation to accommodate the wider wingspan of the robotic arms, whereas smaller platforms such as the da Vinci Xi, the ports can be as close as 4–5 cm if required. With larger platforms such as the da Vinci S and Si, the majority of retroperitoneal surgeries are performed with three robotic ports [19, 54], often referred to as "one-handed surgery" since the other robotic arm is used to retract the kidney, with the surgeon switching between the 2 arms as required. Recent uptake of smaller platforms such as the da Vinci Xi has made 4 arm retroperitoneal renal surgery easier and more popular [54]. The da Vinci Xi also allows for more space for surgical assistant on abdominal side. Marconi et al. suggests that the space limitations of retroperitoneal port placement have contributed to the resistance in uptake of the retroperitoneal approach, as the transperitoneal approach has a wide working space and is more suitable for surgical assistants [7].

20.4.3 Obesity

Elevated BMI is associated with several comorbidities that are associated with poor surgical outcomes and increase peri-operative morbidity [55–57]. The topic of obesity and robotic partial nephrectomy is perplexing to the effect that Kott et al. discuss a BMI paradox [55] where better outcomes are seen in patients who are overweight and mildly obese as compared to "normal" weight patients, with the point of inflection being a BMI of 30 kg/m^2. It is thought that an increase in BMI increases the excess retroperitoneal adipose tissue which increases surgical technical complexity, leading to longer trocars and decreasing the already limited space of the retroperitoneal cavity [3, 19]. In addition, excess perinephric fat in Gerota's fascia can extend medially obscuring anatomic landmarks such as the origin of the renal vessels causing a longer period of dissection and excess lateral retraction during robotic nephrectomy [58]. Some authors argue that an increase in BMI could potentially cause an increase in estimated blood loss and operation time [59], however a multi-centre centre study by Abdullah et al. has found that obesity was not an independent predictor of higher estimated blood loss and operative time with robotic partial nephrectomies, rather a consequence of higher nephrometry score and tumour size [29].

Transperitoneal access and pneumoperitoneum for robotic renal surgery is significantly more difficult in obese patients. However, once access is gained into the abdominal cavity, obesity is not prohibitive to transperitoneal robotic surgery [58]. Kapoor et al. [60] performed a study on transperitoneal laparoscopic radical nephrectomy and found a comparable complication rate between obese and non-obese patients with a longer operative time for the obese cohort. These findings were similar to those of Fugita et al. who also reported no difference in nephrectomy outcomes in obese patients [61].

Retroperitoneoscopic robotic surgery in obese patients provides the advantage of easier camera and port placement compared to transperitoneal surgery, since obese patients are often thinner on their flanks, and their landmarks of ASIS and 12 rib usually palpable [62, 63]. Additionally, the retroperitoneal adipose tissue is easy to separate during retroperitoneoscopic balloon insufflation in obese patients. However, once retroperitoneoscopy is obtained, the excessive adipose tissue of the rectoperineal space may be overwhelming and disorientating.

A study by Ng et al. demonstrated that transperitoneal access was associated with a longer operative time and hospital stay than retroperitoneoscopic approach, which the authors state was probably a result of the larger tumour size and complex pelvicalyceal reconstruction in the transperitoneal group [9]. Colombo et al. demonstrated a shorter stay in hospital for the retroperitoneal group, although subject to the same selection biases in tumour characteristics. The use of robot-assisted renal surgery appears to have exaggerated the differences between the two approaches. Malki et al. demonstrated a significantly shorter operating time, fewer postoperative complications, a shorter hospital stay, less blood loss, lower rates of blood transfusion with the retroperitoneal approach [64]. Ultimately, both approaches appear feasible in the obese patient, and more data is required from large cohort or controlled trials to make any genuine conclusions. It is up to the judgement of the clinician as to which approach is appropriate in each patient.

20.4.4 Paediatric and Petite Patients

The use of robot-assisted renal surgery is an evolving field in paediatric surgery, with very few cases of robotic management of renal tumours reported in the literature to date [65]. The small working space in petite patients, both retroperitoneally and transperitoneally, extends the debate of transperitoneal versus retroperitoneal access to paediatric urology. For radical nephrectomy, both the transperitoneal and retroperitoneal approach have been utilised with similar complication rates. Retroperitoneal approach has the added advantage, or disadvantage, of using two trocars instead of three [66]. The transperitoneal approach is more suitable for bilateral nephrectomies [67]. For partial nephrectomies, the results show a preference for transperitoneal approach due to technical difficulties. Esposito et al. compared the two approaches and found significant differences in operative time, length of stay, and complication rates, and concluded transperitoneal approach was superior [68]. Ultimately, it appears that both approaches are feasible for a radical nephrectomy, and a transperitoneal approach is favoured in partial nephrectomies.

20.4.5 Laterality of Lesion

Right transabdominal robotic renal surgery is often easier than left transabdominal renal surgery. The colonic reflection diverges lower on the right side than the left, usually providing direct visualisation of the right kidney, and sometimes the right renal vein in thin patients. On the left side, the renal vein and artery lay hidden behind the splenic flexure of the colon, requiring additional colonic reflection during left transabdominal renal surgery. Inadvertent dissection and ligation of the tail of the pancreas and the superior mesenteric artery can occur during this dissection if the colonic mesentery is not reflected properly.

Conversely, during retroperitoneal surgery, the left kidney is easier to dissect than the right kidneys. Retroperitoneoscopy on the left provides immediate visualisation of the left renal artery. Retroperitoneoscopy on the right side provides immediate exposure to the IVC and its numerous small lumbar tributaries, which can be a source of bleeding or disorientation for inexperienced surgeons.

20.4.6 Redo Surgeries

Repeat partial nephrectomy is a surgically complex treatment option in someone who has developed a new or recurrent tumour in the same kidney [69]. Repeat surgery is complicated by fibrosis and obliteration of normal peri-renal planes [70]. Although radical nephrectomy is possible [71], partial nephrectomy has its advantages in preserving renal function. This is emphasised by the recurrence of tumours thought due to the bilateral nature and multifocality of the disease, in addition to patients with solitary kidneys, salvage partial nephrectomies and post-ablation surgery [25, 69]. The use of robotic surgery in repeat partial nephrectomies is undergoing continuous development. The intense perinephric fibrosis obscures the tissue planes in a repeat procedure and can increase operation time, blood loss, hospital stay, postoperative urine leak, greater need for postoperative dialysis (pertinent to solitary kidneys) and intraoperative injury to adjacent structures [69, 70, 72, 73]. Autorino et al. [69] removed 12 tumours in 9 patients with a transabdominal approach and found that robot-assisted partial nephrectomy is safe and feasible for repeat partial nephrectomies with two complications. Although the approach is more technically demanding, the robotic platform facilitate key steps in the partial nephrectomy procedure, improving surgical outcomes. Watson et al. [74] found an overall complication rate of 58% and 19% rate of urinary leakage over 26 patients who underwent repeat robotic partial nephrectomy. Martini et al. [75] performed 24 radical salvage nephrectomies and 8 salvage partial nephrectomy and found a 0% complication rate, ascribed to be a reflection of surgical experience and patient selection, as salvage surgery is likely to be offered to the most fit patients and in case of high chance of success.

Repeat surgeries for isolated recurrence of disease has been shown to be safe and feasible for robotic surgery with a retroperitoneal robot-assisted approach [76] and a transabdominal approach [77]. Robotic transabdominal approach has allowed the opportunity to do surgeries that have not been able to be performed laparoscopically [77]. Ghandour et al. [76] demonstrated no positive margins and lack of surgical related admissions within ninety days of the surgery in twelve patients who underwent retroperitoneal robotic excision surgery for retroperitoneal isolated recurrence. This is an evolving field needs further research to declare which approach is appropriate for the management of recurrences and further clarify the role of robotic surgery in the management of simple and complicated tumour recurrences.

During robotic renal surgery following partial nephrectomy, special attention needs to be made preoperatively to the presence and location of surgical sealants, particularly permanent adhesives such as Acrylic glues such as *Glubran* (GEM surgical, Italy). Permanent sealants can obliterate the surgical planes and create permanent adhesions to the flank side wall or critical organs. We do not advocate these adhesives for this reason, but in the event a redo surgery following renal adhesives is required, we advocate a transabdominal approach in the event of local recurrence so that the kidney can be adequately mobilised and inspected.

20.5 Outcomes of Robotic Transperitoneal Versus Robotic Retroperitoneal Approaches

Transperitoneal and retroperitoneal robotic access in renal surgery may influence perioperative and postoperative outcomes for the patient [4, 8, 36]. The choice of transperitoneal or retroperitoneal access in robotic renal surgery and the proposed advantages and outcomes associated with each approach is an issue of ongoing debate.

In recent times, large, matched pair multi-institutional studies and international multicentre studies have attempted to evaluate both transperitoneal and retroperitoneal approaches and compare the intraoperative outcomes, post-operative outcomes, and oncological outcomes, with an aim to demonstrate objective difference in outcomes between the two surgical techniques [4, 7, 23, 31, 33, 36, 78–80].

20.6 Intraoperative Outcomes

The main intraoperative parameters evaluated in current literature are operative time, time to vascular control, warm ischemia time and estimated blood loss.

20.6.1 Operative Time

Retroperitoneal approach allows for a prompt and direct access to renal hilum, allowing for a shorter intraoperative time in comparison to the transperitoneal approach while also reducing the chance of renal pedicle injury [4, 7, 23, 31, 33, 36, 78]. Current literature have shown a shorter operation time associated with retroperitoneal when compared with transperitoneal, with a mean weighted difference ranging from 13 to 48 min [4, 7, 8, 23, 31, 36, 37, 79, 80].

A metanalysis by Fan et al. reported difference of 48 min between retroperitoneal and transperitoneal partial nephrectomy but did not demonstrate any clinically significant difference in operating time with retroperitoneal and transperitoneal approach for radical nephrectomy [36]. Similarly, multiple systematic reviews and meta-analyses all reported significantly shorter operating time with retroperitoneal approach when compared with transperitoneal approach [7, 8, 23,

78, 79]. Analysis by Xia et al. demonstrated a shorter operating time for retroperitoneal surgery with a mean weighted difference of 28 min. Zhu et al. [7, 79] also demonstrated the same with a mean weighted difference 21 min. Contrary to this, a multicentre study by Porpiglia et al. which compared 413 patients that were propensity matched in each group, reported a significantly shorter operative time in the transperitoneal approach (115 min) when compared with retroperitoneal approach (150 min) [81]. This could be because the creation of a virtual retroperitoneal space can sometimes be performed laparoscopically to create a working space for robotic trocars [4]. Meanwhile, some single centre studies reported no difference in mean operating time between retroperitoneal and transperitoneal Techniques [40, 82].

It has also been demonstrated that renal artery and vein control were achieved in a significantly shorter time with the retroperitoneal approach when compared with transperitoneal technique with a weighted mean difference of 68 and 53 min respectively [36]. This can be explained by the transperitoneal approach requiring considerable mobilisation of the renal hilum while retroperitoneal approach offering direct and rapid access to the renal hilum.

20.6.2 Estimated Blood Loss and Warm Ischemia Time

Renal surgery via retroperitoneal access has been proposed to have lower estimated blood loss when compared with transperitoneal approach [37, 40, 83, 84]. This is theorised due to the easier identification and control of the renal hilum and less surgical dissection involved in the retroperitoneal approach and the use of early unclamping technique often used in the transperitoneal procedure [40, 79, 84]. However, numerous large multicentre observational studies have demonstrated no statistically significant difference in estimated blood loss between the transperitoneal and retroperitoneal approaches [4, 7, 23, 31, 33, 36, 37, 40, 78, 79, 82–84]. A meta-analyses demonstrated estimated blood loss is no different between retroperitoneal and transperitoneal robotic renal surgery.

Similarly, there is no significant difference in warm ischemia time in both retroperitoneal and transperitoneal surgical techniques. There were also no significant differences were found in simple enucleation rates and clampless procedures [4].

20.6.3 Operative Duration

Retroperitoneal robotic renal surgery provides a direct and rapid access to the kidney and renal hilum and does not need extensive mobilisation of the bowel or kidney. This can contribute to the shorter time to vascular control and shorter operating time reported in literature. Transperitoneal approaches for posterior tumours are feasible, but require additional time to access the posterolateral surface of the lesion and increase the operative times for transperitoneal surgery [23, 36, 37, 40, 79, 83]. Anterior tumours are rarely addressed by a retroperitoneal approach due to the small working space and possibility of entry into the peritoneal membrane along the anterior renal border, which is another factor why retroperitoneal surgery may be quicker overall.

20.6.4 Intraoperative Injuries

Intraoperative complications are reported to be lower in retroperitoneal robotic surgery compared to transperitoneal [23, 83, 85, 86]. This may be due to the immediate access to the renal pedicle and the avoidance of the intraperitoneal organs associated with transperitoneal approach [4, 36]. Some authors point out there may be a selection bias accounting for the differences in complications, since studies show retroperitoneal robotic surgery is more commonly performed by more experienced surgeons with prior transabdominal robotic experience, and on patients with smaller tumours.

20.7 Postoperative Outcomes

20.7.1 Length of Hospital Stay

Retroperitoneal robotic renal surgery is reported to have a shorter drain duration and earlier return of the bowel function [31, 78, 86]. with a mean weighted difference of 0.8–1 day [36, 37, 79, 83, 86]. Additional analysis by Fan et al. demonstrated a significant difference in length of stay for partial nephrectomy with a mean weighted difference of 1 day between retroperitoneal and transperitoneal approaches but the same study did not demonstrate statistical difference in length of stay for radical nephrectomies [36]. It is however important to note that this particular analysis was limited due to it being observational, having varying protocols, differing levels of surgical expertise and lack of random sequence generation. The lower time of drain maintenance and post-operative hospital stay associated with retroperitoneal surgery may lead to less post-operative analgesic requirements. However most large multi-centre studies and meta-analysis did not show clinically or statistically significant difference in post-operative pain or analgesic requirements [4, 31, 36, 85, 86].

Several studies have shown that transperitoneal renal surgery results in significantly longer length of stays compared to the retroperitoneal approach [4, 37, 40, 79, 82, 83, 86]. It is believed that manipulation of the bowel increases the rates of post-operative ileus. However, there is lack of strong evidence to suggest that this is the cause [85], to the extent that the opposite effect has been cited in some literature [24]. The time to first oral intake is not significantly different between retroperitoneal and transperitoneal techniques [36, 82]. A multivariate analysis by

Kim et al. predicted surgical approach to be an independent predictor of postoperative length of stay [87]. Meanwhile, other studies like Carbonara et al. [78] failed to show significant difference in post operative length of stay between the two approaches [78].

20.7.2 Post-Operative Renal Function

Studies have not demonstrated a difference in serum creatinine in the early postoperative period when contrasting the two approaches [4, 7, 31, 36, 37, 40, 79, 82, 83]. Furthermore, there is no significant difference in median variation of eGFR between baseline levels and in the subsequent follow up time between the retroperitoneal and transperitoneal patient groups [4, 7, 31, 36, 37, 40, 78, 79, 81–83, 87].

20.7.3 Post-Operative Complications

Some authors have reported transperitoneal renal surgery associated with higher surgical complications, and Clavien-Dindo two and above complications when compared with retroperitoneal [4]. However, the majority of the available data report no significant differences in surgical outcomes between transperitoneal and retroperitoneal approaches [7, 8, 23, 31, 33, 78, 79]. Both approaches have shown to have comparable postoperative and overall complication rates [4, 7, 31, 33, 36, 78, 83, 85, 86]. An analysis by Dell'Oglio et al. observed no differences in warm ischemia time, estimated blood loss, postoperative complication rate, post operative eGFR and positive surgical margins in the two surgical techniques. Interestingly, in this analysis the patients had equivalent outcomes after either transperitoneal or retroperitoneal technique regardless of the tumour location [32]. The study also observed no advantage with the different tumour position (anterior versus posterior) and the approach (transperitoneal versus retroperitoneal) used to resect the lesion [32].

20.7.4 Post-Operative Intraabdominal Adhesions

There is no consensus as to when a retroperitoneal approach or a transperitoneal approach should be employed in robot-assisted laparoscopic nephrectomy or partial nephrectomy. However, adhesions in the abdomen appear to be a relative contraindication for some surgeons. It is thought that adhesions due to previous abdominal surgery leads to increase in operation time, estimated blood loss and general increase complications such as longer stay in hospital and conversion to open surgery. However, Abdullah et al. [29] conducted a prospective multicentre study with 1686 patients and compared patients undergoing robot-assisted laparoscopic partial nephrectomy with and without a history of previous major abdominal surgery. They found that there was no difference in operation time, warm ischemia time, length of stay, positive margins, and other perioperative complications between the two groups excluding an increase in estimated blood loss in the prior surgery group that did not translate to higher rates of transfusion [29]. A particular strength of this study was that the two groups were found to not have a statistically significant difference in RENAL nephrometry score, Charlson comorbidities index, tumour size and pre-operative eGFR. These findings were supported by Zargar et al. [88] in their single centre study with 627 patients [88]. Moreover, a study that investigated non-robotic transperitoneal laparoscopic radical nephrectomies shared similar results to the robotic partial nephrectomies although these findings are limited by being a retrospective single centre study with selection bias [89]. However, these studies are observational in nature, and as such limits the conclusions. Ultimately, it appears that prior abdominal surgery and adhesions have a less significant effect on perioperative and intraoperative outcomes than conventionally thought.

20.8 Oncological Outcomes

20.8.1 Local and Distant Recurrence

Robotic renal surgery provides excellent cancer control and high cure rate for treating renal masses [90, 91]. The five-year survival rate after robotic laparoscopic surgery for malignant renal masses has been reported to be 91% [91]. Overall recurrence rate post robotic nephrectomy at 72 months was reported to be at 2.9% [91] No clear difference exists in the overall recurrence rate, local recurrence rate, or distant recurrence rate between transperitoneal and retroperitoneal surgical techniques and both approaches had comparable long-term survival rates [4, 36, 37]. There are no differences recorded in rates of positive surgical margins between transperitoneal or retroperitoneal approach [4, 39, 40, 78–80, 82, 83, 85, 86].

20.8.2 Port Site Recurrence and Crepitus

The incidence of port site recurrence is not well defined in robotic renal cancer surgery, but majority of available literature describe the incidence as rare after laparoscopic resection of renal cell carcinomas, with overall estimated incidence ranging from 0.03 to 0.35% [37, 92–96]. The incidence is higher following robotic surgery for upper tract urothelial cell carcinoma and with retroperitoneal laparoscopic surgery [92, 93, 95, 96]. Risk factors for port site recurrence include positive surgical margins, high grade tumours, ruptured tumours, and no wrap removal [92–94, 96, 97]. Other risks include retroperitoneoscopy, port site air leak, high CO^2 insufflation pressure, aerosolization of tumour cells, and contamination of operative field or port sites [98–101].

Rassweiler et al. demonstrated 1.6% of its 377-patient cohort developed post site recurrence within 12 months after laparoscopic nephroureterectomy. The authors recommended open surgery for patients with advanced tumours of pT3 and higher as a result [93]. A study by Kang et al. reported that air leak during retroperitoneal renal surgery increases the potential risk of port site recurrence in patients with upper tract urothelial carcinoma [92]. The incidence of port site recurrence was 2.8% in patients with renal pelvic tumours and and 0.7% in patients with ureteral tumours in their series, with overall incidence of 1.7% [92]. They stipulated that constant leakage of large volumes of CO_2 alongside the poorly seated retroperitoneal ports increases the concentration of aerosolized tumour cells within the subcutaneous tissue surrounding the ports [92]. Studies by Bouvy et al. [98] reported CO_2 insufflation as a major factor leading to port site recurrences. Some authors also report that subcutaneous emphysema and crepitus are increased following retroperitoneal robotic renal surgery, due to the small working space and larger degree of air leaks around the ports, but studies are still underway. Many retroperitoneoscopic surgeons advocate utilisation of lower insufflation pressures in the retroperitoneum, typically 7–10 cm H_2O pressure in the retroperitoneum, as opposed to 12–15 cm H_2O in the peritoneum, since the retroperitoneal space requires less working volume. Other studies found no significant difference in tumour seeding between the CO_2 pressures and a gasless surgery group [91, 98, 102]. We advocate that port sites should be examined during surveillance follow up and wide local excision considered where appropriate [91]. Recommendations to reduce the incidence include avoiding air leakage, abiding by strict guidelines for proper tumour resection without spillage or aerolisation, and always removing the specimen under direct vision with the use of impermeable specimen bags [91, 92, 103, 104].

20.9 Conclusions

Transperitoneal and retroperitoneal approaches are equally excellent approaches for performing robotic assisted renal surgery. Transperitoneal and retroperitoneal approaches have comparable intraoperative, post-operative outcomes and both approaches have their own merits in select cases [4, 7, 31, 33, 36, 37, 78]. Transperitoneal robotic surgery remains more popular due to the familiar anatomy and larger working volume of the peritoneum. Retroperitoneal robotic renal surgery continues to grow in popularity, particularly for small posterior tumours in the hands of experienced surgeons with access to smaller robotic platforms that can accommodate the smaller working space of the retroperitoneum It is important for surgeons to be confident in both transperitoneal and retroperitoneal approaches, so that they can modulate the choice of approach appropriately to each individual case. The final choice of approach should reflect surgeon experience, tumour anatomy, and the surgeon's understanding of competing advantages and disadvantages of each [4, 24, 39, 105].

References

1. Clayman RV, Kavoussi LR, Soper NJ, Dierks SM, Meretyk S, Darcy MD, Roemer FD, Pingleton ED, Thomson PG, Long SR. Laparoscopic nephrectomy: initial case report. J Urol. 1991;146(2):278–82.
2. Gaur DD, Agarwal DK, Purohit KC. Retroperitoneal laparoscopic nephrectomy: initial case report. J Urol. 1993;149(1):103–5.
3. Cacciamani GE, Medina LG, Gill T, Abreu A, Sotelo R, Artibani W, Gill IS. Impact of surgical factors on robotic partial nephrectomy outcomes: comprehensive systematic review and meta-analysis. J Urol. 2018;200(2):258–74.
4. Porpiglia F, Mari A, Amparore D, Fiori C, Antonelli A, Artibani W, Bove P, Brunocilla E, Capitanio U, da Pozzo L, di Maida F, Gontero P, Longo N, Marra G, Rocco B, Schiavina R, Simeone C, Siracusano S, Tellini R, Terrone C, Villari D, Ficarra V, Carini M, Minervini A. Transperitoneal vs retroperitoneal minimally invasive partial nephrectomy: comparison of perioperative outcomes and functional follow-up in a large multi-institutional cohort (The RECORD 2 Project). Surg Endosc. 2021;35(8):4295–304.
5. Guillonneau B, Jayet C, Tewari A, Vallancien G. Robot assisted laparoscopic nephrectomy. J Urol. 2001;166(1):200–1.
6. Bertolo R, Autorino R, Simone G, Derweesh I, Garisto JD, Minervini A, Eun D, Perdona S, Porter J, Rha KH, Mottrie A, White WM, Schips L, Yang B, Jacobsohn K, Uzzo RG, Challacombe B, Ferro M, Sulek J, Capitanio U, Anele UA, Tuderti G, Costantini M, Ryan S, Bindayi A, Mari A, Carini M, Keehn A, Quarto G, Liao M, Chang K, Larcher A, de Naeyer G, de Cobelli O, Berardinelli F, Zhang C, Langenstroer P, Kutikov A, Chen D, de Luyk N, Sundaram CP, Montorsi F, Stein RJ, Haber GP, Hampton LJ, Dasgupta P, Gallucci M, Kaouk J, Porpiglia F. Outcomes of robot-assisted partial nephrectomy for clinical T2 renal tumors: a multicenter analysis (ROSULA Collaborative Group). Eur Urol. 2018;74(2):226–32.
7. Xia L, Zhang X, Wang X, Xu T, Qin L, Zhang X, Zhong S, Shen Z. Transperitoneal versus retroperitoneal robot-assisted partial nephrectomy: a systematic review and meta-analysis. Int J Surg. 2016;30:109–15.
8. Ren T, Liu Y, Zhao X, Ni S, Zhang C, Guo C, Ren M. Transperitoneal approach versus retroperitoneal approach: a meta-analysis of laparoscopic partial nephrectomy for renal cell carcinoma. PLoS One. 2014;9:e91978.
9. Ng CS, Gill IS, Ramani AP, Steinberg AP, Spaliviero M, Abreu SC, Kaouk JH, Desai MM. Transperitoneal versus retroperitoneal laparoscopic partial nephrectomy: patient selection and perioperative outcomes. J Urol. 2005;174(3):846–9.
10. Ball M, Gorin M, Jayram G, Pierorazio P, Allaf M. Robot-assisted radical nephrectomy with inferior vena cava tumor thrombectomy: technique and initial outcomes. Can J Urol. 2015;22.
11. Liu G, Ma Y, Wang S, Han X, Gao D. Laparoscopic versus open radical nephrectomy for renal cell carcinoma: a systematic review and meta-analysis. Transl Oncol. 2017;10(4):501–10.
12. Porreca A, D'Agostino D, Dente D, Dandrea M, Salvaggio A, Cappa E, Zuccala A, del Rosso A, Chessa F, Romagnoli D, Mengoni F, Borghesi M, Schiavina R. Retroperitoneal approach for robot-assisted partial nephrectomy: technique and early outcomes. Int Braz J Urol. 2018;44(1):63–8.
13. Montisci E, Corona A, Serra S, de Lisa A. Laparoscopic nephrectomy treatment of renal tumors over 7 cm: our experience. Urologia. 2012;79(Suppl 19):91–5.
14. Bird VG, Shields JM, Aziz M, Ayyathurai R, De Los Santos R, Roeter, DH Laparoscopic radical nephrectomy for patients with T2 and T3 renal-cell carcinoma: evaluation of perioperative outcomes. J Endourol. 2009;23(9):1527–33.
15. Laird A, Choy KCC, Delaney H, Cutress ML, O'Connor KM, Tolley DA, McNeill SA, Stewart GD, Riddick ACP. Matched pair analysis of laparoscopic versus open radical nephrectomy for the treatment of T3 renal cell carcinoma. World J Urol. 2015;33(1):25–32.

16. Ganpule AP, Sharma R, Thimmegowda M, Veeramani M, Desai MR. Laparoscopic radical nephrectomy versus open radical nephrectomy in T1–T3 renal tumors: an outcome analysis. Indian J Urol. 2008;24(1):39–43.
17. Ke XW, Zeng X, Wei X, Shen YQ, Gan JH, Tian JH, Hu ZQ. Robotic-assisted laparoscopic nephrectomy with vein thrombectomy: initial experience and outcomes from a single surgeon. Curr Med Sci. 2018;38(5):834–9.
18. Dellaportas D, Arkadopoulos N, Tzanoglou I, Bairamidis E, Gemenetzis G, Xanthakos P, Nastos C, Kostopanagiotou G, Vassiliou I, Smyrniotis V. Technical intraoperative maneuvers for the management of inferior vena cava thrombus in renal cell carcinoma. Front Surg. 2017;4(48).
19. Marconi L, Challacombe B. Robotic partial nephrectomy for posterior renal tumours: retro or transperitoneal approach? Eur Urol Focus. 2018;4(5):632–5.
20. EAU Guidelines. editors. presented at the EAU Annual Congress Milan 2021. ISBN 978-94-92671-13-4.
21. Chopra S, Simone G, Metcalfe C, De Castro Abreu AL, Nabhani J, Ferriero M, Bove AM, Sotelo R, Aron M, Desai MM, Gallucci M, Gill IS. Robot-assisted level II-III inferior vena cava tumor thrombectomy: step-by-step technique and 1-year outcomes. Eur Urol. 2017;72(2):267–74.
22. Yang F, Zhou Q, Li X, Xing N. The methods and techniques of identifying renal pedicle vessels during retroperitoneal laparoscopic radical and partial nephrectomy. World J Surg Oncol. 2019;17(1):38.
23. McLean A, Mukherjee A, Phukan C, Veeratterapillay R, Soomro N, Somani B, Rai BP. Trans-peritoneal vs. retroperitoneal robotic assisted partial nephrectomy in posterior renal tumours: need for a risk-stratified patient individualised approach. A systematic review and meta-analysis. J Robot Surg. 2020;14(1):1–9.
24. Desai MM, Strzempkowski B, Matin SF, Steinberg AP, Ng C, Meraney AM, Kaouk JH, Gill IS. Prospective randomized comparison of transperitoneal versus retroperitoneal laparoscopic radical nephrectomy. J Urol. 2005;173(1):38–41.
25. Shuch B, Linehan WM, Bratslavsky G. Repeat partial nephrectomy: surgical, functional and oncological outcomes. Curr Opin Urol. 2011;21(5):368–75.
26. Raison N, Doeuk N, Malthouse T, Kasivisvanathan V, Lam W, Challacombe B. Challenging situations in partial nephrectomy. Int J Surg. 2016;36:568–73.
27. Nguyen CT, Lane BR, Kaouk JH, Hegarty N, Gill IS, Novick AC, Campbell SC. Surgical salvage of renal cell carcinoma recurrence after thermal ablative therapy. J Urol. 2008;180(1):104–9; discussion 9.
28. Kowalczyk KJ, Hooper HB, Linehan WM, Pinto PA, Wood BJ, Bratslavsky G. Partial nephrectomy after previous radio frequency ablation: the National Cancer Institute experience. J Urol. 2009;182(5):2158–63.
29. Abdullah N, Rahbar H, Barod R, Dalela D, Larson J, Johnson M, Mass A, Zargar H, Allaf M, Bhayani S, Stifelman M, Kaouk J, Rogers C. Multicentre outcomes of robot-assisted partial nephrectomy after major open abdominal surgery. BJU Int. 2016;118(2):298–301.
30. Asali M, Tsivian A. Laparoscopic nephrectomy in xanthogranulomatous pyelonephritis. Central Eur J Urol. 2019;72(3):319–23.
31. Arora S, Heulitt G, Menon M, Jeong W, Ahlawat RK, Capitanio U, Moon DA, Maes KK, Rawal S, Mottrie A, Bhandari M, Rogers CG, Porter JR. Retroperitoneal vs transperitoneal robot-assisted partial nephrectomy: comparison in a multi-institutional setting. Urology. 2018;120:131–7.
32. Dell'Oglio P, de Naeyer G, Xiangjun L, Hamilton Z, Capitanio U, Ripa F, Cianflone F, Muttin F, Schatteman P, D'Hondt F, Ma X, Bindayi A, Zhang X, Derweesh I, Mottrie A, Montorsi F, Larcher A. The impact of surgical strategy in robot-assisted partial nephrectomy: is it beneficial to treat anterior tumours with transperitoneal access and posterior tumours with retroperitoneal access? Eur Urol Oncol. 2021;4(1):112–6.

33. Zhou J, Liu ZH, Cao DH, Peng ZF, Song P, Yang L, Liu LR, Wei Q, Dong Q. Retroperitoneal or transperitoneal approach in robot-assisted partial nephrectomy, which one is better? Cancer Med. 2021;10(10):3299–308.
34. McAllister M, Bhayani SB, Ong A, Jaffe W, Malkowicz SB, Vanarsdalen K, Chow GK, Jarrett TW. Vena caval transection during retroperitoneoscopic nephrectomy: report of the complication and review of the literature. J Urol. 2004;172(1):183–5.
35. Wright JL, Porter JR. Laparoscopic partial nephrectomy: comparison of transperitoneal and retroperitoneal approaches. J Urol. 2005;174(3):841–5.
36. Fan X, Xu K, Lin T, Liu H, Yin Z, Dong W, Huang H, Huang J. Comparison of transperitoneal and retroperitoneal laparoscopic nephrectomy for renal cell carcinoma: a systematic review and meta-analysis. BJU Int. 2013;111(4):611–21.
37. Mittakanti HR, Heulitt G, Li H-F, Porter JR. Transperitoneal vs. retroperitoneal robotic partial nephrectomy: a matched-paired analysis. World J Urol. 2020;38(5):1093–9.
38. Varkarakis IM, Allaf ME, Bhayani SB, Inagaki T, Su LM, Kavoussi LR, Jarrett TW. Pancreatic injuries during laparoscopic urologic surgery. Urology. 2004;64(6):1089–93.
39. Lasser MS, Ghavamian R. Surgical complications of laparoscopic urological surgery. Arab J Urol. 2012;10(1):81–8.
40. Abaza R, Gerhard RS, Martinez O. Feasibility of adopting retroperitoneal robotic partial nephrectomy after extensive transperitoneal experience. World J Urol. 2020;38(11):1087–92.
41. Malkoc E, Ramirez D, Kara O, Maurice MJ, Nelson RJ, Caputo PA, Kaouk JH. Robotic and open partial nephrectomy for localized renal tumors larger than 7 cm: a single-center experience. World J Urol. 2017;35(5):781–7.
42. Anele UA, Marchioni M, Yang B, Simone G, Uzzo RG, Lau C, Mir MC, Capitanio U, Porter J, Jacobsohn K, de Luyk N, Mari A, Chang K, Fiori C, Sulek J, Mottrie A, White W, Perdona S, Quarto G, Bindayi A, Ashrafi A, Schips L, Berardinelli F, Zhang C, Gallucci M, Ramirez-Backhaus M, Larcher A, Kilday P, Liao M, Langenstroer P, Dasgupta P, Challacombe B, Kutikov A, Minervini A, Rha KH, Sundaram CP, Hampton LJ, Porpiglia F, Aron M, Derweesh I, Autorino R. Robotic versus laparoscopic radical nephrectomy: a large multi-institutional analysis (ROSULA Collaborative Group). World J Urol. 2019;37(11):2439–50.
43. Strauss DM, Lee R, Maffucci F, Abbott D, Masic S, Kutikov A. The future of "Retro" robotic partial nephrectomy. Transl Androl Urol. 2021;10(5):2199–208.
44. Luo L, Liu Y-N, Zhang Y, Zhang G-M, Sun L-J, Liu Y, Wang F-M. An easy and effective method to locate renal vein during retroperitoneal laparoscopic radical nephrectomy: single-center experience. Med Sci Monit. 2018;24:5147–51.
45. Yang Q, Du J, Zhao Z-H, Chen X-S, Zhou L, Yao X. Fast access and early ligation of the renal pedicle significantly facilitates retroperitoneal laparoscopic radical nephrectomy procedures: modified laparoscopic radical nephrectomy. World J Surg Oncol. 2013;11(1):27.
46. Porpiglia F, Terrone C, Cracco C, Renard J, Musso F, Grande S, Scarpa RM. Direct access to the renal artery at the level of treitz ligament during left radical laparoscopic transperitoneal nephrectomy. Eur Urol. 2005;48(2):291–5.
47. Choo SH, Lee SY, Sung HH, Jeon HG, Jeong BC, Jeon SS, Lee HM, Choi HY, Seo SI. Transperitoneal versus retroperitoneal robotic partial nephrectomy: matched-pair comparisons by nephrometry scores. World J Urol. 2014;32(6):1523–9.
48. Lim IIP, Honeyman JN, Fialkowski EA, Murphy JM, Price AP, Abramson SJ, Quaglia MPL, Heaton TE. Experience with retroperitoneal partial nephrectomy in bilateral Wilms tumor. Eur J Pediatr Surg. 2015; 25(1):113–7.
49. Benway BM, Wang AJ, Cabello JM, Bhayani SB. Robotic partial nephrectomy with sliding-clip renorrhaphy: technique and outcomes. Eur Urol. 2009;55:592–9.
50. Ryan J, Maccraith E, Davis NF, Mclornan L. A systematic management algorithm for perioperative complications after robotic assisted partial nephrectomy. Can Urol Assoc J. 2019;13(11):E371–E376.
51. Lee RA, Strauss D, Kutikov A. Role of minimally invasive partial nephrectomy in the management of renal mass. Transl Androl Urol. 2020;9(6):3140–8.

52. Kaouk JH, Khalifeh A, Hillyer S, Haber G-P, Stein RJ, Autorino R. Robot-assisted laparoscopic partial nephrectomy: step-by-step contemporary technique and surgical outcomes at a single high-volume institution. Eur Urol. 2012;62(3):553–61.
53. Feliciano J, Stifelman M. Robotic retroperitoneal partial nephrectomy: a four-arm approach. Jsls. 2012;16(2):208–11.
54. Ghani KR, Porter J, Menon M, Rogers C. Robotic retroperitoneal partial nephrectomy: a step-by-step guide. BJU Int. 2014;114:311–3.
55. Kott O, Golijanin B, Pereira JF, Chambers A, Knasin A, Tucci C, Golijanin D. The BMI paradox and robotic assisted partial nephrectomy. Front Surg. 2020;6:74–74.
56. Bogers RP, Bemelmans WJ, Hoogenveen RT, Boshuizen HC, Woodward M, Knekt P, Van Dam RM, Hu FB, Visscher TL, Menotti A, Thorpe RJ, Jamrozik K, Calling S, Strand BH, Shipley MJ. Association of overweight with increased risk of coronary heart disease partly independent of blood pressure and cholesterol levels: a meta-analysis of 21 cohort studies including more than 300 000 persons. Arch Intern Med. 2007;167(16):1720–8.
57. Watanabe J, Tatsumi K, Ota M, Suwa Y, Suzuki S, Watanabe A, Ishibe A, Watanabe K, Akiyama H, Ichikawa Y, Morita S, Endo I. The impact of visceral obesity on surgical outcomes of laparoscopic surgery for colon cancer. Int J Colorectal Dis. 2014;29:343–51.
58. Ioffe E, Hakimi AA, Oh SK, Agalliu I, Ginzburg N, Williams SK, Kao L, Rozenblit AM, Ghavamian R. Effect of visceral obesity on minimally invasive partial nephrectomy. Urology. 2013;82:612–9.
59. Naeem N, Petros F, Sukumar S, Patel M, Bhandari A, Kaul S, Menon M, Rogers C. Robot-Assisted Partial Nephrectomy in Obese Patients. J Endourol. 2011;25(1):101–5.
60. Kapoor A, Nassir A, Chew B, Gillis A, Luke P, Whelan P. Comparison of laparoscopic radical renal surgery in morbidly obese and non-obese patients. J Endourol. 2004;18(7):657–60.
61. Fugita OE, Chan DY, Roberts WW, Kavoussi LR, Jarrett TW. Laparoscopic radical nephrectomy in obese patients: outcomes and technical considerations. Urology. 2004;63(2):247–52.
62. Doublet J, Belair G. Retroperitoneal laparoscopic nephrectomy is safe and effective in obese patients: a comparative study of 55 procedures. Urology. 2000;56(1):63–6.
63. Małkiewicz B, Szydełko T, Dembowski J, Tupikowski K, Zdrojowy R. Laparoscopic radical nephrectomy in extremely obese patients. Central Eur J Urol. 2012;65(2):100–2.
64. Malki M, Oakley J, Hussain M, Barber N. Retroperitoneal robot-assisted partial nephrectomy in obese patients. J Laparoendosc Adv Surg Tech A. 2019;29(8):1027–32.
65. Blanc T, Pio L, Clermidi P, Muller C, Orbach D, Minard-Colin V, Harte C, Meignan P, Kohaut J, Heloury Y, Sarnacki S. Robotic-assisted laparoscopic management of renal tumors in children: preliminary results. Pediatr Blood Cancer. 2019;66(Suppl 3):e27867.
66. Antoniou D, Karetsos C. Laparoscopy or retroperitoneoscopy: which is the best approach in pediatric urology? Transl Pediatr. 2016;5(4):205–13.
67. Valla JS. Retroperitoneoscopic surgery in children. Semin Pediatr Surg. 2007;16(4):270–7.
68. Esposito C, Escolino M, Miyano G, Caione P, Chiarenza F, Riccipetitoni G, Yamataka A, Savanelli A, Settimi A, Varlet F, Patkowski D, Cerulo M, Castagnetti M, Till H, Marotta R, la Manna A, Valla JS. A comparison between laparoscopic and retroperitoneoscopic approach for partial nephrectomy in children with duplex kidney: a multicentric survey. World J Urol. 2016;34:939–48.
69. Autorino R, Khalifeh A, Laydner H, Samarasekera D, Rizkala E, Eyraud R, Haber GP, Stein RJ, Kaouk JH. Repeat robot-assisted partial nephrectomy (RAPN): feasibility and early outcomes. BJU Int. 2013;111(5):767–72.
70. Johnson A, Sudarshan S, Liu J, Linehan WM, Pinto PA, Bratslavsky G. Feasibility and outcomes of repeat partial nephrectomy. J Urol. 2008;180(1):89–93.
71. Abarzua-Cabezas FG, Sverrisson E, de la Cruz R, Spiess PE, Haddock P, Sexton WJ. Oncological and functional outcomes of salvage renal surgery following failed primary intervention for renal cell carcinoma. International Braz J Urol. 2015;41(1):147–54.
72. Simmons MN, Hillyer SP, Lee BH, Fergany AF, Kaouk J, Campbell SC. Functional recovery after partial nephrectomy: effects of volume loss and ischemic injury. J Urol. 2012;187(5):1667–73.

73. Liu NW, Khurana K, Sudarshan S, Pinto PA, Linehan WM, Bratslavsky G. Repeat partial nephrectomy on the solitary kidney: surgical, functional and oncological outcomes. J Urol. 2010;183(5):1719–24.
74. Watson MJ, Sidana A, Diaz AW, Siddiqui MM, Hankins RA, Bratslavsky G, Linehan WM, Metwalli AR. Repeat robotic partial nephrectomy: characteristics, complications, and renal functional outcomes. J Endourol. 2016;30(11):1219–26.
75. Martini A, Turri F, Barod R, Rocco B, Capitanio U, Briganti A, Montorsi F, Mottrie A, Challacombe B, Lagerveld BW, Bensalah K, Abaza R, Badani KK, Mehrazin R, Buscarini M, Larcher A, Okhawere K, Martinez OE, Khene Z.-E, Sonpreet R, Campain N, De Groote R, Dell'oglio P, Grivas N, Goonewardene S, Hemal A, Rivas JG. Salvage robot-assisted renal surgery for local recurrence after surgical resection or renal mass ablation: classification, techniques, and clinical outcomes. Eur Urol. 2021.
76. Ghandour R, Miranda AF, Singla N, Meng X, Enikeev D, Woldu S, Bagrodia A, Cadeddu J, Gahan J, Margulis V. Feasibility and safety of robotic excision of ipsilateral retroperitoneal recurrence after nephrectomy for renal cell carcinoma. Urology. 2020;145:159–65.
77. Gilbert D, Abaza R. Robotic excision of recurrent renal cell carcinomas with laparoscopic ultrasound assistance. Urology. 2015;85(5):1206–10.
78. Carbonara U, Eun D, Derweesh I, Capitanio U, Celia A, Fiori C, Checcucci E, Amparore D, Lee J, Larcher A, Patel D, Meagher M, Crocerossa F, Veccia A, Hampton LJ, Montorsi F, Porpiglia F, Autorino R. Retroperitoneal versus transepritoneal robot-assisted partial nephrectomy for postero-lateral renal masses: an international multicenter analysis. World J Urol. 2021.
79. Zhu D, Shao X, Guo G, Zhang N, Shi T, Wang Y, Gu L. Comparison of outcomes between transperitoneal and retroperitoneal robotic partial nephrectomy: a meta-analysis based on comparative studies. Front Oncol. 2020;10:592193.
80. Fu J, Ye S, Ye HJ. Retroperitoneal versus transperitoneal laparoscopic partial nephrectomy: a systematic review and meta-analysis. Chin Med Sci J. 2015;30(4):239–44.
81. Paulucci DJ, Beksac AT, Porter J, Abaza R, Eun DD, Bhandari A, Hemal AK, Badani KK. A multi-institutional propensity score matched comparison of transperitoneal and retroperitoneal partial nephrectomy for cT1 posterior tumors. J Laparoendosc Adv Surg Tech A. 2019;29(1):29–34.
82. Maurice MJ, Kaouk JH, Ramirez D, Bhayani SB, Allaf ME, Rogers CG, Stifelman MD. Robotic partial nephrectomy for posterior tumors through a retroperitoneal approach offers decreased length of stay compared with the transperitoneal approach: a propensity-matched analysis. J Endourol. 2017;31:158–62.
83. Pavan N, Derweesh I, Hampton LJ, White WM, Porter J, Challacombe BJ, Dasgupta P, Bertolo R, Kaouk J, Mirone V, Porpiglia F, Autorino R. Rc partial nephrectomy: systematic review and cumulative analysis of comparative outcomes. J Endourol. 2018;32(7):591–6.
84. Hughes-Hallett A, Patki P, Patel N, Barber NJ, Sullivan M, Thilagarajah R. Robot-assisted partial nephrectomy: a comparison of the transperitoneal and retroperitoneal approaches. J Endourol. 2013;27(7):869–74.
85. Kim HY, Lee DS, Yoo JM, Lee JH, Lee SJ. Retroperitoneal laparoscopic radical nephrectomy for large (>7 cm) solid renal tumors: comparison of perioperative outcomes with the transperitoneal approach. J Laparoendosc Adv Surg Tech A. 2017;27(4):393–7.
86. Laviana AA, Tan HJ, Hu JC, Weizer AZ, Chang SS, Barocas DA. Retroperitoneal versus transperitoneal robotic-assisted laparoscopic partial nephrectomy: a matched-pair, bicenter analysis with cost comparison using time-driven activity-based costing. Curr Opin Urol. 2018;28(2):108–14.
87. Kim EH, Larson JA, Potretzke AM, Hulsey NK, Bhayani SB, Figenshau RS. Retroperitoneal robot-assisted partial nephrectomy for posterior renal masses is associated with earlier hospital discharge: a single-institution retrospective comparison. J Endourol. 2015;29:1137–42.
88. Zargar H, Isac W, Autorino R, Khalifeh A, Nemer O, Akca O, Laydner H, Brandao LF, Stein RJ, Kaouk JH. Robot-assisted laparoscopic partial nephrectomy in patients with previous abdominal surgery: single center experience. Int J Med Robot. 2015;11(4):389–94.

89. Yanai Y, Takeda T, Miyajima A, Matsumoto K, Hagiwara M, Mizuno R, Kikuchi E, Asanuma H, Oya M. Is transperitoneal laparoscopic radical nephrectomy suitable for patients with a history of abdominal surgery? Asian J Endosc Surg. 2019;12(4):429–33.
90. Peyronnet B, Seisen T, Oger E, Vaessen C, Grassano Y, Benoit T, Carrouget J, Pradère B, Khene Z, Giwerc A, Mathieu R, Beauval JB, Nouhaud FX, Bigot P, Doumerc N, Bernhard JC, Mejean A, Patard JJ, Shariat S, Roupret M, Bensalah K. Comparison of 1800 robotic and open partial nephrectomies for renal tumors. Ann Surg Oncol. 2016;23(13):4277–83.
91. Salkini MW, Idris N, Lamoshi AR. The incidence and pattern of renal cell carcinoma recurrence after robotic partial nephrectomy. Urol Ann. 2019;11(4):353–7.
92. Kang Q, Yu Y, Yang B. Incidence of port site metastasis in laparoscopic radical nephroureterectomy: single-institution experience. Urology. 2019;131:130–5.
93. Rassweiler J, Tsivian A, Kumar AV, Lymberakis C, Schulze M, Seeman O, Frede T. Oncological safety of laparoscopic surgery for urological malignancy: experience with more than 1,000 operations. J Urol. 2003;169(6):2072–5.
94. Tanaka K, Hara I, Takenaka A, Kawabata G, Fujisawa M. Incidence of local and port site recurrence of urologic cancer after laparoscopic surgery. Urology. 2008;71(4):728–34.
95. Muntener M, Schaeffer EM, Romero FR, Nielsen ME, Allaf ME, Brito FA, Pavlovich CP, Kavoussi LR, Jarrett TW. Incidence of local recurrence and port site metastasis after laparoscopic radical nephroureterectomy. Urology. 2007;70(5):864–8.
96. Micali S, Celia A, Bove P, de Stefani S, Sighinolfi MC, Kavoussi LR, Bianchi G. Tumor seeding in urological laparoscopy: an international survey. J Urol. 2004;171(6 Pt 1):2151–4.
97. Shimokihara K, Kawahara T, Takamoto D, Mochizuki T, Hattori Y, Teranishi JI, Miyoshi Y, Chiba S, Uemura H. Port site recurrence after laparoscopic radical nephrectomy: a case report. J Med Case Rep. 2017;11(1):151.
98. Bouvy ND, Marquet RL, Jeekel H, Bonjer HJ. Impact of gas(less) laparoscopy and laparotomy on peritoneal tumor growth and abdominal wall metastases. Ann Surg. 1996;224(6):694–700; discussion 1.
99. Watson DI, Mathew G, Ellis T, Baigrie CF, Rofe AM, Jamieson GG. Gasless laparoscopy may reduce the risk of port-site metastases following laparascopic tumor surgery. Arch Surg. 1997;132(2):166–8; discussion 9.
100. Mathew G, Watson DI, Ellis T, de Young N, Rofe AM, Jamieson GG. The effect of laparoscopy on the movement of tumor cells and metastasis to surgical wounds. Surg Endosc. 1997;11(12):1163–6.
101. Jones DB, Guo LW, Reinhard MK, Soper NJ, Philpott GW, Connett J, Fleshman JW. Impact of pneumoperitoneum on trocar site implantation of colon cancer in hamster model. Dis Colon Rectum. 1995;38(11):1182–8.
102. Ramirez PT, Wolf JK, Levenback C. Laparoscopic port-site metastases: etiology and prevention. Gynecol Oncol. 2003;91(1):179–89.
103. Wang N, Wang K, Zhong D, Liu X, Sun JI, Lin L, Ge L, Yang BO. Port-site metastasis as a primary complication following retroperitoneal laparoscopic radical resection of renal pelvis carcinoma or nephron-sparing surgery: a report of three cases and review of the literature. Oncol Lett. 2016;11(6):3933–8.
104. Castillo OA, Vitagliano G, Díaz M, Sánchez-Salas R. Port-site metastasis after laparoscopic partial nephrectomy: Case report and literature review. J Endourol. 2007;21(4):404-7.
105. Khandwala YS, Jeong IG, Han DH, Kim JH, Li S, Wang Y, Chang SL, Chung BI. Surgeon preference of surgical approach for partial nephrectomy in patients with baseline chronic kidney disease: a nationwide population-based analysis in the USA. Int Urol Nephrol. 2017;49(11):1921–7.
106. Breda A, Anterasian C, Belldegrun A (eds). Management and outcomes of tumor recurrence after focal ablation renal therapy 2010; Larchmont, NY: Liebert.

107. Kallingal GJS, Swain S, Darwiche F, Punnen S, Manoharan M, Gonzalgo ML, Parekh DJ. Robotic partial nephrectomy with the Da Vinci Xi. Adv Urol. 2016;2016:9675095
108. Stefanidis D, Goldfarb M, Kercher KW, Hope WW, Richardson W, Fanelli RD. SAGES guidelines for minimally invasive treatment of adrenal pathology. Surg Endosc. 2013;27(11):3960-80.

Robotic Radical Nephrectomy

21

Riccardo Campi, Selcuk Erdem, Onder Kara, Umberto Carbonara, Michele Marchioni, Alessio Pecoraro, Riccardo Bertolo, Alexandre Ingels, Maximilian Kriegmair, Nicola Pavan, Eduard Roussel, Angela Pecoraro, and Daniele Amparore

Radical nephrectomy is an established surgical procedure with evolving indications. Current guidelines recommend radical nephrectomy as the treatment of choice for larger and/or locally advanced renal tumors not amenable to nephron-sparing surgery. The European Association of Urology (EAU) guidelines is the only one to encourage the use of laparoscopic over open approach for radical nephrectomy owing to similar oncological outcomes but lower perioperative morbidity [1].

R. Campi (✉) · A. Pecoraro
Unit of Urological Robotic Surgery and Renal Transplantation, University of Florence, Careggi Hospital, Florence, Italy
e-mail: riccardo.campi@gmail.com; riccardo.campi@unifi.it

R. Campi
Department of Experimental and Clinical Medicine, University of Florence, Florence, Italy

S. Erdem
Division of Urologic Oncology, Faculty of Medicine, Department of Urology, Istanbul University, Istanbul, Turkey

O. Kara
School of Medicine, Department of Urology, Kocaeli University, Kocaeli, Turkey

U. Carbonara
Andrology and Kidney Transplantation Unit, Department of Emergency and Organ Transplantation-Urology, University of Bari, Bari, Italy

M. Marchioni
Laboratory of Biostatistics, Department of Medical, Oral and Biotechnological Sciences, D'Annunzio University of Chieti-Pescara, Chieti, Italy

Department of Urology, SS Annunziata Hospital, D'Annunzio University of Chieti-Pescara, Chieti, Italy

R. Bertolo
Department of Urology, San Carlo Di Nancy Hospital, Rome, Italy

Technological advances of minimally-invasive techniques with the introduction of the robotic platform arouse early controversy regarding whether or not the robotic is appropriate for performing radical nephrectomy. However, robotic radical nephrectomy showed encouraging outcomes in tackling demanding procedures such as the management of large tumors, aberrant anatomy, or higher tumor stages involving contiguous organ invasion [2]. In 2021, a systematic review of literature and meta-analysis involving 12 studies and a total of 64.221 patients investigated the current role of robotic radical nephrectomy in the management of renal cell carcinoma [3]. Notably, robotic radical nephrectomy seems to offer several advantages compared to open radical nephrectomy, including shorter hospitalization length of stay, and fewer complications. In addition, the robotic approach reported a shorter hospitalization time even compared to laparoscopic radical prostatectomy with no differences in terms of postoperative complications. Moreover, long-term outcomes indicate that minimally invasive and open approaches have equivalent cancer-specific survival [3]. In this scenario, the robotic radical nephrectomy could represent a valid option for the management of renal masses not suitable for nephron-sparing surgery. The higher cost of the robotic is the main limiting factor that encourages the detractors to avoid the spread and the evolving of this surgical approach for radical nephrectomy [4]. Nevertheless, robotic radical nephrectomy might be deemed cost-effective if it can reduce complications, transfusions, conversions, and hospitalization time.

The removal of the entire kidney including Gerota's fascia and regional lymph nodes, as well as the ipsilateral adrenal gland (if the adrenal-sparing approach is not indicated) represent the main steps of the radical nephrectomy even with the robotic approach (Fig. 21.1). Advantages of the robotic radical nephrectomy such as 3D vision, articulated instruments, and a better suture-step compared to laparoscopic surgery allow more thorough retroperitoneal node dissection in appropriate patients, as well as management of complex scenarios such that include vena cava tumor thrombus, invasion of contiguous organs like the liver or pancreas, or for

---

A. Ingels
Department of Urology, University Hospital Henri Mondor, APHP, 51 Avenue du Maréchal de Lattre de Tassigny, 94010 Créteil, France

Biomaps, UMR1281, INSERM, CNRS, CEA, Université Paris Saclay, Villejuif, France

M. Kriegmair
Department of Urology, University Medical Centre Mannheim, Mannheim, Germany

N. Pavan
Urology Clinic, Department of Medical, Surgical and Health Science, University of Trieste, Trieste, Italy

E. Roussel
Department of Urology, University Hospitals Leuven, Leuven, Belgium

A. Pecoraro · D. Amparore
Division of Urology, Department of Oncology, School of Medicine, San Luigi Hospital, University of Turin, Orbassano, Turin, Italy

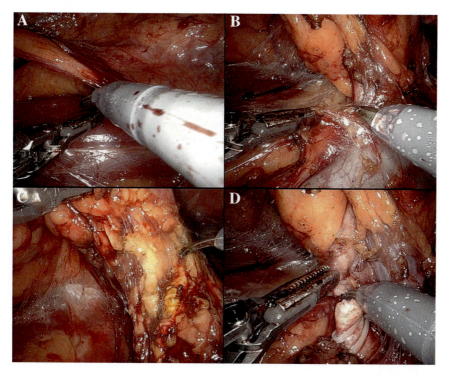

Fig. 21.1 Intraoperative snapshots during robotic right radical nephrectomy. **A** Identification of the psoas muscle plane. **B** Hilar control with 4th arm retraction of the kidney. **C** Dissection with Hem-o-Lok® (Weck Closure Systems, Research Triangle Park, NC, USA) of the renal artery before clipping and dividing the renal vein. **D** Completion of robotic radical nephrectomy and mobilization of the upper pole of the kidney leaving the adrenal gland "in situ"

extremely large tumors over 20 cm or larger [4]. The major challenges of laparoscopic radical nephrectomy for large renal masses are the limited working space, neovascularity requiring extreme care to prevent injury, and difficult access to the renal hilum due to the tumor drooping over the hilum and often the great vessels themselves [4]. The dexterity of the robotic instruments, as well as surgeon control of the scope, allowed to overcome these surgical challenges. The initial robotic experience was mainly based on the use of the *da Vinci* S® or Si® Surgical Systems (Intuitive Surgical®, Sunnyvale, CA, USA) that would typically require a meticulous robotic and assistance port-placement (as triangulation around the kidney of the ports in the upper quadrant particularly) where this can be critical to avoid arm collisions. More recently, the introduction of the Xi® robotic platform further facilitated this approach to minimize instrument clashing, which was certainly a limitation during radical nephrectomy [4].

References

1. Ljungberg B, Albiges L, Bedke J et al. European Association of Urology (EAU) Guidelines on Renal Cell Carcinoma (RCC). Version 2021. Available at: https://uroweb.org/guideline/renal-cell-carcinoma/
2. Petros FG, Angell JE, Abaza R. Outcomes of robotic nephrectomy including highest-complexity cases: largest series to date and literature review. Urol. 2015;85(6):1352–8. https://doi.org/10.1016/j.urology.2014.11.063.
3. Crocerossa F, Carbonara U, Cantiello F et al. Robot-assisted radical nephrectomy: a systematic review and meta-analysis of comparative studies. Eur Urol. 2020;17:S0302-2838(20)30854-X. https://doi.org/10.1016/j.eururo.2020.10.034.
4. Abaza R, Gerhard RS, Martinez O. Robotic radical nephrectomy for massive renal tumors. J Laparoendosc Adv Surg Tech A. 2020;30(2):196–200. https://doi.org/10.1089/lap.2019.0630.
5. Laviana AA, Tan HJ, Hu JC, Weizer AZ, Chang SS, Barocas DA. Retroperitoneal versus transperitoneal robotic-assisted laparoscopic partial nephrectomy: a matched-pair, bicenter analysis with cost comparison using time-driven activity-based costing. Curr Opin Urol. 2018;28(2):108–14.
6. Maurice MJ, Kaouk JH, Ramirez D, Bhayani SB, Allaf ME, Rogers CG, Stifelman MD. Robotic partial nephrectomy for posterior tumors through a retroperitoneal approach offers decreased length of stay compared with the transperitoneal approach: a propensity-matched analysis. J Endourol. 2017;31(2):158–62.
7. Mittakanti HR, Heulitt G, Li HF, Porter JR. Transperitoneal vs. retroperitoneal robotic partial nephrectomy: a matched-paired analysis. World J Urol. 2020;38(5):1093–9.
8. Patel M, Porter J. Robotic retroperitoneal partial nephrectomy. World J Urol. 2013;31(6):1377–82.
9. Patel MN, Kaul SA, Laungani R, Eun D, Bhandari M, Menon M, Rogers CG. Retroperitoneal robotic renal surgery: technique and early results. J Robot Surg. 2009;3(1):1.
10. Paulucci DJ, Beksac AT, Porter J, Abaza R, Eun DD, Bhandari A, Hemal AK, Badani KK. A multi-institutional propensity score matched comparison of transperitoneal and retroperitoneal partial nephrectomy for cT1 posterior tumors. J Laparoendosc Adv Surg Tech A. 2019;29(1):29–34.
11. Stroup SP, Hamilton ZA, Marshall MT, Lee HJ, Berquist SW, Hassan AS, Beksac AT, Field CA, Bloch A, Wan F, McDonald ML, Patel ND, L'Esperance JO, Derweesh IH. Comparison of retroperitoneal and transperitoneal robotic partial nephrectomy for Pentafecta perioperative and renal functional outcomes. World J Urol. 2017;35(11):1721–8.
12. Takagi T, Yoshida K, Kondo T, Kobayashi H, Iizuka J, Okumi M, Ishida H, Tanabe K. Comparisons of surgical outcomes between transperitoneal and retroperitoneal approaches in robot-assisted laparoscopic partial nephrectomy for lateral renal tumors: a propensity score-matched comparative analysis. J Robot Surg. 2021;15(1):99–104.
13. Weizer AZ, Palella GV, Montgomery JS, Miller DC, Hafez KS. Robot-assisted retroperitoneal partial nephrectomy: technique and perioperative results. J Endourol. 2011;25(4):553–7.
14. Zhu D, Shao X, Guo G, Zhang N, Shi T, Wang Y, Gu L. Comparison of outcomes between transperitoneal and retroperitoneal robotic partial nephrectomy: a meta-analysis based on comparative studies. Front Oncol. 2020;10:592193.

Preoperative Setting-Up of Patients Undergoing Robotic Inferior Vena Cava Thrombectomy

22

Raj Kumar, Nima Nassiri, Daniel Park, Vinay Duddalwar, Inderbir Gill, and Giovanni Cacciamani

22.1 Introduction

Between 4 and 10% of renal cancers are associated with tumor thrombus in the inferior vena cava (IVC) [1]. Traditional open IVC thrombectomy remains a physically challenging and technically demanding surgery with significant perioperative morbidity and mortality [2]. However, as robotic techniques continue to evolve, carefully selected patients may have the opportunity to undergo robotic IVC thrombectomy (RIVCT). As a relatively new procedure, RIVCT techniques are growing and improving rapidly. Beginning in 2011, groups began reporting outcomes for level I or II RIVCTs [3]. The first series of robotic level III thrombectomy cases was reported by Gill et al. in 2015, demonstrating the safety

R. Kumar · N. Nassiri · D. Park · I. Gill · G. Cacciamani (✉)
Department of Urology, Keck School of Medicine, University of Southern California, Los Angeles, CA, USA
e-mail: Giovanni.cacciamani@med.usc.edu

R. Kumar
e-mail: rkumar28@uic.edu

N. Nassiri
e-mail: Nima.Nassiri@med.usc.edu

D. Park
e-mail: Daniel.Park@med.usc.edu

I. Gill
e-mail: igill@med.usc.edu

V. Duddalwar · G. Cacciamani
Department of Radiology, Keck School of Medicine, University of Southern California, Los Angeles, CA, USA
e-mail: vinay.duddalwar@med.usc.edu

and feasibility of the procedure [4]. Only a few years later, the first robotic IVC thrombectomy for a level IV thrombus with a mini-thoracotomy for cardiac control was successfully performed [5].

To date, there have not been any prospective randomized trials comparing outcomes of RIVCT to open surgery. However, several series have been published confirming the efficacy of RIVCT. While sample sizes are relatively small due to strict patient selection, the procedure has been generally standardized, creating a uniform and reproducible technique [6]. The approach hinges on minimizing manipulation of the IVC, dissecting tissue away from the great vessel [7]. This "IVC-first, kidney-last" approach has worked to minimize thrombus embolism and major hemorrhage.

For patients without metastatic disease, surgical excision of the tumor and thrombus is the first-line treatment. This provides a 5-year cancer-specific survival of up to 65% [4]. While surgical technique and skill is important, preoperative planning is paramount, and heavily influences RIVCT outcomes. Careful patient selection and evaluation must precede a surgical approach that is tailored to each patient. Preoperative considerations include a battery of testing, imaging, consultations, tumor staging, and preoperative procedures. Strict adhesion to standardized preoperative procedure minimizes complication rate and can drastically improve outcomes.

22.2 Patient Selection

22.2.1 Clinical Staging

Careful patient selection is the cornerstone of successful RIVCT. Perhaps the most important part of preoperative workup involves staging of the tumor thrombus, which should be performed less than a week before surgery. Staging may be performed either by computed tomography (CT) or magnetic resonance imaging (MRI), both of which have excellent sensitivity and specificity for assessing extent of tumor thrombus [8]. The most used staging system was developed by Neves and Zincke at the Mayo Clinic in 1987 [9, 10]. This system describes four levels of tumor thrombus based on cephalad extent within the IVC (Table 22.1). The staging system was modified by Ciancio et al. in 2002 to subdivide a level III thrombus into a further four categories [11].

This staging system may be used in conjunction with the American Joint Committee on Cancer (AJCC) system, which uses the familiar tumor-node-metastases (TNM) method. Regarding tumor thrombus, the AJCC TNM system is classified as follows [12]:

- T3a—Tumor extends into the renal vein, but not beyond Gerota's fascia
- T3b—Tumor extends into the IVC inferior to the diaphragm
- T3c—Tumor extends into the IVC superior to the diaphragm or invades the wall of the IVC.

Table 22.1 Mayo staging system of vena caval thrombectomy

Mayo staging system	Criteria
Level 0	Thrombus extending into the renal vein
Level I	Thrombus extending into the IVC no more than 2 cm superior the renal vein
Level II	Thrombus extending into the IVC more than 2 cm superior to the renal vein, but not to the hepatic vein
Level IIIa	Thrombus extending into the retrohepatic IVC, but inferior to the major hepatic veins
Level IIIb	Thrombus extending into the retrohepatic IVC, reaching the ostia of the major hepatic vessels
Level IIIc	Thrombus extending into the retrohepatic IVC superior to the major hepatic vessels, but inferior to the diaphragm
Level IIId	Supradiaphragmatic thrombus, but inferior to the right atrium
Level IV	Supradiaphragmatic thrombus that extends into the right atrium

Additionally, the degree of IVC lumenal occlusion may be described by the following system proposed by Blute et al. [13], which may be helpful with preoperative surgical planning:

- A—IVC with no occlusion
- B—IVC is partially occluded, distal bland thrombus limited to the pelvis
- C—IVC is partially occluded by tumor thrombus, associated bland thrombus
- D—IVC is completely occluded by tumor thrombus, associated bland thrombus.

22.3 Patient Evaluation

22.3.1 Imaging

Abdominopelvic imaging is vital to surgical approach and technique. Thrombus anatomy should be carefully studied including length, diameter, vessel involvement, arterialization, and bland thrombus presence/extent. Assessment of IVC anatomy should involve diameter, presence of blood flow, wall invasion, and the locations of bilateral renal vasculature. An assessment of hepatic anatomy should include the number and location of short and main hepatic veins, liver size, and involvement as suggested by congestion. Renal anatomy study should include number of renal arteries and veins, venous flow and collaterals, and renal tumor size/stage. Finally, the retroperitoneal anatomy should be carefully considered to assess adenopathy and venous collaterals [4].

As mentioned prior, MRI or CT imaging should be performed less than a week before surgery [8]. If the patient has acceptable renal function, CT is commonly performed. A multi-phasic CT is generally preferred, providing imaging at multiple different times following contrast administration. This method has a high sensitivity (93%) and specificity (97%) for detecting tumor thrombus [14, 15]. Patients with contrast allergies or borderline renal function may receive an MRI with contrast allowing for multi-planar reformatting. CT and MRI imaging is preferred as it describes the extent of the renal tumor into the peri-renal fat, adrenal involvement, intra-abdominal adenopathy, caval flow characteristics, and vascularity of the kidney, including any collateral vessels [16]. A multiplanar review of the multiphase images on a workstation by an experienced abdominal radiologist often leads to a more detailed nuanced mapping of the vasculature. Multiplanar review is important as a single plane review may miss crucial details such as focal IVC wall involvement and variant anatomy. A direct consultation between the urological team and radiologist is critical for surgical planning. Additionally, for patients with level IIId or IV thrombi, a transesophageal echocardiogram is generally warranted to assess involvement of the right atrium.

Occasionally, neither CT nor MRI may be possible, either due to availability or patient intolerance. In such cases, inferior vena cavography may be used for assessment and staging. However, this imaging modality is limited due to its invasive nature, high contrast load, and risk of complications [10, 17]. Abdominal ultrasound may also be used, but results are highly dependent on the position of the thrombus and skill of the ultrasonographer [18]. Studies have shown that ultrasonography has a sensitivity of 68% when detecting thrombi below the level of insertion of the hepatic vein. Additionally, in more than 40% of cases, the IVC is not fully visualized by ultrasound imaging [19].

22.3.2 Additional Pertinent Testing

All patients should receive metastatic workup within 30 days prior to surgery. This should include pertinent laboratory testing such as a complete blood count, comprehensive metabolic panel, serum calcium, liver function tests, and urinalysis [20]. If urothelial carcinoma is within the differential diagnosis or if urinalysis reveals gross or microscopic hematuria, urine cytology or cystoscopy should be considered. Additionally, patients should have a chest CT, bone scan, and brain MRI if possible. If necessary, a pet-CT should be ordered to assess potentially metastatic lesions [16].

Renal function should be assessed prior to surgery. Radionuclide mercaptoacetyltriglycine-3 renal scan and 24-hour urine collection for creatinine clearance, protein excretion, and estimated glomerular filtration rate may be considered as needed [16]. Cardio-pulmonary clearance and lower extremity duplex Doppler ultrasonography should be ordered prior to surgery.

22.4 Preoperative Procedures

22.4.1 Angioembolization

Reliable preoperative renal artery angioembolization (RAE) is immensely helpful for RIVCT, particularly for left-sided thrombi. This is because intraoperatively the left renal vein is ligated well before control of the left renal artery is achieved. Therefore, RAE helps to minimize blood control and allows for early ligation of the renal vein [4].

Studies have shown that the efficacy of RAE varies by the tumor size, tumor vascularity, and the completeness of embolization [21, 22]. In patients with large, high level tumor thrombi, RAE may help downsize or partially regress the tumor thrombus prior to surgery, which can optimize surgical approach and outcomes [2, 23]. Additionally, preoperative RAE can induce local edema that can improve cleavage between the infarcted kidney and other surrounding tissues [24]. This may help with plane dissection, and the effect appears to be most pronounced at 72 hours following RAE [25]. However, this improved dissection must be weighted against the risk of collateral vessel development. As a result, the recommended time between RAE and surgery is less than 24 hours to 2 days [1, 26–29].

It has also been suggested that delaying the time between RAE and surgery may stimulate the production of tumor antibodies as a result of extensive tumor necrosis [24, 30]. This delay is suggested to act as a kind of autovaccination to provide specific active immunotherapy that may be protective against metastases. Though studies have shown mixed results, this hypothesis is far from proven [31–33].

22.4.2 Placement of IVC Filter

An additional consideration involves consulting interventional radiology to place a preoperative IVC Greenfield filter. Preoperative placement may be useful in patients who present with pulmonary emboli despite administration of anticoagulation or in patients for whom anticoagulation is contraindicated. Additionally, if the IVC is completely and chronically occluded prior to surgery, placement of a filter may be indicated. Due to the risk of decreased flow caused by collateral vessels, the IVC should be placed inferior to the contralateral vessel [34]. If an IVC filter must be placed, it should be done less than 48 hours before surgery [17, 35]. It should also be placed suprarenal through a superior approach [35].It should be noted that if a patient presents with an IVC thrombus presents following a pulmonary embolism, the appropriate treatment is often urgent nephrectomy rather than placement of an IVC filter. Filters are often avoided because the thrombus often incorporates the filter into itself as it grows [13, 34]. This can unnecessarily complicate surgical complexity and adversely affect outcomes. Intraoperatively, placement of a filter may be considered if distal bland thrombus exists that is not associated with tumor thrombus. This may be indicated to prevent the propagation of bland thrombus, achieve negative surgical margins, or clear vena cava wall invasion [13].

22.5 Preoperative Considerations

22.5.1 Preoperative Medical Therapy

Generally, RIVCT patients are referred for surgical therapy without prior medical therapy [8]. There has been little success with systemic immunotherapy trials [36]. Recently however, there has been growing interest in the use of systemic kinase inhibitors to downsize tumor thrombus level prior to surgery [8, 28]. Several retrospective studies have produced variable results, showing decreased thrombus levels in between 7 and 19% of cases [37–39].

It should be noted that—though it is possible to decrease tumor level with targeted medical therapy—this does not always change surgical approach. Additionally, some tumor thrombi may continue to grow despite medical therapy. Therefore, if a tumor thrombus is resectable at presentation, it may be prudent to refer for surgery rather than administer systemic medical therapy.

22.5.2 Anti-coagulation

In the setting of RIVTC, anti-coagulation is sometimes given as treatment/prophylaxis for pulmonary embolism. Tumor thrombi generally consist of non-friable tumor tissue that is unlikely to cause a pulmonary embolism [8]. However, when a pulmonary embolism occurs mortality is immensely high. An assessment of eight series of a total of 803 IVC thrombectomy patients showed that despite an incidence of 1.49%, overall mortality from preoperative pulmonary embolism was 75% [40–45]. Therefore, in cases of preoperative pulmonary embolism, anti-coagulation may be administered. Anti-coagulation may also be appropriate if preoperative imaging reveals significant bland thrombus.

22.5.3 Consultations

Prior to surgery various consultations may be appropriate based on patient circumstances and characteristics. Anesthesia and cardiothoracic surgical consultations are recommended for patients older than 50 years of age as well as patients who will receive cardiopulmonary bypass [20, 35]. An anesthesiologist familiar with rapid fluid shift, cardiopulmonary bypass, and transesophageal echocardiogram is preferred [10]. Particularly for level II to IV thrombi, transesophageal echocardiogram (TEE) monitoring can be immensely helpful. It is recommended that such patients receive TEE preoperatively following induction of anesthesia [46]. The

TEE may be performed as a continuous intraoperative monitoring measure at the discretion of the surgeon and the anesthesiologist. This can be helpful to assist in dissection, monitor patient volume responsiveness and cardiac performance, assess intraoperative complications (such as intraoperative embolism) in real-time, and ensure complete resection of tumor thrombus.

Hepatobiliary consultation is warranted for tumor thrombi particularly of level III and IV. A skilled hepatobiliary team typically assists with mobilization of the liver intraoperatively. This involves disconnection of the perihepatic ligaments, including the falciform ligaments, the right and left triangular ligaments, and the coronary ligaments [47]. This allows for the vessel tourniquet to be placed in the suprahepatic and infradiaphragmatic IVC, superior to the proximal IVC thrombus.

Cardiology should be consulted if the patient has two or more risk factors for coronary artery disease [35]. Consultation with vascular surgery may also be warranted if the surgeon does not have expertise with complex vascular reconstruction. An experienced hospitalist or intensivist should be consulted for perioperative management. Finally, a skilled surgical oncologist should be consulted and prepared in the case of conversion to open surgery.

Given the potential medical complexity of renal tumors with caval involvement, the involvement of medical hospitalists or intensivists teams in the coordination of multi-disciplinary care is recommended. Patients with high level tumor thrombi are at risk for sudden conversion to a variety of medical maladies, including sudden onset hepatopathy and Budd-Chiari Syndrome, with resultant coagulopathy and a classical clinical triad of pain, ascites, and hepatomegaly. Such medical sequelae are often poor prognostic harbingers, and a vigilant eye for the development of these must be maintained. The post-operative recovery of these patients is also often challenging, and intensivist care in the acute post-operative setting, followed by hospitalist involvement as the patient transitions to the ward, remains critical.

Bland thrombus distal to the tumor thrombus may develop from the venous stasis secondary to chronic luminal occlusion of the IVC and the hypercoagulability of malignancy. As such, and evaluation of the extent of bland thrombus burden in the lower extremities using duplex ultrasonography of the bilateral lower extremities starting from the groin and extending distally may guide pre-operative, intra-operative, and post-operative strategies. For instance, the utilization and extent of pre-operative anticoagulation may be in part guided by the extent of distal bland thrombus. Intraoperatively, both tumor involvement within the wall of the IVC firstly, and extent of distal bland thrombus, secondly, may guide the decision to perform inferior vena cavectomy. Lastly, extent of bland thrombus will certainly play a role in the anticoagulation approach in the post-operative setting. One study recommended intraoperative placement of a IVC filter in patients with evidence of distal tumor thrombus that is not associated with tumor thrombus. The same study stated that IVC filters must never be placed superior to tumor thrombus due to the possibility of tumor incorporating into the filter [13]. In such a case, it may be worth consulting with an experienced vascular surgeon or interventional radiologist.

Lastly, even within the urologic team in charge of the patient's care, the active participation of specialists with both minimally invasive and open surgical skills is a must. The potential for catastrophic intraoperative complications such as tumor embolism increases with the extent of IVC involvement and the risk of conversion to open surgery has a similar correlation. As such, we recommend that surgical teams discuss the possibility of open conversion well in advance, and have a practiced, set plan for rapid undocking and open conversion should the need arise.

References

1. Kundavaram C, et al. Advances in robotic vena cava tumor thrombectomy: intracaval balloon occlusion, patch grafting, and vena cavoscopy. Eur Urol. 2016;70(5):884–90.
2. Blute ML, et al. The Mayo Clinic experience with surgical management, complications and outcome for patients with renal cell carcinoma and venous tumour thrombus. BJU Int. 2004;94(1):33–41.
3. Masic S, Smaldone MC. Robotic renal surgery for renal cell carcinoma with inferior vena cava thrombus. Transl Androl Urol. 2021;10(5):2195–8.
4. Gill IS, et al. Robotic level III inferior vena cava tumor thrombectomy: initial series. J Urol. 2015;194(4):929–38.
5. Gill IS, et al. Renal cancer with extensive level IV intracardiac tumour thrombus removed by robot. Lancet. 2020;396(10262): e88.
6. Campi R, et al. Techniques and outcomes of minimally-invasive surgery for nonmetastatic renal cell carcinoma with inferior vena cava thrombosis: a systematic review of the literature. Minerva Urol Nefrol. 2019;71(4):339–58.
7. Chopra S, et al. Robot-assisted level II–III inferior vena cava tumor thrombectomy: step-by-step technique and 1-year outcomes. Eur Urol. 2017;72(2):267–74.
8. Agochukwu N, Shuch B. Clinical management of renal cell carcinoma with venous tumor thrombus. World J Urol. 2014;32(3):581–9.
9. Neves RJ, Zincke H. Surgical treatment of renal cancer with vena cava extension. Br J Urol. 1987;59(5):390–5.
10. Ghoreifi A, Djaladat H. surgical tips for inferior vena cava thrombectomy. Curr Urol Rep. 2020;21(12):51.
11. Ciancio G, et al. Management of renal cell carcinoma with level III thrombus in the inferior vena cava. J Urol. 2002;168(4 Pt 1):1374–7.
12. Swami U, et al. Revisiting AJCC TNM staging for renal cell carcinoma: quest for improvement. Ann Transl Med. 2019;7(Suppl 1):S18.
13. Blute ML, et al. Results of inferior vena caval interruption by greenfield filter, ligation or resection during radical nephrectomy and tumor thrombectomy. J Urol. 2007;178(2):440–5; discussion 444.
14. Nazim SM, et al. Accuracy of multidetector CT scans in staging of renal carcinoma. Int J Surg. 2011;9(1):86–90.
15. Renard AS, et al. Is multidetector CT-scan able to detect T3a renal tumor before surgery? Scand J Urol. 2019;53(5):350–5.
16. Sun Y, de Castro Abreu AL, Gill IS. Robotic inferior vena cava thrombus surgery: novel strategies. Curr Opin Urol. 2014;24(2):140–7.
17. Lawindy SM, et al. Important surgical considerations in the management of renal cell carcinoma (RCC) with inferior vena cava (IVC) tumour thrombus. BJU Int. 2012;110(7):926–39.
18. Guo HF, Song Y, Na YQ. Value of abdominal ultrasound scan, CT and MRI for diagnosing inferior vena cava tumour thrombus in renal cell carcinoma. Chin Med J (Engl). 2009;122(19):2299–302.

19. Trombetta C, et al. Evaluation of tumor thrombi in the inferior vena cava with intraoperative ultrasound. World J Urol. 2007;25(4):381–4.
20. Psutka SP, Leibovich BC. Management of inferior vena cava tumor thrombus in locally advanced renal cell carcinoma. Ther Adv Urol. 2015;7(4):216–29.
21. Bakal CW, et al. Value of preoperative renal artery embolization in reducing blood transfusion requirements during nephrectomy for renal cell carcinoma. J Vasc Interv Radiol. 1993;4(6):727–31.
22. Subramanian VS, et al. Utility of preoperative renal artery embolization for management of renal tumors with inferior vena caval thrombi. Urology. 2009;74(1):154–9.
23. Schwartz MJ, et al. Renal artery embolization: clinical indications and experience from over 100 cases. BJU Int. 2007;99(4):881–6.
24. Kalman D, Varenhorst E. The role of arterial embolization in renal cell carcinoma. Scand J Urol Nephrol. 1999;33(3):162–70.
25. Muller A, Rouviere O. Renal artery embolization-indications, technical approaches and outcomes. Nat Rev Nephrol. 2015;11(5):288–301.
26. Sauk S, Zuckerman DA. Renal artery embolization. Semin Intervent Radiol. 2011;28(4):396–406.
27. Murphy C, Abaza R. Complex robotic nephrectomy and inferior vena cava tumor thrombectomy: an evolving landscape. Curr Opin Urol. 2020;30(1):83–9.
28. Peng C, et al. Role of presurgical targeted molecular therapy in renal cell carcinoma with an inferior vena cava tumor thrombus. Onco Targets Ther. 2018;11:1997–2005.
29. Li Q, et al. Role of intraoperative ultrasound in robotic-assisted radical nephrectomy with inferior vena cava thrombectomy in renal cell carcinoma. World J Urol. 2020;38(12):3191–8.
30. Wallace S, et al. Embolization of renal carcinoma. Radiology. 1981;138(3):563–70.
31. Nakano H, Nihira H, Toge T. Treatment of renal cancer patients by transcatheter embolization and its effects on lymphocyte proliferative responses. J Urol. 1983;130(1):24–7.
32. Ekelund L, et al. Occlusion of renal arterial tumor supply with absolute ethanol. Experience with 20 cases. Acta Radiol Diagn (Stockh). 1984;25(3): p. 195-201.
33. Kato T, et al. The role of embolization/chemoembolization in the treatment of renal cell carcinoma. Prog Clin Biol Res. 1989;303:697–705.
34. Pouliot F, et al. Contemporary management of renal tumors with venous tumor thrombus. J Urol. 2010;184(3):833–41; quiz 1235.
35. Woodruff DY, et al. The perioperative management of an inferior vena caval tumor thrombus in patients with renal cell carcinoma. Urol Oncol. 2013;31(5):517–21.
36. Zisman A, et al. Renal cell carcinoma with tumor thrombus extension: biology, role of nephrectomy and response to immunotherapy. J Urol. 2003;169(3):909–16.
37. Cost NG, et al. The impact of targeted molecular therapies on the level of renal cell carcinoma vena caval tumor thrombus. Eur Urol. 2011;59(6):912–8.
38. Bigot P, et al. Neoadjuvant targeted molecular therapies in patients undergoing nephrectomy and inferior vena cava thrombectomy: is it useful? World J Urol. 2014;32(1):109–14.
39. Fukuda H, et al. Limited benefit of targeted molecular therapy for inferior vena cava thrombus associated with renal cell carcinoma. Int J Clin Oncol. 2017;22(4):767–73.
40. Lambert EH, et al. Prognostic risk stratification and clinical outcomes in patients undergoing surgical treatment for renal cell carcinoma with vascular tumor thrombus. Urology. 2007;69(6):1054–8.
41. Ciancio G, Livingstone AS, Soloway M. Surgical management of renal cell carcinoma with tumor thrombus in the renal and inferior vena cava: the University of Miami experience in using liver transplantation techniques. Eur Urol. 2007;51(4):988–94; discussion 994-5.
42. Bissada NK, et al. Long-term experience with management of renal cell carcinoma involving the inferior vena cava. Urology. 2003;61(1):89–92.
43. Jibiki M, et al. Surgical strategy for treating renal cell carcinoma with thrombus extending into the inferior vena cava. J Vasc Surg. 2004;39(4):829–35.
44. Nesbitt JC, et al. Surgical management of renal cell carcinoma with inferior vena cava tumor thrombus. Ann Thorac Surg. 1997;63(6):1592–600.

45. Shuch B, et al. Intraoperative thrombus embolization during nephrectomy and tumor thrombectomy: critical analysis of the University of California-Los Angeles experience. J Urol. 2009;181(2):492–8; discussion 498–9.
46. Calderone CE, et al. The role of transesophageal echocardiography in the management of renal cell carcinoma with venous tumor thrombus. Echocardiography. 2018;35(12):2047–55.
47. Wang B, et al. Robot-assisted level III–IV inferior vena cava thrombectomy: initial series with step-by-step procedures and 1-yr outcomes. Eur Urol. 2020;78(1):77–86.

23

Renal Cell Carcinoma with Tumor Thrombus: A Review of Relevant Anatomy and Surgical Techniques for the General Urologist

Christian A. Dewan, Joseph P. Vaughan, Ian C. Bennie, and Maurizio Buscarini

23.1 Introduction

Renal cell carcinoma (RCC) is estimated to account for 4.1% of all new cancer diagnoses and 2.4% of all cancer deaths in 2020 according to the National Cancer Institute SEER database. This will likely total 73,000 new cases and 15,000 deaths [1]. RCC is one of the most lethal of the common cancers urologists will encounter with a 5-year relative survival of 75.2% [1]. Renal cell carcinoma is one of a small subset of malignancies that are associated with tumor thrombus formation, which is tumor extension into a blood vessel. An estimated 4–10% of patients with RCC will have some degree of tumor thrombus extending into the renal vein or inferior vena cava at the time of diagnosis [2]. Tumor thrombi change the staging of RCC and therefore are an important part of initial patient workup. It is known that such tumors are more aggressive with higher Fuhrman grades, N+ or M+ at time of surgery and have higher probability of recurrence with lower cancer-specific survival [3]. Aggressive surgical intervention with radical nephrectomy and thrombectomy can be performed with survival benefits. Therefore, a thorough

C. A. Dewan (✉) · J. P. Vaughan · I. C. Bennie · M. Buscarini
Department of Urology, The University of Tennessee Health Science Center, 910 Madison Avenue, Memphis, TN 38163, USA
e-mail: cdewan@uthsc.edu

J. P. Vaughan
e-mail: jvaugha7@uthsc.edu

I. C. Bennie
e-mail: ibennie@uthsc.edu

M. Buscarini
e-mail: mbuscari@uthsc.edu

understanding of the surgical anatomy and approaches for varying levels of RCC tumor thrombus is of utmost importance when treating these patients.

RCC tumor thrombi are classified according to the extent to which they invade the inferior vena cava. The Mayo Clinic RCC Tumor Thrombus Classification System divides tumor thrombi into four categories ranging from level one to level four.

Level zero thrombi are limited to the renal vein. Level one thrombi extend into the inferior vena cava but less than two centimeters above the renal vein orifice. Level two thrombi are more than two centimeters above the orifice but below the hepatic vein. Level three thrombi extend above the hepatic vein but below the diaphragm, and finally level four thrombi are above the diaphragm [4]. Classifying the level of the tumor thrombus becomes vitally important in surgical planning as it will dictate the surgical approach. Level zero thrombi may be amenable to simple renal vein ligation while level four can require thoracotomy and possible open heart surgery with coordination of many surgical teams.

Here we will review the anatomy associated with each level of tumor thrombus and attempt to construct an outline for surgical techniques that may be used. We aim to give a concise overview so that general urologists may use it to understand these potentially complicated cases.

23.2 Anatomy of the IVC and Tributaries Related to Renal Surgery

Adequate knowledge of the normal anatomy of the inferior vena cava, its tributaries relevant to renal surgery, and common variations is essential in minimizing adverse events associated with complex radical nephrectomies and thrombectomy. The inferior vena cava ascends along the anterolateral border of the vertebral column to the right of the abdominal aorta where it enters the thoracic cavity at the level of T8 through the vena caval foramen of the central tendon of the diaphragm.

It is sometimes accompanied by the phrenic nerve through its foramen [5]. Cases of left-sided IVC and bilateral IVCs have been reported and should be identified pre-operatively [6]. Other important relations include the duodenum and head of the pancreas anteriorly at the level of the kidney, the hepatoduodenal ligament anteriorly at the level of the liver, the right renal artery passing posteriorly, and the root of the mesentery and right gonadal artery anteriorly [7].

The IVC tributaries relevant to renal surgery and classification of invasion of thromboses include right and left renal veins, right suprarenal vein, hepatic veins, and right and left inferior phrenic veins [8]. The renal veins drain into the IVC laterally at the level of L2. Thromboses of the renal veins constitute a level zero invasion [4]. The right suprarenal vein empties into the IVC laterally and slightly superior to the right renal vein also at L2 [9]. It formed an anastomosis with an accessory hepatic vein before emptying into the IVC in 20% of 440 patients in a study performed by Omura et al. [10]. The accepted normal anatomy of hepatic drainage is that the left, middle, and right hepatic veins empty into the IVC at the level of T8 immediately before the IVC enters the thorax [9]. However, a study by Fang et al. found that 61% of 200 cadavers' middle and left hepatic veins combined to form a common trunk that then emptied into the IVC. Additionally, it was not uncommon for additional, accessory veins to be present [11]. The hepatic veins also separate levels one and two from level three thrombotic invasions. Lastly, the inferior phrenic veins travel along the inferior aspect of the diaphragm and empty into the IVC as the IVC enters the vena caval foramen at T8 [9].

They are also highly variant in their course. The right inferior phrenic vein emptied into the right hepatic vein in 8% of cadavers in a 2005 study by Loukas et al. The left inferior phrenic vein was more highly variable being found emptying into the IVC (37%), left suprarenal vein (25%), left renal vein (15%), and left hepatic vein (14%) [12].

The kidneys are typically drained solely by the renal veins. However, there are many clinically significant variations in course and anastomoses [13]. The right renal vein is typically shorter in length at 2–2.5 cm and less commonly has anastomoses as compared to the left renal vein, but it still drains the right suprarenal vein in 6% of cases and the ascending lumbar vein in 3% of cases.

The left renal vein is typically 8.5 cm in length and drains the left suprarenal vein and left gonadal vein. It also commonly has additional tributaries from lumbar veins or the ascending lumbar vein. As it courses medially towards the IVC, it passes anteriorly to the aorta and inferiorly to the superior mesenteric artery, which creates a possible site of constriction commonly leading to a left-sided varicocele. Invasion of RCC into the left renal vein can also cause a left-sided varicocele if it obstructs the drainage of the left gonadal vein [14]. Cases of right-sided varicoceles caused by RCC invasion into the right renal vein have also been reported [15]. Other common variations of renal veins include multiple renal veins and a circumaortic left renal vein.

23.3 Kidney and Liver Venous Drainage and Anatomy

As mentioned previously, the kidneys are drained solely by the renal veins, but can have variations in course and anatomy [13]. The renal venous system has what is called a "free anastomosis" system in place due to extensive collateral communication through venous collars around minor calyceal infundibula, which allows venous blood to communicate and flow freely throughout all segments of the kidney [13, 16]. Venous drainage in the kidney begins as the interlobular veins that progresses as the arcuate, interlobar, lobar, and segmental veins.

A group of segmental veins then unite to form a tributary that becomes the renal vein. Having a group of segmental veins uniting to form the renal vein allows for extensive collateral venous drainage of the kidney, and occlusion of a segmental venous branch will have little effect on venous outflow [16]. The right and left renal veins lie anterior to their respective renal arteries as they drain into the IVC. An important anatomical difference to consider between the renal veins is the fact that the right renal vein measures approximately 2 to 4 cm long while the left renal vein is 6 to 10 cm [16]. The left renal vein receives drainage superiorly from the left suprarenal (adrenal) vein and drainage inferiorly from the left gonadal (testicular or ovarian) vein. In approximately 75% of the population, the left renal vein has the possibility of also receiving additional tributaries that can be clinically significant in size and are highly variable [13]. These anatomical variants are important considerations due to possibility of avulsion during a surgical procedure. The left renal vein exits the kidney and travels medially traversing the angle formed between the superior mesenteric artery anteriorly and the aorta posteriorly. The left renal vein can be compressed between these two structures, known as nutcracker syndrome. The right renal vein differs from the left in its course as it travels towards the IVC, as well as the fact that it does not have extrarenal vessels join its course before it enters the IVC [13].

Large RCC tumor thrombi have the potential to extend cephalically to a subhepatic level interfering with venous drainage from the liver; therefore, knowledge of hepatic venous drainage proves important role. Hepatic venous blood is returned to the IVC via the hepatic veins.

There are three major hepatic veins: the right, middle (central), and left hepatic vein that pass in a posterosuperior direction through the liver to empty into the IVC which lies posterior to the surface of the liver [17]. A variable number of small, accessory veins run from the liver directly into the IVC below the level of the main hepatic veins [17]. During the course of radical nephrectomies with subdiaphragmatic or intrathoracic tumor thrombus, it may be necessary to use liver transplant techniques to mobilize the right lobe of the liver and access the retrohepatic vena cava [18]. Knowledge of the anatomical relationships among these short hepato-caval vessels is key to assure optimal vascular control and prevent uncontrolled bleeding.

23.4 Supra-Diaphragmatic Vena Cava Anatomical Relations

An important surgical consideration for RCC tumor extending into the inferior vena cava is control of the distal end of the tumor thrombus [19]. For surgical removal of tumor thrombi extending above the level of the diaphragm, the suptradiaphragmatic vena cava must be exposed. On average the length of the supradiaphragmatic IVC (from right atrial appendage to diaphragm) was 20.6 mm and width 28.7 mm [19]. Relevant vascular anatomy in relation to the supradiaphragmatic IVC includes the phrenic veins, diaphragmatic veins, and the right phrenic nerve. The diaphragmatic veins and their location for insertion into the supradiaphragmatic vena cava, as well as the phrenic veins and right phrenic nerve in relation to the supradiaphragmatic IVC are important surgical considerations. Different approaches have been elucidated to gain access to the supradiagphragmatic IVC when performing a thrombectomy. Careful consideration must be taken with the abdominal approach as to not transect any of the important vasculature encountered when dissecting the IVC from the diaphragm.

23.5 Key Retroperitoneal Anatomical Landmarks Relevant to Renal Surgery (Diaphragm, Cysterna Chili, Lymph Nodes, Pleura)

The cisterna chyli is a saccular lymphatic structure located at the L1-L2 vertebral body level in an area known as the retrocrural space, located just beneath the abdominal aorta [20].

The cisterna chyli receives lymphatic drainage from intestines and lower body structures and anastomoses with other lumbar and intestinal lymphatics as it continues in the cephalic direction as the thoracic duct [21, 22]. Anatomical variations of the cisterna chyli are highly prevalent, and complex variations can result in a plexus configuration as opposed to a single identifiable duct [22]. This is a large ductal system that carries a significant amount of lymphatic fluid, and inadvertent intraoperative injury to this structure could potentially lead to postoperative chylous fistuli, chylothoraces, and refractory chylous leakage.

Therefore, identification and preservation of the cisterna chyli is critical during RCC tumor thrombus removal and lymph node dissection.

23.6 Modern Imaging, Role of CT, MRI, and US in RCC with Vein Thrombus

Imaging plays a vital role in the management of RCC from diagnosis, to staging of disease, as well as assessment of response to medical or surgical therapy. Evaluation of the proximal extent, volume of tumor thrombus, and potential caval wall invasion are all necessary information for pre-operative planning considerations [23]. A clear pre-operative understanding of the tumor burden and thrombus may also direct the need for multidisciplinary surgical approaches [23]. Historically, Inferior Vena Cavography was used for the detection and evaluation of tumor thrombi, however, this procedure was limited by its invasive nature and procedural complications [23], Rossi 2018. Revolutions in imaging throughout the past decade have had a significant impact on the ability to manage kidney cancer; conversely, new surveillance protocols combined with serial imaging and advances in cross-sectional imaging have enhanced the ability to grade and stage kidney cancer [24]. With respect to RCC with venous thrombus, the imaging modality used must reliably identify any infra- or suprahepatic as well as intra-cardial extension of the thrombus [25]. Pre-operative determination of the tumor thrombus stage and the cranial extent of the thrombus is used to guide pre-operative planning for surgical approach to resection [25]. Different modalities that are currently used for pre-operative planning include MRI, CT, and ultrasound. CT remains the most appropriate imaging modality for classification of RCC thrombus. While RCC can appear as iso-, hyper-, and hypodense lesions on non-contrast CT, it usually demonstrates significant contrast enhancement and areas of necrosis following intravenous contrast application [25]. When compared to CT, MRI has superior soft tissue contrast resolution and ultrasound has found increasing utilization for repeated scanning and surveillance of tumors. While ultrasound is a non-invasive and commonly used way to evaluate patients with RCC, this method is largely dependent on the ultrasonographer and the position of the thrombus. It has been shown that the use of ultrasound to detect tumor thrombus location below the level of the insertion of the hepatic vein has a sensitivity of 68% [23]. Several studies have shown that a multiparametric imaging approach is most likely to yield the highest diagnostic accuracy [25]. While perioperative imaging for tumor thrombus removal is essential, intraoperative imaging can also be performed with transesophageal echocardiography (TEE), which gives the surgeon a real-time view of the tumor. The use of TEE has been studied and has proved effective as a technique to monitor the tumor thrombus position intra-operatively. This imaging modality is used most often as a way to delineate the uppermost rim of the tumor thrombus for higher stage tumors, such as those that extend into the atrium of the heart [26].

23.7 Surgical Approaches

After determining the level of tumor thrombus, the surgeon should begin to formulate a surgical plan. One of the first decisions the surgeon will make is the approach the he or she will take for the operation. This decision should not be overlooked as there are many described approaches and advantages and disadvantages to consider for each. Here we will discuss different incision types and the appropriate times for their use. The most commonly used incisions in renal surgery, including IVC thrombectomy, are flank, subcostal, midline, and thoracoabdominal.

The flank incision, while commonly used for access and exposure of the kidney and renal hilum in nephrectomies and partial nephrectomies may be inadequate in providing exposure to the IVC, thus, its utility in these operations is limited [23]. The subcostal incision is a popular approach as it gives excellent exposure to the renal hilum and the IVC. The incision can be extended laterally (chevron incision) in the case of bilateral disease and can also be extended superiorly for a sternotomy in the case of level IV thrombi. Subcostal incisions are associated with a high degree of postoperative pain [27]. The midline incision is an attractive approach for these complex surgeries as it also provides excellent IVC exposure as well as access to bilateral kidneys and renal hila. The midline incision can be extended cephalad for sternotomy. The disadvantage to this approach is that it may limit the ability to manipulate the liver and have access to the retrohepatic IVC should this be necessary [27]. The thoracoabdominal incision can also be considered. This incision may provide the best exposure to the hepatic vessels and retrohepatic IVC, however, this advantage must be balanced with the possible complications. These include severe post-operative pain, pneumothroax, phrenic nerve injury, impairing diaphragmatic function, splenic injury, as well as requirement of a chest tube postoperatively [28].

23.8 Liver Transplant Techniques

When a tumor thrombus extends into the inferior vena cava above the hepatic vessels (level III and IV tumor thrombus), liver transplant surgical techniques will likely need to be employed for proper control. Mobilization of the liver (Langenbuch maneuver) is necessary to obtain access to the retrohepatic IVC. This begins with dividing the triangular ligamentous attachments as well as the falciform ligament.

The small hepatic veins draining the caudate lobe are also ligated. This technique will allow for excellent visualization of the retrohepatic IVC [27]. Care must be taken to preserve the left, right, and middle hepatic veins as these are the primary venous drainage sources of the liver and cannot be sacrificed [29].

During liver mobilization, a Pringle maneuver may also be performed to decrease the amount of vascular congestion and bleeding from the liver. This is only necessary when a vascular clamp is placed above the hepatic vessels. In the pringle maneuver, the surgeon first identifies the Foramen of Winslow and then the hepatoduodenal ligament, which includes the hepatic artery, portal vein and the common bile duct. The hepatoduodenal ligament is then clamped.

Care must be taken to minimize the amount of time the hepatoduodenal ligament is clamped as splenic congestion, portal vein thrombosis, and ischemic liver injury can occur if the clamp times exceeds 60 min [30].

In some instances, tumors of the left kidney may require further exposure to the left retroperitoneum. To do this, the surgeon may perform the Mattox maneuver, which is commonly used in trauma surgery to control bleeding in the left retroperitoneum. Interestingly, this technique was first described by a chief surgery resident, Dr. Kenneth Mattox, working with a second year urology resident during a trauma case at Baylor College of Medicine. During the case, they needed to quickly mobilize the viscera to obtain access to the retroperitoneum as the patient was bleeding and the source was suspected to be either the aorta or IVC. Since that time, the maneuver has carried his name [31]. The maneuver begins by incising the peritoneum along the White Line of Toldt from the splenic flexure to the sigmoid colon. Once this is done, the spleen, tail of pancreas, left kidney, and the stomach may be mobilized.

23.9 Extracorporeal Circulation and Combined Cardiothoracic Approaches

When the IVC is completely occluded, a bypass mechanism must be used to ensure venous return to the heart. This has historically been done with two different methods: cardiopulmonary bypass (CPB) and venovenous bypass (VVB). If these techniques must be used, it is important to have assistance from a cardiothoracic surgeon and anesthesia team with experience in these cases. The level of extension of the tumor thrombus will dictate the bypass technique that is used. For level IV thrombi, a CPB will be necessary prior to atriotomy. During a CPB, the femoral vein and superior vena cava are cannulated as well as the right subclavian artery. An oxygenator is utilized to return oxygenated blood back to the arterial system.

The patient will require systemic heparinization as well as deep hypothermic circulatory arrest (DHCA), which allows the bypass circuit and heart to be stopped once hypothermia is achieved. CPB carries a high risk of stroke and perioperative mortality [27].

Venovenous bypass (VVB) can be used when the tumor thrombus extends above the diaphragm but not into the right atrium. During this procedure, the IVC is controlled above the level of the tumor thrombus, possible in the intracaval section, and the inferiorly below the renal veins. The IVC, or more commonly the femoral vein, is the cannulated as well as the SVC. This allows venous bypass around the clamped IVC.

23.10 Robotic RCC Thrombus Removal

As discussed in previous sections, traditionally surgery for renal cell carcinoma with tumor thrombus has been performed via an open approach requiring large thoracoabdominal incisions. However, in recent years there have been advances in the use of laparoscopic and robotic-assisted approaches for these complex cases, including level III thrombi. In 2000, Savage and Gill reported the first case report of a planned laparoscopic nephrectomy and tumor thrombectomy extending into the renal vein (level I thrombus) with good success [32]. Following this report, Desai et al. published a case series in 2003 showing the feasibility of a laparoscopic approach in patients with level I tumor thrombi [33]. In 2014, Shao et al. published a report of successful laparoscopic radical nephrectomy and thrombectomy in 11 patients with right-sided RCC, including six with level II thrombi and five with level IV thrombi. No major intraoperative or postoperative complications occurred showing the feasibility of a minimally invasive technique even in the most difficult patients.

Since that time, some major advancements have been made in the field of minimally invasive surgery including the widespread implementation of robotic-assisted laparoscopic surgery. Urologists were among the earliest adopters of robotic surgery and in 2000 the first procedure performed on the da Vinci system in the USA was a prostatectomy [34]. The robot has continued to be an important tool utilized in urologic procedures and is now commonplace in renal cancer surgery. In 2011, Abaza published the first case series involving robotic-assisted nephrectomy with tumor thrombectomy. In this series, five patients had this procedure with a mean operative time of 327 min, mean estimated blood loss of 170 cc, and mean length of stay of 1.2 days. The tumor thrombi extended into the IVC 1, 2, 4, and 5 cm as well as one patient that had two tumor thrombi extending 3 and 2 cm. The tumor thrombi extending 5 cm into the IVC reached the level of the liver, which would classify this as level III, however, this classification was not noted in the paper. There were no complications, transfusions or readmissions for these patients and all patients required opening of the IVC as well as either tangential clamp or cross clamp of the IVC [35]. In 2015, Gill et al. published the first case series reporting nine patients that underwent level III tumor thombectomy. They were able to perform the entire procedure, including intrahepatic IVC control, IVC repair, radical nephrectomy, retroperitoneal lymphadenectomy completely intracoporeal utilizing a 7-port technique. The median operative time was 4.9 h, average estimated blood loss was 375 cc, and average hospital stay was 4.5 days. There were no intraoperative complications and 1 Clavien 3b postoperative complication [36]. Other groups have been able to replicate this procedure with good outcomes [37] and it seems that the robot may be poised to play a bigger role in RCC with tumor thrombus in the coming years.

References

1. Cancer of the kidney and renal pelvis-cancer stat facts. SEER;2021. https://seer.cancer.gov/statfacts/html/kidrp.html.
2. Martínez-Salamanca JI et al. Prognostic impact of the 2009 UICC/AJCC TNM staging system for renal cell carcinoma with venous extension. Eur Urol. 2011;59:120–127.
3. Moinzadeh A, Libertino JA. Prognostic significance of tumor thrombus level in patients with renal cell carcinoma and venous tumor thrombus extension. Is all T3b the same? J Urol. 2004;171, 598–601.
4. Quencer KB, Friedman T, Sheth R, Oklu R. Tumor thrombus: incidence, imaging, prognosis and treatment. Cardiovasc Diagn Ther. 2017;7 S165-S177–S177.
5. Shahid Z, Burns B. Anatomy, abdomen and pelvis, diaphragm. StatPearls. Treasure Island (FL): StatPearls Publishing;2020.
6. Nishibe T, et al. Abdominal aortic aneurysm with left-sided inferior vena cava. Report of a case. Int Angiol. 2004;23(4):400–2.
7. Gray H, et al. Gray's anatomy: the anatomical basis of clinical practice. Edinburgh; New York: Elsevier Churchill Livingstone;2005.
8. Drake RL, et al. Gray's anatomy for students. Philadelphia, PA: Churchill Livingstone/Elsevier;2015.
9. Tucker WD, et al. Anatomy, abdomen and pelvis, inferior vena cava. StatPearls. Treasure Island (FL): StatPearls Publishing;2020.
10. Omura K, et al. Anatomical variations of the right adrenal vein: concordance between multidetector computed tomography and catheter venography. Hypertension. 2017;69(3):428–34.
11. Fang CH, et al. Anatomical variations of hepatic veins: three-dimensional computed tomography scans of 200 subjects. World J Surg. 2012;36(1):120–4.
12. Loukas M, Louis RG, Hullett J, Loiacano M, Skidd P, Wagner T. An anatomical classification of the variations of the inferior phrenic vein. Surg Radiol Anat. 2005;27(6):566–74.
13. Bowdino CS, et al. Anatomy, abdomen and pelvis, renal veins. StatPearls. Treasure Island (FL): StatPearls Publishing;2020.
14. Pinals RS, Krane SM. Medical aspects of renal carcinoma. Postgrad Med J. 1962;38(443):507–19.
15. Ryan JW, et al. A rare testicular vein anatomical variant contributes to right-sided varicocoele formation and leads to the diagnosis of renal cell carcinoma. BMJ Case Rep. 2017;2017.
16. Kavoussi LR, Peters C, Partin AW, Dmochowski RR. Campbell-Walsh-Wein urology. [Electronic Resource], 12th ed. Elsevier;2021. http://search.ebscohost.com/login.aspx?direct=true&db=cat06193a&AN=uthsc.55852&site=eds-live. Accessed May 12, 2021.
17. Mahadevan V. Anatomy of the liver. Surgery (Oxford). 2020;38(8):427-431. https://doi.org/10.1016/j.mpsur.2014.10.004.

18. Ciancio G, Livingstone AS, Soloway M. Surgical management of renal cell carcinoma with tumor thrombus in the renal and inferior vena cava: the university of Miami experience in using liver transplantation techniques. Eur Urol. 2007;51:988–95.
19. Shchukin D, Lesovoy V, Garagatiy I, Khareba G, Hsaine R. Surgical approaches to supradiaphragmatic segment of IVC and right atrium through abdominal cavity during intravenous tumor thrombus removal. Adv Urol. 2014;2014(924269):9. https://doi.org/10.1155/2014/924269.
20. Loukas M, Wartmann CT, Louis RG, Tubbs RS, Salter EG, Gupta AA, Curry B. Cisterna chyli: a detailed anatomic investigation. Clin Anat. 2007;20:683–8.
21. Dogan NU, Dogan S, Erol M, Uzun BT. Cisterna chyli: an important landmark in laparoscopic paraaortic lymphadenectomy. Gynecol Oncol. 2020;156(2):511. https://doi.org/10.1016/j.ygyno.2019.12.004.
22. Pinto PS, Sirlin CB, Andrade-Barreto OA, Brown MA, Mindelzun RE, Mattrey RF. Cisterna chyli at routine abdominal MR imaging: a normal anatomic structure in the retrocrural space. Radiographics. 2004;24:809–17.
23. Lawindy SM. Important surgical considerations in the management of renal cell carcinoma (RCC) with inferior vena cava (IVC) tumour thrombus. BJU Int. 2012;110:926–39.
24. Krajewski KM, Pedrosa I. Imaging advances in the management of kidney cancer [published online ahead of print, 2018 Oct 29]. J Clin Oncol. 2018;36(36):JCO2018791236.https://doi.org/10.1200/JCO.2018.79.1236.
25. Heidenreich A, Ravery V. European society of oncological urology. Preoperative imaging in renal cell cancer. World J Urol. 2004;22(5):307–315. https://doi.org/10.1007/s00345-004-0411-2.
26. Hallscheidt PJ, Fink C, Haferkamp A, Bock M, Luburic A, Zuna I, Noeldge G, Kauffmann G, et al. Preoperative staging of renal cell carcinoma with inferior vena cava thrombus using multidetector CT and MRI: prospective study with histopathological correlation. J Comput Assist Tomogr. 2005;29(1):64–68. Cited in: Journals@Ovid Full Text at http://ovidsp.ovid.com/ovidweb.cgi?T=JS&PAGE=reference&D=ovftg&NEWS=N&AN=00004728-200501000-00012. Accessed May 22, 2021.
27. Pouliot F, Shuch B, LaRochelle JC, Pantuck A, Belldegrun AS. Contemporary management of renal tumors with venous tumor thrombus. J Urol. 2010;184:833–41.
28. Venkat S, Matteliano A, Drachenberg D. Thoracoabdominal approach for large retroperitoneal masses: case series and review. Case Rep Urol. 2019;2019.
29. Blute ML, Inman BA, Gelpi FJ. Hinman's atlas of urologic surgery, Chapter 11;2019. p. 97–111.
30. Olumi Aria F, Blute ML. Campbell-Walsh-Wein urology, Chapter 101;2020. p. 2248–78.
31. Aseni P, Grande AM, Romani F, Birindelli A, Di Saverio S. Basic operative techniques in abdominal injury. In: Aseni P, De Carlis L, Mazzola A, Grande AM, editors. Operative techniques and recent advances in acute care and emergency surgery. Cham: Springer;2019.
32. Savage SJ, Gill IS. Laparoscopic radical nephrectomy for renal cell carcinoma in a patient with level i renal vein tumor thrombus. J Urol. 2000;163:1243–4.
33. Desai MM, Gill IS, Ramani AP, Matin SF, Kaouk JH, Miguel CJ. Laparoscopic radical nephrectomy for cancer with level I renal vein involvement. J Urol. 2003;169:487–91.
34. Leal GT, Campos CO. 30 years of robotic surgery. World J Surg. 2016;40:2550–7.
35. Abaza R. Initial series of robotic radical nephrectomy with vena caval tumor thrombectomy. Eur Urol. 2011;59:652–6.
36. Ramirez D, Maurice MJ, Cohen B, Krishnamurthi V, Haber G-P. Robotic level III IVC tumor thrombectomy: duplicating the open approach. Urology. 2016;90:204–7.
37. Gill IS, Charles M, Andre A, Vinay D, Sameer C, Mark C, Duraiyah T, Osamu U, Raj S, Andrew H, et al. Robotic level III inferior vena cava tumor thrombectomy: initial series. J Urol. 2015;194:929–38.

Cytoreductive Nephrectomy in Metastatic Renal Cell Carcinoma

24

Roser Vives Dilme, Juan Gómez Rivas, Riccardo Campi, Javier Puente, and Jesús Moreno Sierra

24.1 Introduction

Renal cell carcinoma (RCC) is responsible for more than 30,000 deaths per year in Europe, accounting for 3% of all cancer diagnoses and 2% of all cancer deaths worldwide [12, 20]. Approximately, 15–18% of patients present with metastatic disease at the time of diagnosis and up to 40% of patients with initially localized disease will develop metastases during follow-up [40].

Cytoreductive nephrectomy (CN) is the surgical removal of the kidney and primary tumour in the setting of metastatic disease. CN was considered the gold standard treatment for metastatic RCC (mRCC) during the cytokine therapy era based on two randomized phase 3 trials comparing CN plus interferon alfa-2b

---

R. Vives Dilme (✉) · J. Gómez Rivas · J. Moreno Sierra
Department of Urology, Hospital Clínico San Carlos, Complutense University of Madrid, Madrid, Spain
e-mail: roser.vives@salud.madrid.org

J. Moreno Sierra
e-mail: jmorenos@salud.madrid.org

R. Campi
Unit of Urological Robotic Surgery and Renal Transplantation, Careggi Hospital, University of Florence, Florence, Italy
e-mail: riccardo.campi@unifi.it

Department of Experimental and Clinical Medicine, University of Florence, Florence, Italy

European Association of Urology (EAU) Young Academic Urologists (YAU) Renal Cancer Working Group, Arnhem, The Netherlands

J. Puente
Medical Oncology Department, Hospital Clínico San Carlos, Instituto de Investigación Sanitaria del Hospital Clínico San Carlos (IdISSC), CIBERONC, Madrid, Spain

(IFNα-2b) versus IFNα-2b alone in treatment of mRCC, showing an increase in median overall survival (OS) for patients who underwent CN (13.6 vs. 7.8 months) [13, 14, 28].

Subsequently, since the advent of systemic targeted therapies in 2005, the role of CN in the treatment of mRCC has been questioned. Several retrospective studies demonstrated an overall survival benefit in patients treated with targeted therapy who underwent CN [5], whereas the recent randomized phase 3 CARMENA trial showed the noninferiority of systemic tyrosine kinase inhibitors (TKI) therapy alone compared to upfront CN plus systemic TKI therapy in intermediate-risk and poor-risk mRCC patients [27]. Moreover, current advances have shown improved oncological outcomes from immune checkpoint inhibitors (ICI) as compared to standard TKI monotherapy [31, 32, 37].

However, despite recent developments in systemic therapies, surgery remains a key component in mRCC treatment. According to the rapidly changing mRCC treatment scenario, patient selection, surgical approach and treatment sequence are some of the aspects currently under evaluation. In this context, recent studies introduce the use of a minimally invasive approach for CN with the aim of reducing the morbidity associated with this procedure.

24.2 Evidence for Cytoreductive Nephrectomy in the New Era of Systemic Therapy

CN was adopted as the standard of care in mRCC treatment in the cytokine era. In 2001, two randomized clinical trials (EORTC 30,947, SWOG 8949) demonstrated the therapeutic benefit of CN in mRCC patients [13, 28]. Later, a combined analysis of both trials (n = 331) showed an overall survival (OS) of 13.6 months for patients undergoing CN prior to IFNα versus 7.8 months for patients receiving systemic treatment with IFNα alone (HR 0.69; 95% CI 0.55–0.87, p = 0.002) [14].

In recent years, the introduction of the new targeted therapies replacing the standard systemic cytokine treatment led to question the role of CN. Several retrospective studies were conducted to evaluate the benefit of CN in mRCC treatment, demonstrating improved OS associated with surgery in these patients [7, 17, 19]. Interestingly, when patients were stratified according to the International Metastatic Renal Cell Carcinoma Database Consortium (IMDC) prognostic factors [18], the subgroup analysis showed the absence of significant benefit in OS in those patients belonging to the poor prognosis risk group who underwent CN (HR 0.67, 95% CI 0.44–1.01, p = 0.06) [7] and OS 6 versus 5.4 months (p > 0.1) [19]. Recently, Bhindi et al. [5] performed a systematic review of the current available evidence, which demonstrated improved OS associated with CN in mRCC patients (HR ranged from 0.39 to 0.68) and identified good performance status (PS) and good/intermediate IMDC or Memorial Sloan Kettering Cancer Center (MSKCC) [30] risk classification as the most important predictive factors of

OS benefit with CN. In this regard, careful patient selection appears to be a key factor to identify those mRCC patients who may benefit from surgery.

On the other hand, recent prospective randomized trials have challenged this evidence. The CARMENA trial [27] compared upfront CN followed by sunitinib therapy (226 patients) to sunitinib therapy alone (224 patients) in 450 intermediate-risk and poor-risk mRCC patients according to MSKCC criteria. Noninferiority of sunitinib therapy alone compared to CN plus sunitinib was demonstrated (OS 18.4 vs. 13.9 months, HR 0.89). However, the trial had some limitations such as significant crossover, with 17% of patients in the sunitinib alone arm undergoing subsequent CN and 7% of patients in the CN plus sunitinib arm not receiving surgery, and the inclusion of only poor-risk MSKCC (43%) and intermediate-risk MSKCC (57%) patients when previous studies had already shown the absence of OS benefit from CN in these subgroups of mRCC patients [7, 19]. Furthermore, in the setting of new and more effective systemic therapies for mRCC treatment, it is being questioned whether surgery could delay the initiation of these therapies in mRCC patients. The SURTIME trial [4] compared 50 patients receiving immediate CN followed by sunitinib therapy to 49 patients who received sunitinib followed by deferred CN, showing a significant increased median OS in patients who underwent deferred CN after initial systemic treatment (32.4 vs. 15 months, HR 0.57, $p < 0.03$). While being underpowered according to poor accrual, the SURTIME trial demonstrated a survival benefit of deferred CN in intermediate-risk patients in whom initial systemic therapy is essential and who were candidates to undergo surgery. These results supported the finding from the CARMENA trial related to the absence of benefit of immediate CN in intermediate-risk patients requiring systemic treatment.

More recently, immune checkpoint inhibitors (ICI) have been established as first-line therapy in mRCC patients [23]. The CheckMate-214 (nivolumab plus ipilimumab vs. sunitinib), KEYNOTE-426 (pembrolizumab plus axitinib vs. sunitinib) and JAVELIN Renal 101 (avelumab plus axitinib vs. sunitinib) trials have demonstrated improved oncological outcomes of ICI combined therapy compared to standard TKI monotherapy [31, 32, 37]. As a noteworthy fact, more than 80% of mRCC patients included in these randomized trials underwent prior nephrectomy [6]. In this setting, Singla et al. [39] presented a retrospective study of a National Cancer Database cohort (n = 391) comparing 221 patients treated with immunotherapy plus CN and 170 patients who received immunotherapy alone, showing an improved OS of the ICI therapy plus CN compared to the ICI therapy alone (HR 0.23, $p < 0.001$). At the present time, three randomized prospective trials are ongoing (NORDIC-SUN, SWOG1931 and PROBE), designed with the aim of reassessing the role of CN in the new immunotherapy era.

In summary, given the rapidly evolution of systemic therapies, the role of CN needs to be redefined. Currently, CN should be considered as a component of the multimodal mRCC treatment in carefully selected patients. Surgical treatment still has a role in mRCC patients with good risk prognosis and good PS, patients with favourable response after systemic therapy and patients requiring palliation of symptoms [5]. Future prospective studies are needed to assess the optimal treatment sequence and to evaluate the CN benefit in the era of immunotherapy.

24.3 Patient Selection for Cytoreductive Nephrectomy

In the current targeted therapy era, patient selection for CN has become of paramount importance. In the setting of mRCC, two prognostic models allow patient risk stratification: Memorial Sloan Kettering Cancer Center (MSKCC) and International mRCC Database Consortium (IMDC) risk scores [18, 30].

Firstly, the MSKCC score classifies mRCC patients in favourable (MSKCC score 0), intermediate (MSKCC score 1–2) and poor (MSKCC score ≥ 3) risk categories related to following criteria: Karnofsky PS < 80%, time from diagnosis to systemic treatment, hemoglobin concentration below the lower limit of normal, calcium > 10 mg/dl and lactate dehydrogenase (LDH) > 1.5 times the upper limit of normal. On the other hand, the IMDC risk score classifies mRCC patients in favourable (IMDC score 0), intermediate (IMDC score 1–2) and poor (IMDC score ≥ 3) risk categories according to the same criteria presented in the MSKCC prognostic model except for increased LDH and adding two new prognostic variables: neutrophils and platelets above the upper limit of normal. However, although these prognostic scores are used to predict OS in mRCC patients, they were not originally designed for this purpose and are limited by the lack of control of tumour burden [41]. In this regard, some retrospective studies have been conducted to identify potential preoperative predictor factors of improved survival after CN, although all of them currently require external validation [9, 24, 26]. Other authors have evaluated independent risk factors, identifying sarcomatoid histology, high metastatic burden, high neutrophil/lymphocyte ratio, high C-reactive protein and progression on presurgical targeted therapies as poor prognostic variables [21]. Abel et al. [1] analyzed a retrospective series of 466 mRCC patients with tumor thrombus undergoing CN and thrombectomy, showing no CN benefit in patients with supradiaphragmatic involvement. Finally, CN in symptomatic patients has been associated with an improvement of local symptoms or signs in 95% of cases [21, 22].

In summary, the new targeted therapy era establishes the need to define validated prognostic scores to optimize the process of patient selection. Currently, based on the available evidence, poor MSKCC/IMDC risk patients, poor PS patients and patients with high metastatic burden appear not to benefit from upfront CN and should be candidates for systemic treatment (Fig. 24.1).

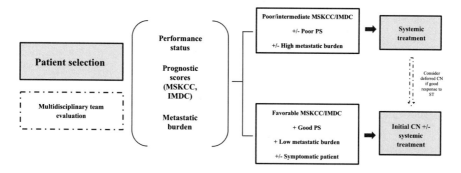

CN = cytoreductive nephrectomy; IMDC = International mRCC Database Consortium risk classification; MSKCC = Memorial Sloan Kettering Cancer Center risk classification; PS = performance status; ST = systemic treatment.

Fig. 24.1 Patient selection for cytoreductive nephrectomy or systematic treatment

24.4 Minimally Invasive Surgery for Cytoreductive Nephrectomy

Minimally invasive surgery is well-established for the treatment of localized RCC. In the setting of mRCC, laparoscopic and robotic surgical approaches have been recently evaluated with the aim of reducing the morbidity related to CN. CN is associated with non-negligible morbidity and mortality rates in mRCC patients, with a perioperative mortality risk of 0–13%, an overall postoperative complication rate of 12–55% and a major complication rate of 3–36% [21, 38].

Several retrospective studies analyzed perioperative outcomes of minimally invasive CN compared to open surgery. Rabets et al. [36], compared laparoscopic CN (22 patients) versus open CN (42 patients), showing benefit of laparoscopic CN in length of hospital stay (2.3 versus 6.1 days, p < 0.001) and operative blood loss (288 versus 1228 ml, p < 0.001). These findings were corroborated in a subsequent retrospective analysis by Matin et al. [25], including 38 patients who underwent laparoscopic CN. Ganeshappa et al. [15], presented a retrospective series (n = 43) comparing laparoscopic and open CN showing decreased blood loss (277 vs. 816 ml, p < 0.001) and length of hospital stay (3.2 vs. 5.1 days, p = 0.001) in the laparoscopic CN group. Finally, the largest retrospective series (n = 120) analyzing laparoscopic CN outcomes showed a postoperative complication rate of 23.3, 28.6% of which were classified as major complications (Clavien-Dindo $\geq$ 3), and a blood transfusion rate of 9.2% [33]. Therefore, based on the reported studies laparoscopic CN is considered a safe and feasible surgical technique in selected patients, although no prospective data are available to date.

The increasing use of robotic surgery in the last decade has led to consider the potential benefit of this surgical technique in the treatment of advanced or mRCC. Robotics provides advantages such as wristed instruments, tremor suppression, 3D vision and a less demanding learning curve compared to laparoscopic CN [3]. In this setting, Anele et al. [2] performed a multi-institutional retrospective study comparing robotic radical nephrectomy (RN) with laparoscopic RN in large renal masses. The analysis showed longer operative duration (185 vs. 126 min, p < 0.001) and shorter length of stay (3 vs. 5 days, p < 0.001) for robotic RN, with no significant differences in perioperative complications (p = 0.2). Remarkably, the robotic RN group presented more advanced disease ($\geq$pT3), histologic grade and nodal involvement, suggesting that surgeons preferred robotic surgery in more complex and surgically challenging cases. Therefore, although studies evaluating the role of robotic CN in the mRCC scenario are needed, recent evidence outline its potential benefit in the treatment of complex RCC cases such as locally advanced RCC or inferior vena cava thrombosis.

Moreover, in the current targeted therapy era, significant postoperative morbidity may delay the initiation of systemic treatment with a consequent detrimental effect on patient management. About 13–30% of patients who underwent upfront CN do not receive systemic therapy due to disease progression or perioperative complications [5, 16]. Gershman et al. [16] conducted a retrospective study of a series of 294 mRCC patients undergoing CN, showing on the multivariable analysis a significant association between laparoscopic approach and earlier administration of systemic therapy (HR 5.05, p < 0.001).

Furthermore, the safety of targeted therapies and ICI prior to surgery needs to be assessed. The SURTIME trial [4] showed no differences in surgical complications between immediate and deferred CN arms in a post-hoc analysis [11]. Pignot et al. [35] presented the first retrospective series (n = 11) evaluating surgical characteristics of mRCC patients undergoing delayed CN after systemic treatment with ICI. The authors described the presence of adhesions and inflammatory tissue reaction in 81.8% of patients. Recently, a retrospective study of a series of 391 mRCC patients receiving ICI plus CN or ICI alone [39] evaluated the safety of performing CN after ICI therapy, showing no prolonged length of stay, 30-day readmissions and positive surgical margins in patients undergoing surgery.

In summary, prospective studies are needed to assess the benefit of minimally invasive CN in the setting of mRCC, although its role appears to be relevant in reducing perioperative morbidity in these patients. Moreover, the impact on perioperative outcomes of new systemic treatments prior to CN needs further evaluation.

24.5 Metastasectomy

Distant metastases in RCC occur most often in the lungs (60–75%), lymph nodes (60–65%), liver (19–40%), bone (40%) and brain (5–7%) [7]. Surgical resection of metastatic sites has been associated with improved outcomes in patients undergoing CN. Although no prospective data are available, retrospective studies showed better cancer-specific and overall survival in patients who underwent complete metastasectomy [29].

Dabestani et al. [10] performed a systematic review of the available evidence, including 16 retrospective studies which demonstrated a survival benefit associated with complete metastasectomy and better symptom control related to local treatment (including pain relief in bone metastases) compared to patients treated with either incomplete or no metastasectomy. Later, a systematic review and meta-analysis were conducted by Zaid et al. [42], analyzing eight cohort studies which showed an improved median OS (36.5–142 vs. 8.4–27 months) and reduced risk of all-cause mortality (HR 2.37, 95% CI 2.03–2.87, $p < 0.001$) in patients undergoing complete surgical metastasectomy compared to those receiving incomplete or no metastasectomy. Finally, Ouzaid et al. [34] presented a systematic review corroborating these findings. The authors analyzed eight comparative studies identifying complete surgical metastasectomy as a significant predictor of overall survival in mRCC patients (HR 0.66, 95% CI 0.46–0.95, $p = 0.03$). Surgical candidates for metastasectomy were those with good PS, limited burden of metastatic disease, metachronous metastases with long interval of disease-free survival and feasible total removal of metastatic disease.

Therefore, in light of the lack of prospective studies, complete metastasectomy remains the appropriate local treatment in selected mRCC patients who are surgical candidates, given the improved overall and cancer-specific survival associated with this procedure.

24.6 Conclusions

The role of CN on mRCC treatment is still object of debate. In carefully selected patients, CN remains an important option as a component of a multimodal therapeutic approach. Recent advances in systemic therapy have challenged the benefits of surgery in mRCC patients. In this setting, future studies are needed to define the optimal sequence of treatment, validated prognostic models to better select patients for CN, benefits of minimally invasive surgery in the mRCC scenario and the therapeutic role of CN in the new immunotherapy era.

References

1. Abel EJ, Spiess PE, Margulis V, et al. Cytoreductive nephrectomy renal cell carcinoma patients with venous tumor thrombus. J Urol. 2017;198:281–8.
2. Anele UA, Marchioni M, Yang B, et al. Robotic versus laparoscopic radical nephrectomy: a large multi-institutional analysis (ROSULA Collaborative Group). World J Urol. 2019;37(11):2439–50.
3. Becher E, Jericevic D, Huang WC. Minimally invasive surgery for patients with locally advanced and/or metastatic renal cell carcinoma. Urol Clin N Am. 2020;47:389–97.
4. Bex A, Mulders P, Jewett M, et al. Comparison of immediate vs deferred cytoreductive nephrectomy in patients with synchronous metastatic renal cell carcinoma receiving sunitinib. The SURTIME Randomized Clinical Trial. JAMA Oncol. 2019;5(2):164–70.
5. Bhindi B, Abel EJ, Albiges L, et al. Systematic review of the role of cytoreductive nephrectomy in the targeted therapy era and beyond: an individualized approach to metastatic renal cell carcinoma. Eur Urol. 2019;75(1):111–28.
6. Bhindi B, Graham J, Wells C, et al. Deferred cytoreductive nephrectomy in patients with newly diagnosed metastatic renal cell carcinoma. Eur Urol. 2020;78:615–23.

7. Bianchi M, Sun M, Jeldres C, Shariat SF, Trinh QD, Briganti A, et al. Distribution of metastatic sites in renal cell carcinoma: a population-based analysis. Ann Oncol. 2012;23:973–80.
8. Choueiri TK, Motzer RJ. Systemic therapy for metastatic renal-cell carcinoma. N Engl J Med. 2017;376:354–66.
9. Culp SH, Tannir NM, Abel EJ, et al. Can we better select patients with metastatic renal cell carcinoma for cytoreductive nephrectomy? Cancer. 2010;116:3378–88.
10. Dabestani S, Marconi L, Hofmann F, Stewart F, Lam TBL, Canfield SE, et al. Local treatment for metastases of renal cell carcinoma: a systematic review. Lancet Oncol. 2014;15:549–61.
11. De Bruijn RE, Mulders P, Jewett MA, et al. Surgical safety of cytoreductive nephrectomy following sunitinib: results from multicentre, randomised controlled trial of immediate versus deferred nephrectomy (SURTIME). Eur Urol. 2019;76(4):437–40.
12. Ferlay J, Colombet M, Soerjomataram I, et al. Cancer incidence and mortality patterns in Europe: estimates for 40 countries and 25 major cancers in 2018. Eur J Cancer. 2018;103:356.
13. Flanigan RC, Salmon SE, Blumenstein BA, et al. Nephrectomy followed by interferon alfa-2b compared with interferon alfa-2b alone for metastatic renal-cell cancer. N Engl J Med. 2001;345:1655–9.
14. Flanigan RC, Mickisch G, Sylvester R, et al. Cytoreductive nephrectomy in patients with metastatic renal cancer: a combined analysis. J Urol. 2004;171:1071–6.
15. Ganeshappa A, Sundaram C, Lerner MA, et al. Role of the laparoscopic approach to cytoreductive nephrectomy in metastatic renal-cell carcinoma: does size matter? J Endourol. 2010;24:1289–92.
16. Gershman B, Moreira DM, Boorjian SA, et al. Comprehensive characterization of the perioperative morbidity of cytoreductive nephrectomy. Eur Urol. 2016;69:84–91.
17. Hanna N, Sun M, Meyer CP, et al. Survival analyses of patients with metastatic renal cancer treated with targeted therapy with or without cytoreductive nephrectomy: a national cancer data base study. J Clin Oncol. 2016;34:3267–75.
18. Heng DY, Xie W, Regan MM, et al. External validation and comparison with other models of the international metastatic renal-cell carcinoma database consortium prognostic model: a population-based study. Lancet Oncol. 2013;14:141–8.
19. Heng DY, Wells JC, Rini BI, et al. Cytoreductive nephrectomy in patients with synchronous metastases from renal cell carcinoma: results from the international metastatic renal cell carcinoma database consortium. Eur Urol. 2014;66:704–10.
20. Hsieh JJ, Purdue MP, Signoretti S, et al. Renal cell carcinoma. Nat Rev Dis Primers. 2017;3:17009.
21. Larcher A, Wallis C, Bex A, et al. Individualised indications for cytoreductive nephrectomy: which criteria define the optimal candidates? Eur Urol Oncol. 2019;4:365–78.
22. Larcher A, Fallara G, Rosiello G, et al. Cytoreductive nephrectomy in metastatic patients with signs or symptoms: implications for Renal Cell Carcinoma Guidelines. Eur Urol. 2020;78(3):321–6.
23. Ljungberg B, Albiges L, Bensalah K, et al. European association of urology guidelines on renal cell carcinoma: the 2020 update. Eur Urol. 2020.
24. Marchioni M, Kriegmair M, Heck M, et al. Development of a novel risk score to select the optimal candidate for cytoreductive nephrectomy among patients with metastatic renal cell carcinoma. Results from a Multi-institutional Registry (REMARCC). Eur Urol Oncol. 2020;S2588–9311(20)30218.
25. Matin SF, Madsen LT, Wood CG. Laparoscopic cytoreductive nephrectomy: the M.D. Anderson Cancer Center experience. Urology. 2006;68(3):528–32.
26. McIntosh AG, Umbreit EC, Holland LC, et al. Optimizing patient selection for cytoreductive nephrectomy based on outcomes in the contemporary era of systemic therapy. Cancer. 2020;126(17):3950–60.
27. Méjean A, Ravaud A, Thezenas S, et al. Sunitinib alone or after nephrectomy in metastatic renal-cell carcinoma. N Engl J Med. 2018;379(5):417–27.

28. Mickisch GH, Garin A, van Poppel H, et al. Radical nephrectomy plus interferon-alfa-based immunotherapy compared with interferon alfa alone in metastatic renal-cell carcinoma: a randomised trial. Lancet. 2001;358:966–70.
29. Mir MC, Matin SF, Bex A, et al. The role of surgery in the management of metastatic kidney cancer: an evidence-based collaborative review. Minerva Urol Nefrol. 2018;70:109–25.
30. Motzer RJ, Bacik J, Schwartz LH, et al. Prognostic factors for survival in previously treated patients with metastatic renal cell carcinoma. J Clin Oncol. 2004;22:454–63.
31. Motzer RJ, Tannir NM, McDermott DF, et al. Nivolumab plus ipilimumab versus sunitinib in advanced renal-cell carcinoma. N Engl J Med. 2018;378:1277–90.
32. Motzer RJ, Penkov K, Haanen J, et al. Avelumab plus axitinib versus sunitinib for advanced renal-cell carcinoma. N Engl J Med. 2019;380:1103–15.
33. Nunez Bragayrac L, Hoffmeyer J, Abbotoy D, et al. Minimally invasive cytoreductive nephrectomy: a multi-institutional experience. World J Urol. 2016;34:1651–6.
34. Ouzaid I, Capitanio U, Staehler M, et al. Surgical metastasectomy in renal cell carcinoma: a systematic review. Eur Urol Oncol. 2019;2(2):141–9.
35. Pignot G, Thiery-Vuillemin A, Walz J, et al. Nephrectomy after complete response to immune checkpoint inhibitors for metastatic renal cell carcinoma: a new surgical challenge? Eur Urol. 2020;77(6):761–3.
36. Rabets JC, Kaouk J, Fergany A, Finelli A, Gill IS, Novick AC. Laparoscopic versus open cytoreductive nephrectomy for metastatic renal cell carcinoma. Urology. 2004;64(5):930–4.
37. Rini BI, Plimack ER, Stus V, et al. Pembrolizumab plus axitinib versus sunitinib for advanced renal-cell carcinoma. N Engl J Med. 2019;380:1116–27.
38. Roussel E, Campi R, Larcher A, et al. Rates and predictors of perioperative complications in cytoreductive nephrectomy: analysis of the registry for metastatic renal cell carcinoma. Eur Urol Oncol. 2020;4:523–9.
39. Singla N, Hutchinson RC, Ghandour RA, et al. Improved survival after cytoreductive nephrectomy for metastatic renal cell carcinoma in the contemporary immunotherapy era: An analysis of the National Cancer Database. Urol Oncol. 2020;38:604.e9–e17.
40. Sorbellini M, Bratslavsky G. Renal cell carcinoma and prognostic factors predictive of survival. Urology. 2010;17:362–3.
41. Westerman ME, Shapiro DD, Tannir NM, et al. Survival following cytoreductive nephrectomy: a comparison of existing prognostic models. BJU Int. 2020;126(6):745–53.
42. Zaid HB, Parker WP, Safdar NS, et al. Outcomes following complete surgical metastasectomy for patients with metastatic renal cell carcinoma: a systematic review and meta-analysis. J Urol. 2017;197(1):44–9.

Printed in the United States
by Baker & Taylor Publisher Services